PICTORIAL ATLAS
OF ACUPUNCTURE

© 2005 KVM Dr. Kolster GmbH Original
title: *Bildatlas der Akupunktur*
ISBN 978-3-932119-35-4

Concept: KVM Dr. Kolster und Co. Produktions- und Verlags-GmbH, Marburg
Projekt Coordinator: Miriam Rodriguez Startz
Editing: KVM Verlag
Layout and typesetting: Prinz und Partner, Marburg
Graphics: iAS Marburg; Gerda Raichle
Photos: Peter Mertin

© 2019 for this English edition:
h.f.ullmann publishing GmbH
Special edition

The English edition has been reviewed by Dr. Chun-Yan Chen and Dr. Hans P. Ogal.

Translation from German: Colin Grant in association with Goodfellow and Egan
Editor: Robin Campbell in association with Goodfellow and Egan
Project management: Karen Baldwin for Goodfellow and Egan Publishing Management, Cambridge
Project coordination: Alex Morkramer
Cover design: Simone Sticker
Front cover photo: © Visuals Unlimited/Getty Images
Back cover photos: Graphics: iAS Marburg/Photography: Peter Mertin

Overall responsibility for production:
h.f.ullmann publishing GmbH, Rolandsecker Weg 30,
53619 Rheinbreitbach, Germany

Printed in India, 2019

ISBN 978-3-8480-0236-8

10 9 8 7 6

www.ullmann-publishing.com

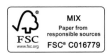

Yu-Lin Lian, Chun-Yan Chen, Michael Hammes, Bernard C. Kolster

PICTORIAL ATLAS
OF ACUPUNCTURE

An illustrated manual of acupuncture points

Edited by Hans P. Ogal and Wolfram Stör

with a preface by
Prof. Dr. Dr. Thomas Ots

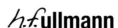

Preface

Knowledge of the exact status and relevance of acupuncture points is an essential tool for the acupuncture therapist. The novice may worry that he will have to learn all the acupuncture points by heart. But experience shows that only about one third of these points at most are actually used in treatment. For this reason the value of an atlas that provides information about a currently important, but seldom used, point cannot be stressed enough.

This comprehensive atlas, beautifully produced with great graphic clarity, is the result of unique collaboration between German and Chinese experts.

The atlas is also noteworthy for the courage of the editors, authors, and the publisher in limiting the indications of the various points to their application uses. This is an area in which the importance of the points has undergone great diversification. These indications have been examined in a meticulous discussion process and redundant or dubious findings discarded.

This pioneering initiative means a substantial gain in practical use, which can only benefit the reader in the practice of acupuncture.

Prof. Dr. Dr. Thomas Ots   Graz

Publisher's Note

Since there is an ongoing discussion regarding the English translation of Chinese names for the various acupuncture points and a standard nomenclature, the publisher has used the translations which come closest to the original German edition and which conform to common English usage.

Foreword

Acupuncture is part of the traditional Chinese approach to medicine. It has also gained popularity among both patients and physicians in western medicine. The success of treatment speaks for itself. In the case of functional disturbances in particular, including various symptoms of pain, acupuncture therapy can help.

This atlas originated in a project to illustrate the full range of the acupuncture points of the primary channels, the Extraordinary vessels Ren Mai and Du Mai, and the most important extraordinary points, in a readily comprehensible way.

Each point is illustrated by means of three pictures. A graphic indicates location in the body, an overview illustrates the point in the context of its pathways, and a photograph shows the acupuncture needle in place. The visual approach enables the systematic study of the various points.

The atlas is designed for everyone with an interest in acupuncture. Beginners can obtain an overview of the most important acupuncture points, whereas experienced practitioners can also learn about less frequently used points and extend their repertoire.

The theoretical foundations of acupuncture as they are based on Traditional Chinese Medicine (TCM) will not be detailed here. Where appropriate, the authors refer the reader to recognised reference works. The emphasis here is placed firmly on the systematic illustration of the channels and points. In this way the atlas offers a meaningful complement to existing acupuncture literature.

An additional aim of this book was to revise the names, properties, and application examples of the individual points. A combination of Chinese sources with the authors' experiences in therapy made it possible to concentrate only on the most significant indications and adapt them to practical needs. The team of Chinese and German authors creates a bridge between oriental and western views of acupuncture.

In order to keep the strain of those models who volunteered for needling demonstration at acceptable levels, very often finer needles than those needed for practice were used. The principal aim of needling of all the points remains the illustration of the topographical location. The correct needling depth and direction are presented in the text that precedes each point.

The authors hope that this atlas will make a contribution to further training in acupuncture and cordially invite specialist comments.

Bad Birnbach, Tianjin, Munich, Marburg, Giessen

Acknowledgements

The completion of this pictorial atlas in this form would be inconceivable without the help of a large number of collaborators and supporters. We wish to express our gratitude to all of them here.

Particular mention must be made of the support provided by the SEIRIN company, which has consistently supported the recognition and integration of acupuncture in university medicine. For this reason the SEIRIN Acupuncture Award was established. It is awarded each year to personalities for exceptional achievement in acupuncture. Laureates to date include: Prof. Dr. J. Bischko (Austria), Prof. Dr. B. Pomeranz (Canada), Dr. J. Gleditsch (Germany), Dr. M.O. Smith (USA), Dr. T. Yamamoto (Japan), Prof. Dr. Dr. Unschuld (Germany), and Prof. J. Bossy (France).

A further vote of thanks must go to the models Patrizia Bartolomeo, Simone Heim, Peter Düsing, and Jürgen Roth for the courage with which they endured needling in photographic sessions that lasted over a period of weeks and thus demonstrated insertion locations in situ. The commitment, patience, and wisdom of the photographer Peter Mertin is also worthy of mention – without him this atlas could never have come about.

However, work itself began after the photographs had been taken. Graphic artists spent many months illustrating the channels, points, and measurements on the photographs. Particular mention should be made here of Kai Naumann who devoted great care and precision to this project over many days and nights. Gratitude is also due to his collaborators Katrin Wiesmeier, Kathrin Ahrens, Matthias Dahmen, and Henrik Heil.

Special thanks are also due to Mrs Sonja Becker for her contribution to the overall project and the collation and editorial evaluation of most texts.

We wish also to thank Thomas Ots for his advice and collaboration in the selection of the 131 most important points.

The three-dimensional illustration of the graphics was fraught with many technical problems. Thomas Kramer, Christoph Krasowski, and Thomas Turtiainen played a key role in graphic layout and production.

Marion Prinz was responsible for layout and typesetting. It is due to her great patience and care that this atlas now lies before you in its current form.

We wish also to thank Mrs Mercedes Creydt for her critical reading of the manuscript and the British Acupuncture Council for the reading of the English edition.

Not least we should also like to thank our families and friends who made many sacrifices during the genesis of this project and who also encouraged us to complete it.

Finger Index

Contents

2.3 The Points of the Extraordinary Vessels Du Mai and Ren Mai 260

2.4 Further Acupuncture Points (Extraordinary Points) 300

3 APPENDIX 344

List of Abbreviations

A., Aa.	Arteria, Arteriae
Bl	Bladder Channel
C	Cervical spinal segment
Du-Mai	Du-Mai (The Governing Vessel)
Ex	Extraordinary Points
Ex-AH	Extraordinary Points Arm and Hand
Ex-B	Extraordinary Point Back
Ex-CA	Extraordinary Points Chest and Abdomen
Ex-HN	Extraordinary Points Head and Neck
Ex-LF	Extraordinary Points Leg and Foot
GB	Gall Bladder Channel
He	Heart Channel
ICS	Intercostal Space
Ki	Kidney Channel
L	Lumbar Spinal Segment
LI	Large Intestine Channel
Lu	Lung Channel
Lv	Liver Channel
M., Mm.	Musculus, Musculi
P	Pericardium Channel
Proc.	Process
Ren	Ren Mai (The Conception Channel)
SJ	San Jiao Channel
SI	Small Intestine Channel
Sp	Spleen Channel
St	Stomach Channel
TCM	Traditional Chinese Medicine
Th	Thoracic Spinal Segment
V., Vv.	Vena, Venae

1 The Basic Principles

1.1 Acupuncture Measurements

In acupuncture the body is measured not in absolute units, but in the relative, proportional units of a given patient. The distances are determined by anatomical-topographical landmarks. The basic unit of measurement in Chinese acupuncture is the cun.

Finger measurements

The finger measurements are obtained from the measurements of the thumb and fingers of a patient. The width of the index and middle fingers at the level of the interphalangeal joint is 1.5 cun.

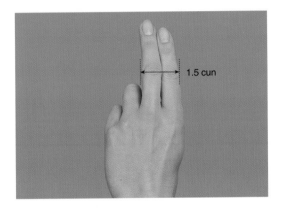

Thumb measurement

The width of the thumb at the level of the interphalageal joint is 1 cun.

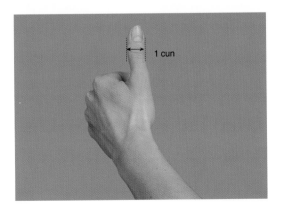

Middle finger measurement

When the tip of the middle finger is placed on the tip of a (moderately stretched) thumb, the distance between the creases of the two interphalangeal joints of the middle finger is also 1 cun.

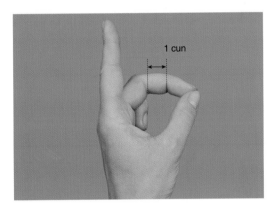

Cross finger measurement

The width of the four fingers held together (at the level of the proximal interphalangeal joint of the longer fingers) is 3 cun.

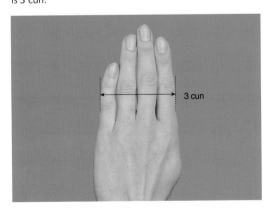

Body measurements

Body measurements, which may differ from finger measurements, are measured as shown below:

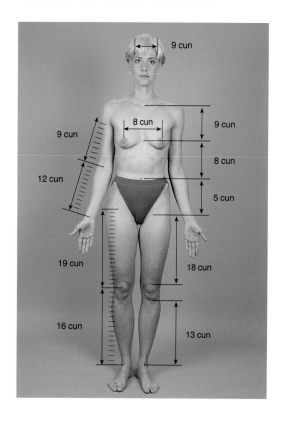

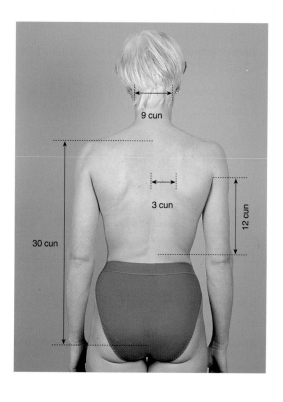

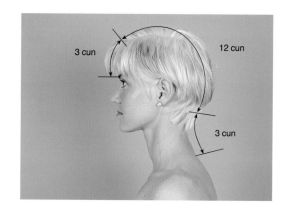

LIMIT POINTS	DISTANCE
Head/Neck	
Distance from St 8 of the one side to St 8 of the other side	9 cun
Distance between centre of eyebrows (Ex-Hn 3) and the centre of the ideal anterior hairline	3 cun
Distance between middle of the ideal anterior hairline and the middle of the ideal posterior hairline	12 cun
Distance between middle of ideal posterior hairline and the inferior border of the spinous process of C7 (Du 14)	3 cun
Distance between the mastoid processes	9 cun
Body	
Distance between the nipples (St 17)	8 cun
Distance between middle of Fossa suprasternalis (Ren 22) and xiphisternal joint (Ren 16)	9 cun
Distance between xiphisternal joint (Ren 16) and umbilicus (Ren 8)	8 cun
Distance between umbilicus (Ren 8) and superior border of pubic symphysis	5 cun
Distance between medial axillary line from centre of axilla to the inferior free end of the 11th rib (Lv 13)	12 cun
Distance in neutral position between the medial edge of the scapula to the line of the spinous process	3 cun
Distance between inferior border of Th1 to tip of coccyx	30 cun
Upper Extremity	
Distance between superior end of anterior axillary crease and cubital crease with straightened arm	9 cun
Distance between cubital crease and inferior wrist crease	12 cun
Lower Extremity	
Distance between superior border of pubic symphysis and superior tip of patella	18 cun
Distance between the lateral prominence of the greater trochanter and popliteal crease	19 cun
Distance between popliteal crease and lateral malleous	16 cun
Distance between medial tibiacondylus and medial malleous	13 cun
Distance between gluteal fold (Bl 36) and popliteal crease (Bl 40)	14 cun

1.2 Acupuncture Techniques

Positioning the patient

Successful acupuncture treatment requires the comfortable and relaxed positioning of the patient. Appropriate positioning can in most cases prevent collapsed needling and any resulting complications. The patient is usually treated lying on his back or stomach but also on his side when the needling of specific points (for example lumboischialgia) is required. When needling affects the stomach or back, the patient is repositioned once the appropriate needling has been performed.

Needling techniques

Any needling is preceded by the appropriate disinfection of the skin.

Basic grip

The grip of the needle is secured between the thumb and index finger of the needling hand. The tip of the middle finger supports the needle and assists in insertion. The second hand can either secure the needling area or help in insertion.

Needling in taut skin

The thumb and index finger or thumb and middle finger of the guiding hand tighten or stretch the main area surrounding the acupuncture point. This technique facilitates needling, in particular where a point is located in soft tissue – such as in the abdominal region.

Needling using nail pressure

Moderate pressure is exerted with the nail of the thumb or index finger into the intended needling point. Needling takes place against the nail, which helps to guide the needle and fix the acupuncture point. This technique may reduce needling pain and is useful in muscles where tissue is not particularly flexible.

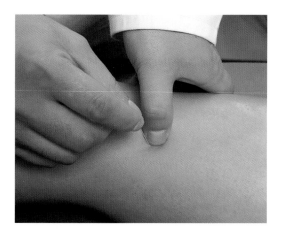

Insertion with a guiding hand

The needling of deeper points requires the use of longer needles. In order to prevent deviation from the direction of insertion or needle bending, the second hand is used to guide the needle. Here, the needle shaft is secured between two sterile swabs. This technique is applied in points located deep inside the muscle (for example GB 30).

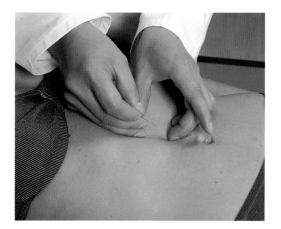

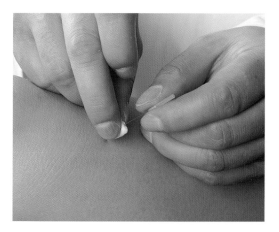

Insertion using guiding tubes

Guide tubes help to reduce pain of needling. The tube is placed on the intended needling point. The needle, which protrudes from the tube by a matter of millimeters, is then tapped into the skin. In China, this method is often used in treating children.

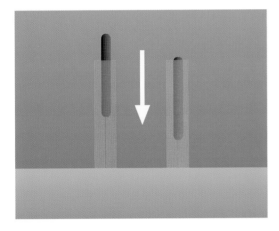

Insertion into pinched skin

The skin at the intended point is nipped between thumb and index finger while the other hand inserts the needle. This technique is appropriate for points where there is little subcutaneous tissue, those located directly above osseous structures such as the Extraordinary Point Ex-HN 3.

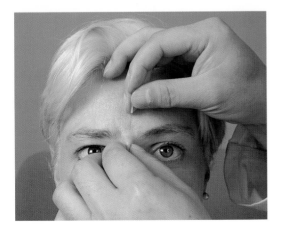

Needling depth

The depth of needling depends on the anatomical location of the point and the anticipated location of the structure which is to be stimulated by the needling of that point. Here, the physical build, constitution, and dysfunction profile will also play a role. As a result, the needling depths indicated can only offer general guidelines. In the treatment of children and slim patients for example, more shallow needling is indicated, whereas in the case of well-built, athletic or adipose patients, greater needling depth is recommended. Where a patient displays only moderate or acute pain, more superficial needling usually suffices. By contrast, severe or chronic disease profiles or paralyses tend to require deeper needling. Anatomical and topographical knowledge are essential in acupuncture, especially in the case of greater needling depths.

The needling depths indicated in this atlas are based on the instructions of appropriate Chinese teaching books.

Needling direction

The angle of insertion depends on the topography of the intended point and the structure to be treated. Various angles are possible for one acupuncture point depending on the intended effect. The most frequently used insertion angles are used in this atlas.

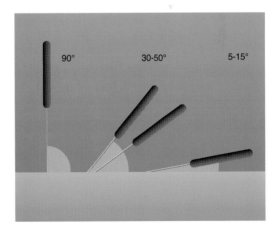

Perpendicular Needling

Perpendicular needling is usually applied to muscular or adipose areas in the body. The needle is inserted at a 90 degree angle to the skin surface.

Oblique needling

The needle is inserted at an angle of between 30 and 50 degrees to the skin surface. Oblique needling is used where the soft tissue is thinner, where pneumothorax is to be avoided, where the needle is to be directed away from the pleura, and where the structure to be treated is located at an oblique angle to the insertion point. As a result, the oblique insertion is often used in the head and chest areas.

Tranverse needling

Here, the needle is inserted at an angle between 5 and 15 degrees to the skin surface. This technique is applied to areas with a very thin, soft tissue layer, for example the skull.

The Qi sensation

Once the insertion area of the acupuncture point has been correctly located, patients experience a characteristic feeling, particularly in Muscular points in the direction and depth of insertion, known in Chinese literature as the arrival of Qi sensation (deqi). This sensation usually differs from the pain of insertion itself and is described as "dull ache," "electrical-tingling," "being tensed up," "heaviness" or "warmth." When this sensation extends along the needled channel we can speak of a PSC-phenomenon (Propagated Sensation along the Channel). This sensation cannot be reproduced in every acupuncture point and varies within the individual and between individuals.

Needle stimulation

Certain needle guidance techniques – such as the moderate pushing or lifting or needle rotation in the region to be treated – provoke Qi sensation. Once a patient experiences this sensation additional techniques can be applied primarily to the selected points, which are aimed at influencing the disease profile in a specific way. These techniques depend on the assessment of the disease profile according to the Chinese criteria of a state of fullness or emptiness. In states of fullness, Xie (sedating) techniques are used; in states of emptiness, Bu (tonifying) techniques are used. The most frequently used techniques are needle twisting and lifting/depressing.

Rotating the needle

The movement of the needle is described here according to its two main components: amplitude and frequency. A twisting movement with low amplitude (rotation of the needle in a rotation arc of < 90 degrees) and high frequency (about 4–8 Hz) is known as a **tonifying technique**.

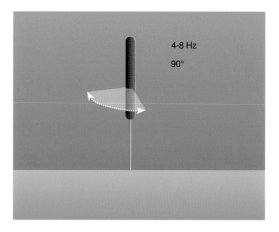

A twisting movement with high amplitude (rotation of the needle in a rotation arc of >180 degrees) and low frequency (about 1–2 Hz) is known as a **sedating technique**.

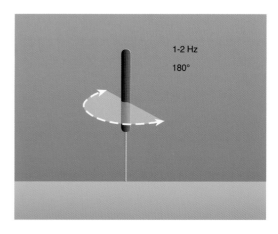

Important Note: The sedating and tonifying processes that are described here are possible only after the arrival of Qi sensation (deqi).

Lifting and depressing the needle

A lifting and lowering movement with low amplitude (< 1 mm) and high frequency (about 4–8 Hz) is known as a **tonifying technique**.

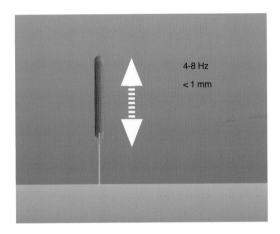

4-8 Hz
< 1 mm

A lifting and lowering movement with high amplitude (> 2 mm) and low frequency (about 1–2 Hz) is known as a **sedating technique**.

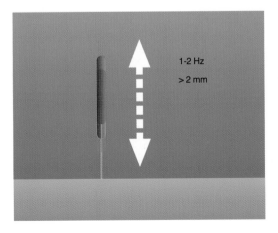

1-2 Hz
> 2 mm

Using breathing

Where the needle is further inserted when the patient exhales and slightly removed when the patient inhales, this is a **tonifying technique**. Where the needle is further inserted when the patient inhales and slightly removed on exhalation, this is known as a **sedating technique**.

Further techniques

Other aspects, such as insertion in or against the course of the channel, the quick covering of the insertion point with a swab after the removal of the needle, or leaving the point "open" after needle removal, play only a minor role in clinical applications and are, therefore, given no further consideration here.

Acupuncture needles

In acupuncture, throwaway sterile needles made of steel are to be recommended. The material of the needle grip is of minor significance, although moxibustion can only be applied with metal grips. Depending on the anatomical and topographical circumstances of the needling point, and the constitution and the dysfunction profile of the patient, needle length and width vary. In the acra and facial regions extremely fine, thin needles with low trauma effect are generally used (e.g. 0.15 x 15 mm).

In China needles measuring 0.22 x 25 mm are used in these regions. The most frequently used size measures 0.25 x 40 mm, occasionally 0.25 x 50 mm. Needles measuring over 75 mm should have a strength of at least 0.30 mm, as otherwise the risk of needle bending will be too high.

2 Channels and Points

2.1 Point Characteristics and Clinical Applications

A description of the point characteristics according to TCM (Traditional Chinese Medicine) does not primarily claim to cover all aspects. Instead, it emphasizes the particular quality of a given acupuncture point.

Details relating to point characteristics should always be considered in the context of areas of clinical application. Here, a description of the characteristics of a point explain how a given acupuncture point affects a given dysfunction in accordance with TCM. It is then possible to indicate a TCM diagnosis for the most appropriate treatment of a given dysfunction.

Information relating to the clinical application of a given acupuncture point takes account of dysfunctions for which a given point can typically be selected. The sequence of clinical applications named should indicate a type of hierarchy. This hierarchy is not, however, absolute, but constitutes a provisional finding for a general medical dysfunction.

Information relating to the clinical applications of the points takes account of both classical sources and the findings of more recent Chinese investigations. Care has been taken to ensure that findings correspond to the actual clinical practice of the authors. Theoretical insights derived from point characteristics do not perform any major role in this book.

In consequence, the tonifying and sedating points derived from the five Shu-points and five phase points are not considered as such. This is particularly true in view of the contradiction with clinical experience resulting from the fact that these points frequently do not possess the characteristics inferred from the theory.

Information about needling depth aims only to provide a point of reference, this allows for individual deviation from the ranges given.

Location and depth of needling

Details relating to acupuncture points and needling depth are based on the authorised standard work published in China entitled *The Acupuncture Points*.

Channel pathways

Illustrations of the channel pathways are based on the reference works listed below (cf. the bibliography in the Appendix):

Beijing College of Traditional Chinese medicine, Shanghai College of Traditional Chinese Medicine, Nanjing College of Traditional Chinese Medicine, The Acupuncture Institute of the Academy of Traditional Chinese Medicine (eds.): *Essentials of Chinese Acupuncture*. Foreign Languages Press, Beijing, 1980

Cheng Xin-nong (ed.): *Chinese Acupuncture and Moxibustion*. Foreign Languages Press, Beijing, 1987

Li Ding: *Acupuncture, Meridian Theory, and Acupuncture points*. Foreign Languages Press, Beijing, 1990

Li Shi-hua (ed.): Yue Han-zhen (Qing). *Jingxuejie. Zhang Can-jia, Zha Chang-hua dianjiao*. Renmin weisheng chubanshe, Beijing, 1990

Liu Gong-wang, Akira Hyodo (eds.): *Fundamentals of Acupuncture and Moxibustion*. Tianjin Science and Technology Translation and Publishing Corporation, Tianjin, 1994

Sun Yon-xian: *JingLuo kaobian*. Qingdao chubanshe, Qingdao, 1989

Point categories

● Back-Shu-points (Bei Shu Xue)

Synonyms: concordance points, transporting points, Shu-points

These acupuncture points lie along the Bladder channel on the back and have a segmental relation to one of the twelve organs in TCM.

Bl 13 (Lung)	Bl 21 (Stomach)
Bl 14 (Pericardium)	Bl 22 (Sanjiao)
Bl 15 (Heart)	Bl 23 (Kidney)
Bl 18 (Liver)	Bl 25 (Large Intestine)
Bl 19 (Gall Bladder)	Bl 27 (Small Intestine)
Bl 20 (Spleen)	Bl 28 (Bladder)

● Mu (gathering) points (Mu Xue)

Synonyms: Alarm points, Herold points, Mu points

These acupuncture points are located on the chest or abdomen along various channels. They have a segmental relation to one of the twelve organs in TCM.

Lu 1 (Lung)	Ren 12 (Stomach)
Ren 17 (Pericardium)	Ren 5 (Sanjiao)
Ren 14 (Heart)	GB 25 (Kidney)
Lv 14 (Liver)	St 25 (Large Intestine)
GB 24 (Gall Bladder)	Ren 4 (Small Intestine)
Lv 13 (Spleen)	Ren 3 (Bladder)

● Qi-source-points (Yuan Xue)

Synonyms: Source points, Qi points, Yuan points

Each of the twelve primary channels possesses a Qi or source point. On the Ying channel this point coincides with the third of the five Shu-points and is, therefore, always distally the third point. According to classical Chinese belief these points should distribute the Qi-source along the channel.

Lu 9	Bl 64
LI 4	Ki 3
St 42	P 7
Sp 3	SJ 4
He 7	GB 40
SI 4	Lv 3

● Connecting points (Luo Xue)

Synonyms: Passage-, Connecting-, Luo points

Each of the twelve primary channels, the Dumai, Ren Mai, and the great Luo-connecting point of the spleen has one connecting point. According to traditional Chinese belief, network vessels branch off such points as these. These vessels in turn are held to connect the coupled channels with each other.

Lu 7	P 6
LI 6	SJ 5
St 40	GB 37
Sp 4	Lv 5
He 5	Du 1
SI 7	Ren 15
Bl 58	Sp 21 (the great Luo-connecting
Ki 4	point of the spleen)

● Confluent points (Ba Mai Jiao Hui Xue)

Synonyms: Tuning points, Cardinal points

Of these eight acupuncture points, four are located on the upper and four on the lower extremity, four on the Yin and four on the Yang channels. According to classical Chinese belief they develop their effect in relation to the eight Extraordinary Vessels.

SI 3 (Du Mai)	Bl 62 (Yang Qiao Mai)
Lu 7 (Ren Mai)	Ki 6 (Yin Qiao Mai)
SJ 5 (Yang Wei Mai)	GB 41 (Dai Mai)
P 6 (Yin Wei Mai)	Sp 4 (Chong Mai)

The five Shu-points (Wu Shu Xue)

Synonym: Five ancient points

Each of the twelve channels possesses five especially classified acupuncture points. Classical Chinese sources compare the channels with water courses in nature. The pathway of the "water" in the principal channels is always conceived as flowing from the acren to the trunk. From the acren to both the knee and elbow-joint five stations are passed through (see below).

● Jing (well) points (Jing Xue)

Synonym: 1st ancient points

These are the first of the five Shu-points at which "water" still lies as if deep in a well.

Lu 11	Bl 67
LI 1	Ki 1
St 45	P 9
Sp 1	SJ 1
He 9	GB 44
SI 1	Lv 1

● Xing (spring) points (Xing Xue)

Synonym: 2nd ancient points

This is the second group of the five Shu-points, at which "water" runs as if from a spring.

Lu 10	Bl 66
LI 2	Ki 2
St 44	P 8
Sp 2	SJ 2
He 8	GB 43
SI 2	Lv 2

● Shu (stream) points (Shu Xue)

Synonym: 3rd Ancient Points

This is the third group of the five Shu-points, through which the water flows at accelerated speed – as if through rapids. On the Yin channels these are also the Qi-source-points.

Lu 9	Bl 65
LI 3	Ki 3
St 43	P 7
Sp 3	SJ 3
He 7	GB 41
SI 3	Lv 3

● Jing (river) points (Jing Xue)

Synonym: 4th ancient points

This is the fourth group of the five Shu-points, past which the water flows like a river.

Lu 8	Bl 60
LI 5	Ki 7
St 41	P 5
Sp 5	SJ 6
He 4	GB 38
SI 5	Lv 4

● He (sea) points (He Xue)

Synonym: 5th ancient points

This is the fifth group of the five Shu-points, at which the "water" flows as if over a river delta in the sea.

Lu 5	Bl 40
LI 11	Ki 10
St 36	P 3
Sp 9	SJ 10
He 3	GB 34
SI 8	Lv 8

Lower He (sea) points (Xia He Xue)

Synonym: Lower points of influence

According to classical Chinese belief the He points should be used especially to treat disorders of the organ of a particular channel. However, the points of the large intestine, small intestine and Sanjiao channel demonstrate no effect on their organs. This role is played by the points on the lower extremity of the stomach and bladder channel, known as the Lower He points.

St 37 (Large Intestine) St 39 (Small Intestine)	Bl 39 (Sanjiao)

Cleft (Xi) points (Xi Xue)

Synonym: Border points, Xi points

Each of the twelve channels possesses a cleft point. Only a certain number of the cleft points find frequent clinical use.

Lu 6	Bl 63
LI 7	Ki 5
St 34	P 4
Sp 8	SJ 7
He 6	GB 36
SI 6	Lv 6

Meeting (master) points (Ba Hui Xue)

Synonym: Master points, Points of influence

According to classical Chinese belief these eight acupuncture points develop their influence in specific regions of the body or in regions with specific functions.

Lv 13 (Zang Organs)	Lu 9 (vessels)
Ren 12 (Fu Organs)	Bl 11 (bones)
Ren 17 (Qi)	GB 34 (tendons)
Bl 17 (blood)	GB 39 (marrow)

The principal acupuncture points

The point categories outlined in chapter 2.1 and in the footer indexes of the following chapters are color-coded for ease of clarity. Neither this code nor the sequence of the list reflect the value of the acupuncture points, but instead describe the specifics of a given point.

Not all the points given systematic illustration below receive the same application. In practice certain points are more frequently used than others. The principal acupuncture points are summarised on this basis. The authors and editors of this book selected a total of 131 points that play a major role in their practical activities. An analysis of these point categories reveals all the key points and many back Shu-points, Mu (gathering) points, Hui-meeting (cardinal) points, connecting points and Qi-source-points (especially located on the Yin channel). Some of the Shu-points, e.g. the He (sea) point, and the Lower He (sea) points are named, whereas only a limited number of cleft points is given importance.

The lung channel (Lu):

Lu 5, Lu 7, Lu 11

The large intestine channel (LI):

LI 4, LI 10, LI 11, LI 14, LI 15, LI 20

The stomach channel (St):

St 2, St 4, St 6, St 7, St 8, St 18, St 21, St 25, St 28, St 29, St 35, St 36, St 37, St 38, St 39, St 40, St 44, St 45

The spleen channel (Sp):

Sp 3, Sp 4, Sp 6, Sp 8, Sp 9, Sp 10

The heart channel (He):

He 1, He 3, He 5, He 7

The small intestine channel (SI):

SI 1, SI 3, SI 6, SI 10, SI 11, SI 14, SI 18, SI 19

The bladder channel (Bl):

Bl 2, Bl 10, Bl 13, Bl 14, Bl 15, Bl 17, Bl 18, Bl 19, Bl 20, Bl 21, Bl 23, Bl 24, Bl 25, Bl 26, Bl 27, Bl 32, Bl 37, Bl 39, Bl 40, Bl 54, Bl 57, Bl 58, Bl 60, Bl 62, Bl 67

The kidney channel (Ki):

Ki 1, Ki 3, Ki 6, Ki 7, Ki 12, Ki 13, Ki 14

The pericardium channel (P):

P 4, P 6

The San Jiao channel (SJ):

SJ 3, SJ 5, SJ 6, SJ 14, SJ 15, SJ 17, SJ 21

The gall bladder channel (GB):

GB 2, GB 12, GB 14, GB 20, GB 21, GB 26, GB 30, GB 31, GB 34, GB 37, GB 39, GB 40, GB 41, GB 43

The liver channel (Lv):

Lv 2, Lv 3, Lv 5, Lv 8

The Du Mai (Du):

Du 3, Du 4, Du 9, Du 14, Du 16, Du 20, Du 23, Du 26

The Ren Mai (Ren):

Ren 3, Ren 4, Ren 6, Ren 8, Ren 10, Ren 12, Ren 13, Ren 14, Ren 17, Ren 24

Extraordinary points (Ex):

Ex-HN 1, Ex-HN 3, Ex-HN 5, Ex-CA 1, Ex-B 2, Ex-B 8, Ex-AH 9, Ex-LF 5, Ex-LF 10

2.2 Acupuncture points of the principal channels

Note

Many published works on acupuncture define the principal channels as being simply a sequence of points. However, the pathway described in traditional Chinese literature can deviate from such a definition even in the surface sections of the channels. The illustrations selected here essentially adopt the findings of the classical reference work in Chinese medicine, the *Huangdi Neijing* (Great Fundamentals of the Yellow Emperor).

2.2.1　The lung channel (Lu)

Synonyms

- lung-meridian
- hand-taiyin-lung channel

Channel pathway

There are 11 acupuncture points in the surface pathway of the lung channel.

The inner pathway begins in the central Sianjiao and descends the spine in order to connect with the large intestine. The return pathway passes through the cardiac orifice of the stomach and traverses the diaphragm. The channel penetrates the lung, the organ which belongs to it. After the pathway ascends the trachea and connects with the larynx and the pharynx, the channel leaves the chest cavity beneath the clavicle at point Lu 1.

The surface pathway of the lung channel passes over the outer part of the inner upper arm to the elbow and runs over the radial area of the inner forearm and the thumb to the radial side of the thumbnail.

Branch vessels run to the large intestine channel and to the index finger at point Lu 7.

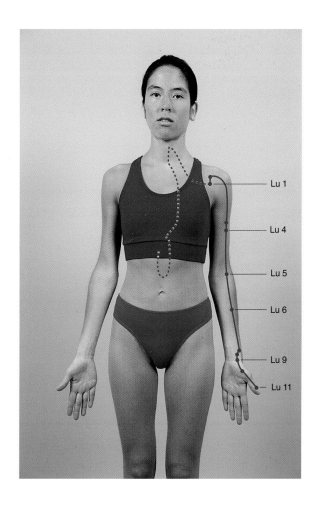

Lu 1

Lu 4

Lu 5

Lu 6

Lu 9

Lu 11

Lu

Lu 1 Zhong Fu   Middle Palace

L: at the level of the 1st ICR, 6 cun lateral to the midline, 1 cun inferior to the fossa clavicularis (Lu 2)

T: 0.5–0.8 cun at 45 degrees oblique to lateral; moxibustion

P: disseminates and descend lung Qi, alleviates coughing and wheezing

A: dysfunctions of the lung and the trachea

Pec: Mu (gathering) point of the lung
CAUTION, AVOID PNEUMOTHORAX!

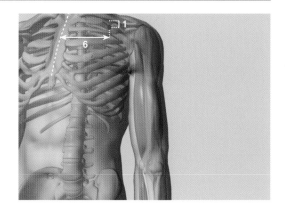

Lu 2 Yun Men   Cloud Gate

L: 6 cun from the midline in the Fossa clavicularis, above the coracoid process

T: 0.5–0.8 cun at 45 degrees oblique laterally; moxibustion

P: disseminates and descends lung Qi, alleviates coughing and wheezing

A: dysfunctions of the lung and the trachea

Pec: CAUTION, AVOID PNEUMOTHORAX!

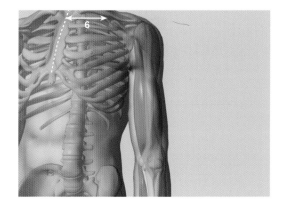

Lu 3 Tian Fu   Heavenly Palace

L: on the antero-lateral aspect of the upper arm, 3 cun inferior to the axillar fold on the radial edge of the biceps brachii muscle

T: 0.3–0.5 cun perpendicular; moxibustion

P: disseminates lung Qi and dissipates harmful influences, clears heat and cools the blood

A: 1. coughing and other dysfunctions of the trachea
2. epistaxis, spitting or coughing blood

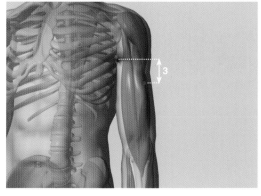

L: Location   **T:** Insertion Technique   **P:** Properties   **A:** Clinical Applications   **Pec:** Peculiarities

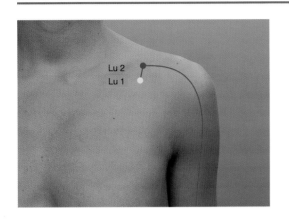

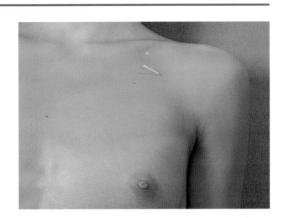

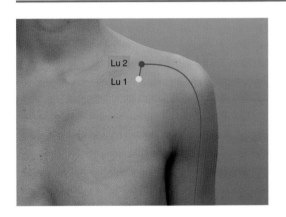

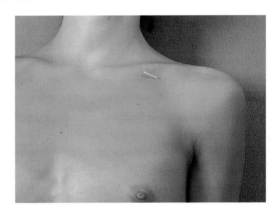

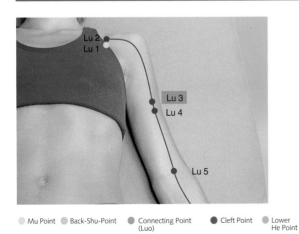

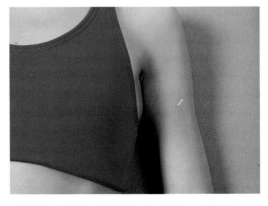

○ Mu Point ○ Back-Shu-Point ● Connecting Point (Luo) ● Cleft Point ● Lower He Point ● Qi-Source-Point (Yuan) ● Confluent Point ● Converging Point

27

Lu

Lu 4 Xia Bai Clasping the White

L: on the antero-lateral aspect of the upper arm, 4 cun inferior to the axillary fold or 5 cun superior to the cubital crease on the radial edge of the biceps brachii muscle

T: 0.5–0.8 cun perpendicular; moxibustion

P: disseminates and descends lung Qi, regulates Qi, and expands the chest

A: 1. dysfunctions of the lung and the trachea
2. thoracic pain, feeling of thoracic fullness

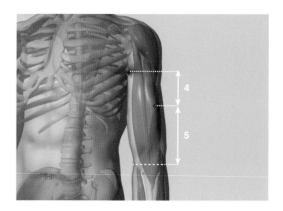

Lu 5 Chi Ze Cubit Marsh

L: in the cubital fold in the depression at the radial side of the biceps brachii muscle

T: 0.5–0.8 cun perpendicular; prick for blood; moxibustion

P: disseminates and descends lung Qi, enriches the yin and moistens the lung

A: 1. coughing, difficulty in breathing, infectious diseases of the superior trachea
2. infectious diseases of the lung

Pec: He (sea) point (5th Shu-point)

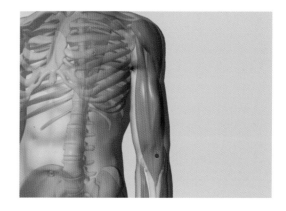

Lu 6 Kong Zui Maximum Opening

L: 7 cun above the inferior wrist crease on the radial inner side of the forearm on the connecting line between Lu 5 and Lu 9

T: 0.5–0.8 cun perpendicular; moxibustion

P: disseminates and descends lung Qi, cools, and soothes blood

A: 1. coughing, shortness of breath, and other dysfunctions of the trachea
2. bleeding from the lung

Pec: cleft (Xi) point

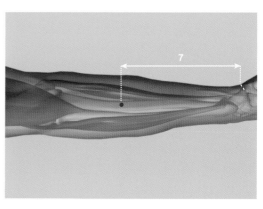

L: Location   T: Insertion Technique   P: Properties   A: Clinical Applications   Pec: Peculiarities

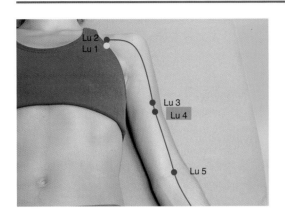
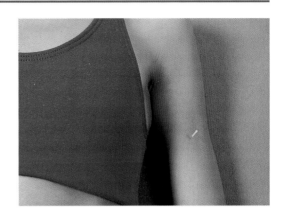

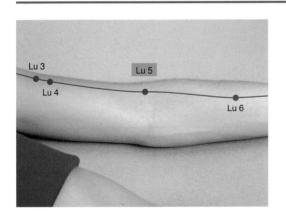
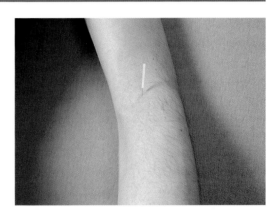

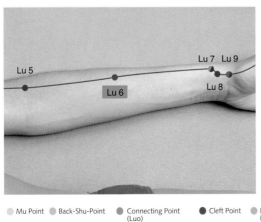
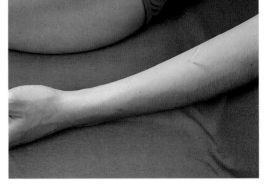

● Mu Point　● Back-Shu-Point　● Connecting Point (Luo)　● Cleft Point　● Lower He Point　● Qi-Source-Point (Yuan)　● Confluent Point　● Converging Point

Lu

Lu 7 Lie Que Broken sequence

L: 1.5 cun above the wrist crease in the depression below the radial styloid, in the cleft between the tendons of the M. brachioradialis and M. abductor pollicis longus

T: 0.5–0.8 cun transverse proximally; moxibustion

P: disseminates lung Qi and dissipates harmful influences, decongests and activates the main channel, regulates the Ren Mai

A: 1. coughing and other diseases of the trachea
2. paralyses and pain in the lower arm
3. acute infections of the urinary tract, micturation dysfunctions

Pec: connecting point (Luo), confluent point (Ba Mai Jiao Hui) of the Ren Mai
command point for neck and rear of head

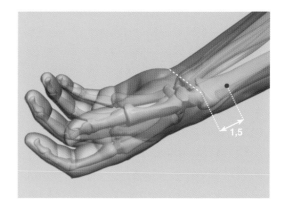

Lu 8 Jing Qu Channel Gutter

L: 1 cun above the inferior wrist crease in the depression between the radial styloid and A. radialis

T: 0.2–0.3 cun perpendicular;
no moxibustion

P: cleanses the lung and alleviates coughing

A: coughing, shortness of breath, and other diseases of the trachea

Pec: Jing (river) point (4th Shu-point)

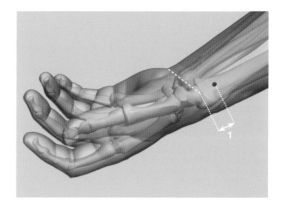

Lu 9 Tai Yuan Supreme Abyss

L: on the radial end of the inferior wrist crease, to the outside of the A. radialis, ulnar to the tendon of the abductor pollicis longus muscle

T: 0.2–0.3 cun perpendicular;
moxibustion

P: soothes coughing and transforms phlegm

A: coughing, shortness of breath, and other diseases of the trachea

Pec: Shu (stream) point (3rd Shu-point), Qi-source-point (Yuan), meeting (master) point (Hui) of the vessels

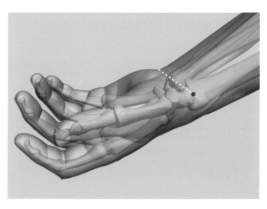

L: Location   T: Insertion Technique   P: Properties   A: Clinical Applications   Pec: Peculiarities

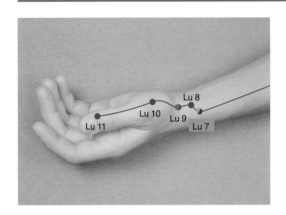

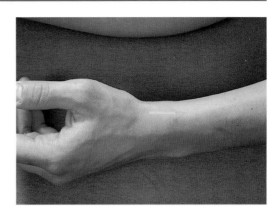

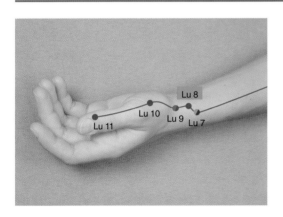

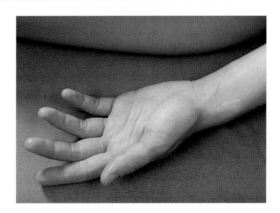

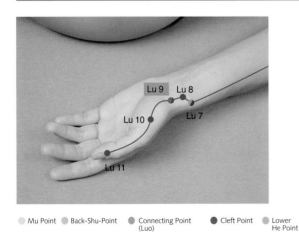

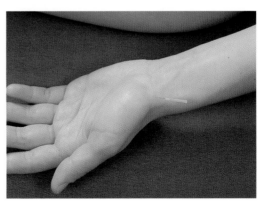

○ Mu Point ○ Back-Shu-Point ○ Connecting Point (Luo) ● Cleft Point ○ Lower He Point ● Qi-Source-Point (Yuan) ● Confluent Point ● Converging Point

Lu 10 Yu Ji Fish Border

L: in the depression above the metacarpophalangeal joint in the centre of the first metacarpal bone, on the border between red and white flesh

T: 0.5–0.8 cun perpendicular; moxibustion

P: clears the lung and soothes coughing, enriches the Yin, and relieves the pharynx

A: 1. coughing, coughing or spitting blood, and other diseases of the trachea
2. painful swelling in the throat and pharynx

Pec: Xing (spring) point (2nd Shu-point)

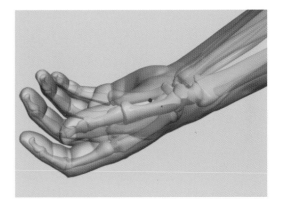

Lu 11 Shao Shang Lesser Shang

L: 0.1 cun superior to and to the side of the corner of the thumbnail

T: 0.1 cun perpendicular; prick to bleed; moxibustion

P: clears the lung and relieves the pharynx, clears the brain, and opens the tendons

A: 1. painful swelling in the throat and pharynx
2. coughing, shortness of breath, and other diseases of the trachea
3. apoplexy, heat-stroke, disturbances in consciousness accompanied by high temperatures

Pec: Jing (well) point (1st Shu-point)

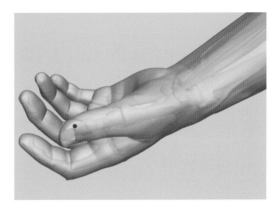

L: Location   T: Insertion Technique   P: Properties   A: Clinical Applications   Pec: Peculiarities

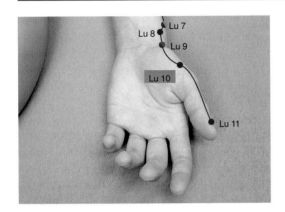

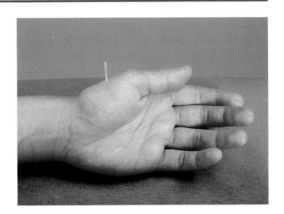

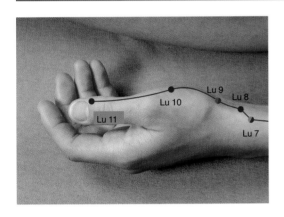

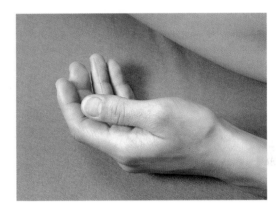

Mu Point   Back-Shu-Point   Connecting Point (Luo)   Cleft Point   Lower He Point   Qi-Source-Point (Yuan)   Confluent Point   Converging Point

LI

2.2.2   The large intestine channel (LI)

Synonyms

• Large intestine meridian

• Hand-Yangming-large intestine channel

Channel pathway

There are 20 points in the surface pathway of the large intestine channel.

The channel begins at the radial side of the tip of the index finger, passes through the interspace between the first and second metacarpal bones, through the anatomical snuffbox and over the superior part of the lateral aspect of the forearm, to the lateral aspect of the elbow. The shoulder is reached via the lower part of the lateral aspect of the upper arm. From this point the channel branches behind the acromion to the seventh cervical vertebra (Du 14) and from there runs on to the supraclavicular fossa.

From the seventh cervical vertebra (Du 14) the channel runs through the supraclavicular fossa and enters the ribs where it there connects with the lung. After traversing the diaphragm the channel reaches its organ, the large intestine.

The surface pathway of the channel leads laterally from the supraclavicular fossa past the lower neck to the corners of the mouth, crossing the meridian line at the philtrum and onto the naso-labial groove opposite (LI 20).

From this point the channel enters into contact with the branches of the stomach channel. At the corners of the mouth two branches run off the pathway to the gums of the lower jaw.

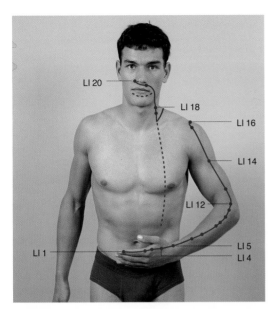

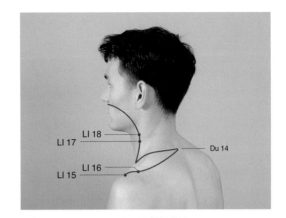

LI

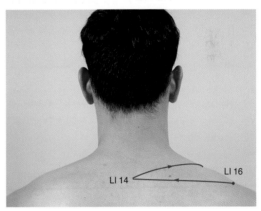

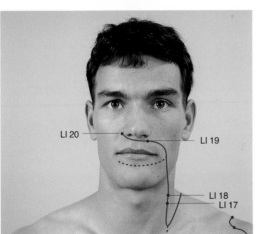

LI 1 Shang Yang   Jing-well and metal point of the large intestine channel

L: 0.1 cun from the corner of the radial border of the nail of the index finger

T: 0.1 cun perpendicular; prick to bleed; moxibustion

P: clears heat and removes inflammation, opens the senses and recovers clarity of spirit

A: 1. acute inflammation in the region of the face, mouth, and pharynx e.g. pharyngitis, tonsillitis, parotitis, parodontis
2. loss of consciousness, coma (complementary or emergency measure)

Pec: Jing (well) point (1st Shu-point)

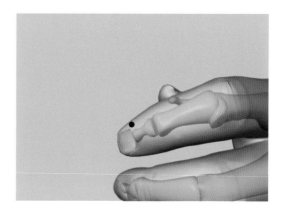

LI 2 Er Jian   Second Space

L: in the depression just distal to the side of the second metacarpo-phalangeal joint of a loosely clenched fist

T: 0.2–0.3 cun perpendicular; moxibustion

P: clears heat and removes inflammation

A: acute inflammation in the region of the head, face, ENT, eyes, and mouth

Pec: Xing (spring) point (2nd Shu-point)

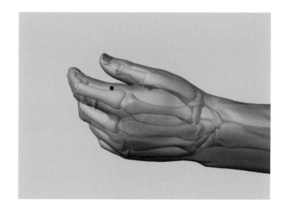

LI 3 San Jian   Third space

L: in the depression just proximal to the second metacarpo-phalangeal joint of a loosely clenched fist

T: 0.3–0.5 cun perpendicular; moxibustion

P: clears heat and removes inflammation

A: 1. acute inflammation in the region of the head, face, ENT, eyes, and mouth
2. pains and lack of finger movement

Pec: Shu (stream) point (3rd Shu-point)

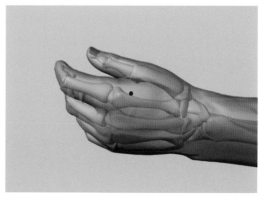

L: Location   **T:** Insertion Technique   **P:** Properties   **A:** Clinical Applications   **Pec:** Peculiarities

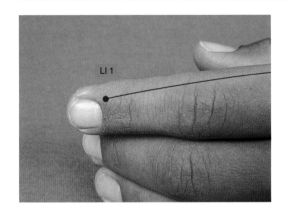

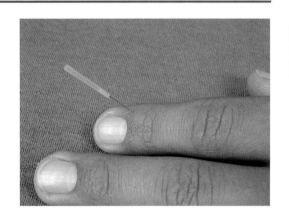

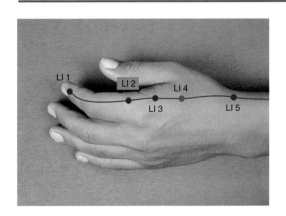

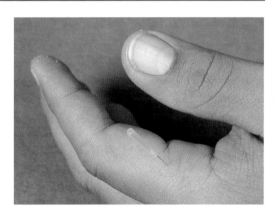

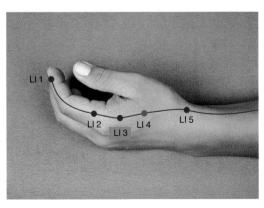

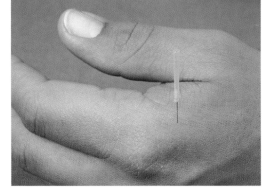

● Mu Point ● Back-Shu-Point ● Connecting Point (Luo) ● Cleft Point ● Lower He Point ● Qi-Source-Point (Yuan) ● Confluent Point ● Converging Point

LI 4 He Gu Joining Valley

L: on the dorsum of the hand, to the side of the midpoint of the second metacarpal bone, in the adductor pollicis muscle

T: 0.5–0.8 cun perpendicular; moxibustion

P: clears heat and releases the surface, decongests and activates the five sensory organs

A: 1. temperature, headaches, painful swelling in the throat and pharynx accompanying "colds"
2. acute inflammation in the region of the neck and the head
3. insufficient or excessive sweating
4. pains and limited movement in the region of the wrist and fingers
5. can promote contractions in the lower musculature

Pec: Qi-source-point (Yuan); CAUTION, STRONG MANI-PULATION INDUCES CONTRACTIONS IN PREGNANCY!

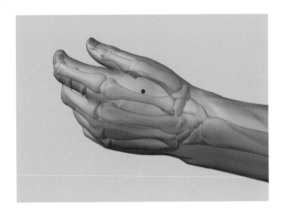

LI 5 Yang Xi Yang Stream

L: on the radial side of the dorsal wrist crease, in the centre of the hollow formed between the tendons of the extensor pollicis longus and brevis muscles, when the thumb is erect (fossa radialis, anatomical snuffbox)

T: 0.3–0.5 cun perpendicular; moxibustion

P: clears and decongests the five sensory organs (ears, eyes, mouth, nose, tongue), relaxes the tendons, and alleviates pain

A: 1. acute inflammation in the region of the head, face, ENT, eyes, and mouth
2. diseases of the ear e.g. tinnitus, deafness
3. wrist pain

Pec: Jing (river) point (4th Shu-point)

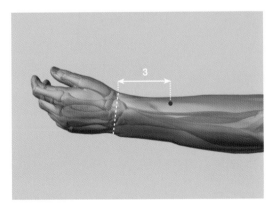

LI 6 Pian Li Veering Passage

L: 3 cun proximal to the dorsal wrist crease on the lateral aspect of the lower arm on the connection line between LI 5 and LI 11 with a slightly bent elbow

T: 0.3–0.7 cun perpendicular; moxibustion

P: clarifies eyesight and sharpens hearing

A: 1. deafness, tinnitus
2. conjunctivitis and other acute inflammations of the eye
3. facial paresis

Pec: connecting point (Luo)

L: Location   T: Insertion Technique   P: Properties   A: Clinical Applications   Pec: Peculiarities

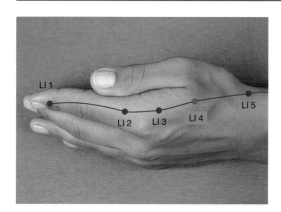

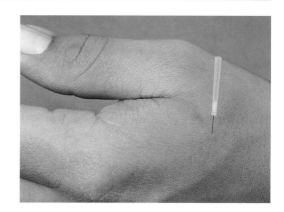

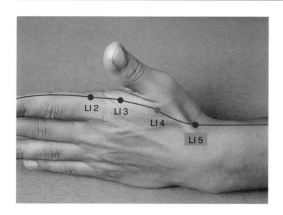

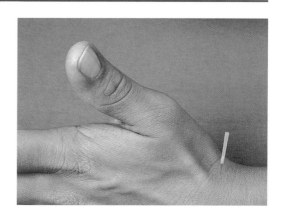

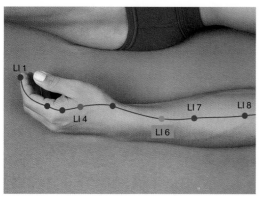

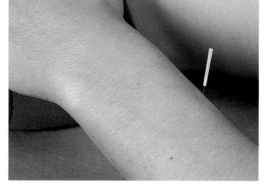

● Mu Point ● Back-Shu-Point ● Connecting Point (Luo) ● Cleft Point ● Lower He Point   ● Qi-Source-Point (Yuan) ● Confluent Point ● Converging Point

LI

LI 7 Wen Liu   Warm flow

L: 5 cun proximal to the dorsal wrist crease, on the lateral aspect of the forearm, on the connection line between LI 5 and LI 11 with a slightly bent elbow

T: 0.5–0.8 cun perpendicular; moxibustion

P: clears heat and removes inflammation

A: 1. acute inflammation in the region of the ENT, eyes, and mouth e.g. laryngitis, pharyngitis, stomatitis, rhinitis

    2. epistaxis

Pec: cleft (Xi) point

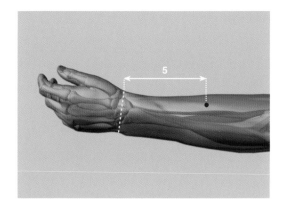

LI 8 Xia Lian   Lower Angle

L: 4 cun distal to LI 11, on the line connecting LI 5 and LI 11

T: 0.5–0.8 cun perpendicular; moxibustion

P: activates the channel and alleviates pain

A: 1. headache; dizziness and numbness

    2. pain in the region of the elbow joint and lower arm

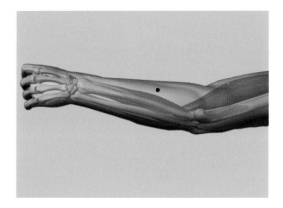

LI 9 Shang Lian   Upper Angle

L: 3 cun distal to LI 11 on the connecting line between LI 5 and LI 11

T: 0.5–0.8 cun perpendicular; moxibustion

P: decongests and activates the channel and its vessels

A: 1. headache

    2. pain and paralyses in the region of the elbow joint and lower arm

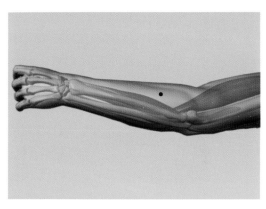

L: Location   T: Insertion Technique   P: Properties   A: Clinical Applications   Pec: Peculiarities

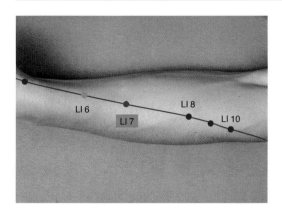
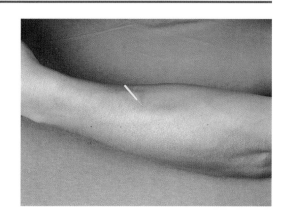

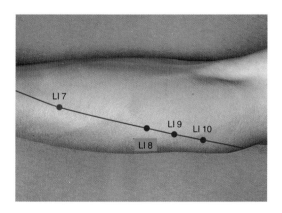
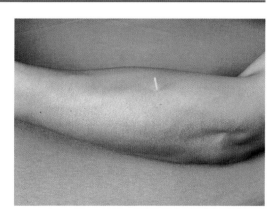

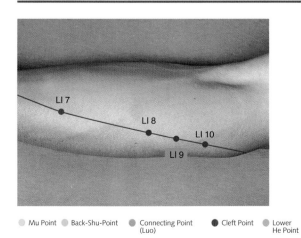
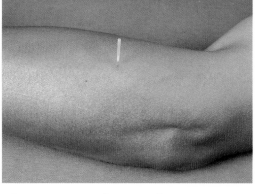

● Mu Point   ● Back-Shu-Point   ● Connecting Point (Luo)   ● Cleft Point   ● Lower He Point   ● Qi-Source-Point (Yuan)   ● Confluent Point   ● Converging Point

LI

LI 10 Shou San Li Arm Three Miles

L: 2 cun distal to LI 11 on the line which connects LI 5 and LI 11

T: 0.5–0.8 cun perpendicular; moxibustion

P: decongests and activates the channel and its vessels

A: pain and restricted movement in the pathway of the large intestine e.g. arm paresis after apoplexy, pain in the elbow joint, pain and cramp in the forearm and hand

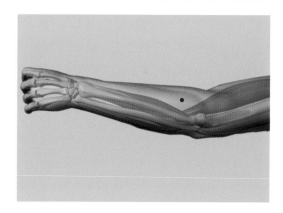

LI 11 Qu Chi Pool at the Crook

L: with elbow bent to 90 degrees, between the lateral end of the cubital crease and the lateral epicondyle of the humerus

T: 0.5–1.2 cun perpendicular; moxibustion

P: expels wind, soothes nausea, clears heat, decreases swelling in edemas, and soothes pain

A: 1. acute inflammation in the region of the head and neck accompanied by temperature and headaches
2. urticaria
3. pains in the region of elbow and lower arm
4. hypertonus
5. psychological and psychosomatic disorders

Pec: He (sea) point (5th Shu-point) symptomatic point in allergies

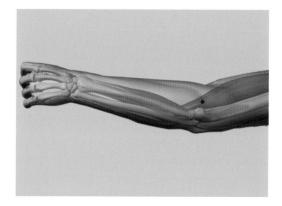

LI 12 Zhou Liao Elbow Crevice

L: with elbow flexed to 90 degrees, 1 cun proximal to LI 11, to the lateral aspect of the edge of the humerus

T: 0.5–0.8 cun perpendicular; moxibustion

P: activates the channel

A: Epicondylitis humeri radialis (Tennis elbow)

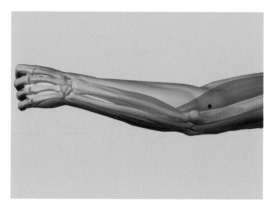

L: Location **T:** Insertion Technique **P:** Properties **A:** Clinical Applications **Pec:** Peculiarities

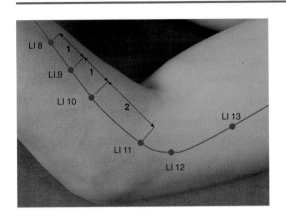

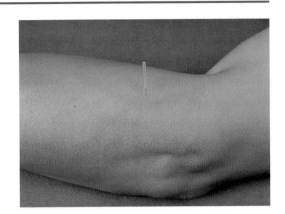

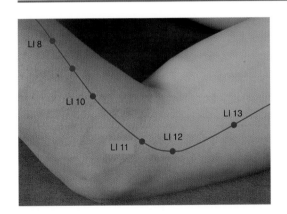

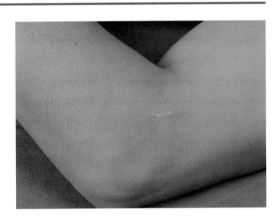

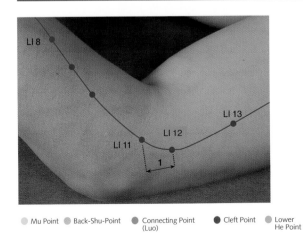

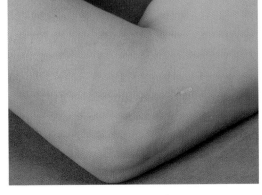

● Mu Point ● Back-Shu-Point ● Connecting Point (Luo) ● Cleft Point ● Lower He Point ● Qi-Source-Point (Yuan) ● Confluent Point ● Converging Point

LI

LI 13 Shou Wu Li   Arm Five Miles

L: 3 cun proximal to LI 11, on the lateral side of the humerus, on the connecting line between LI 11 and LI 15

T: 0.5–0.8 cun perpendicular; moxibustion

P: decongests and activates the channel

A: pain and restricted movement in the upper arm

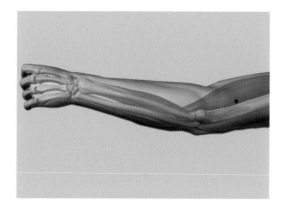

LI 14 Bi Nao   Upper Arm

L: 7 cun proximal to LI 11, on the lateral aspect of the upper arm, on the connecting line between LI 11 and LI 15, at the beginning of the deltoid muscle

T: 0.5–0.8 cun perpendicular or 1–1.5 oblique proximally; moxibustion

P: activates the channel and alleviates pain, removes lymph swelling and sharpens eyesight

A: 1. pain in the region of the deltoid muscle and biceps brachii muscle
2. dysfunctions in the lymphatic outlet in unspecific lymphademitis and lymphadenitis tuberculosa in the neck, throat, and armpit regions
3. diseases of the eye

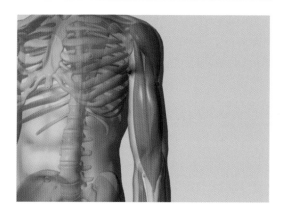

LI 15 Jian Yu   Shoulder bone

L: when the arm is abducted horizontally, between the front and middle parts of the deltoid muscle, in the anterior and inferior depression of the acromion

T: 0.5–1.2 cun perpendicular or oblique distally; moxibustion

P: decongests and activates the channel, expels wind and nausea

A: 1. pain and restricted movement in the region of the shoulder joint and superior extremity
2. urticaria

Pec: CAUTION, AVOID SPREADING GERMS TO THE SHOULDER JOINT!

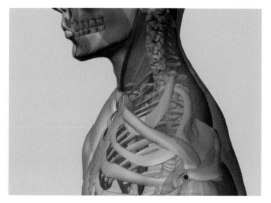

L: Location   **T:** Insertion Technique   **P:** Properties   **A:** Clinical Applications   **Pec:** Peculiarities

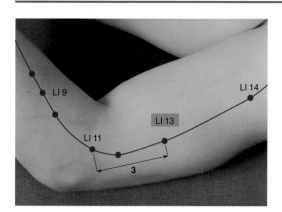

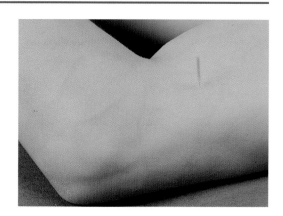

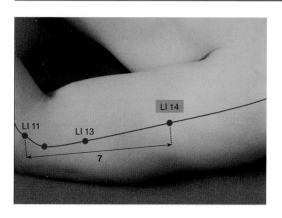

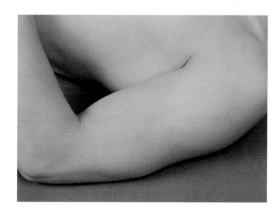

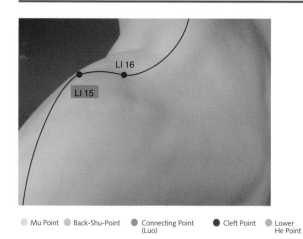

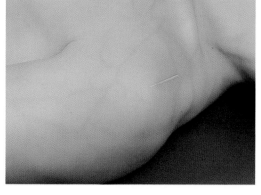

● Mu Point ● Back-Shu-Point ● Connecting Point (Luo) ● Cleft Point ● Lower He Point ● Qi-Source-Point (Yuan) ● Confluent Point ● Converging Point

LI

LI 16 Ju Gu Great Bone

L: in the depression between the lateral end of the
clavicle and the scapular spine

T: 0.4–0.6 cun perpendicular;
moxibustion

P: activates the channel and alleviates pain

A: 1. pain and restricted movement in the shoulder
joint, back, and upper extremity
2. diseases of the thyroid gland e.g. euthyreote
struma (goitre), hyperthyreosis (hyperthyroidism)

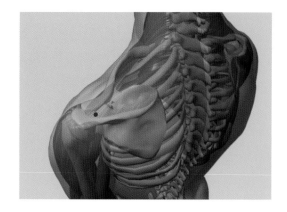

LI 17 Tian Ding Heaven's Tripod

L: on the posterior border of the sternocleidomastoid
muscle, 1 cun inferior to LI 18

T: 0.3–0.5 cun perpendicular;
moxibustion

P: relieves heat and decreases swelling of edema

A: acute inflammation in the region of the pharynx and
throat e.g. pharyngitis, tonsilitis, inflammation of the
vocal cords

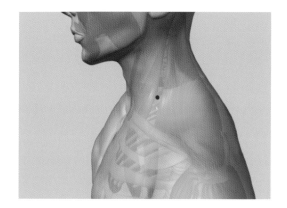

LI 18 Fu Tu Support the Prominence

L: between the two muscle heads of the
sternocleidomastoid muscle, 3 cun lateral to the
laryngeal prominence, 1 cun cranial to LI 17

T: 0.5–0.8 cun perpendicular;
moxibustion

P: relieves heat, decreases edema, soothes coughing,
and relieves breathing difficulty

A: 1. acute inflammation in the region of the pharynx
and throat
2. coughing and asthmatic diseases in diseases of
the trachea

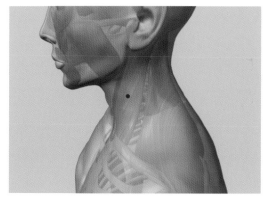

L: Location   **T:** Insertion Technique   **P:** Properties   **A:** Clinical Applications   **Pec:** Peculiarities

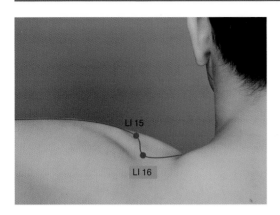

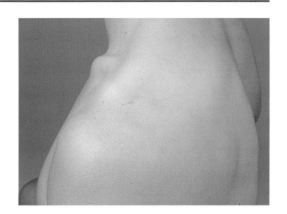

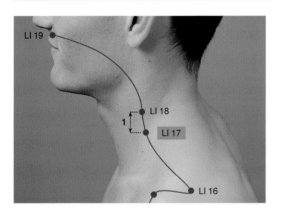

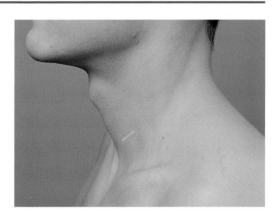

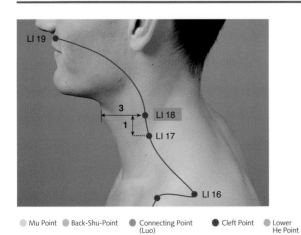

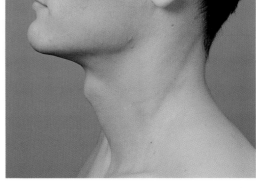

● Mu Point   ● Back-Shu-Point   ● Connecting Point (Luo)   ● Cleft Point   ● Lower He Point   ● Qi-Source-Point (Yuan)   ● Confluent Point   ● Converging Point

LI 19 Kou He Liao Mouth Grain Crevice

L: cranial to the upper lip, directly below the lateral edge of the nostril, at the height of Du 26

T: 0.2 cun perpendicular;
no moxibustion

P: clears the lung and decongests the nose

A: 1. diseases of the nose
2. facial paresis

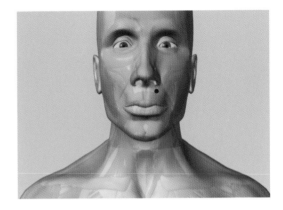

LI 20 Ying Xiang Welcome Fragrance

L: in the naso-labial groove, near the midpoint of the lateral border of the ala nasi.nose

T: 0.2–0.4 cun perpendicular or 0.3–0.5 cun oblique cranially;
no moxibustion

P: clears the lung and decongests the nose, dispels wind, and activates the channel

A: 1. diseases of the nose
2. facial paresis
3. paraestheses in the face

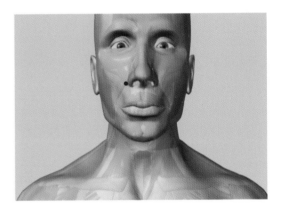

L: Location   T: Insertion Technique   P: Properties   A: Clinical Applications   **Pec:** Peculiarities

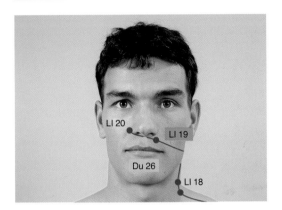

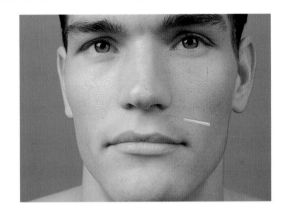

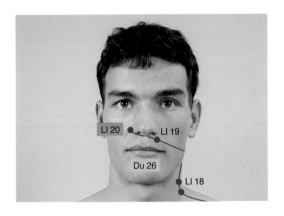

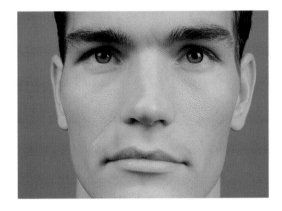

○ Mu Point   ○ Back-Shu-Point   ○ Connecting Point (Luo)   ● Cleft Point   ○ Lower He Point   ● Qi-Source-Point (Yuan)   ● Confluent Point   ● Converging Point

2.2.3   The stomach channel (St)

Synonyms

• Stomach meridian

• Foot Yangming stomach channel

St

Channel pathway

There are 45 acupuncture points in the surface stomach channel pathway.

The surface pathway starts at the lateral side of the nostril and ascends the nose to the inner medial canthus, where it meets the bladder channel. From here the channel runs to its first point on the lower edge of the eye socket and then perpendicular to the corner of the mouth. From this section of the channel branches provide for the gums of the upper jaw, circle the lips, and then meet the Extraordinary Vessel Ren Mai in the groove of the chin.

From the corner of the mouth the channel descends to the lower jaw and as a facial branch to the corner of the jaw, from where it ascends via the zygomatic arch to the level of the temples and the region of the "Head's Binding" (St 8) in front of the ear. A branch runs to Du Mai (Du 24).

The main pathway of the channel extends from the lower jaw over the side of the neck and carotid artery to the upper clavicular fossa. Here the channel starts its inner pathway, which runs down from the diaphragm to its organ, the stomach and the spleen. Connections with the deeper layers of the points Ren 12 and Ren 13 are located here.

From the upper clavicular fossa the surface pathway of the channel runs over the chest and nipple to the abdomen, where the channel runs to the side of the straight abdominal muscle and past the umbilicus to the groin. An inner branch runs from the pyloric orifice of the stomach to point St 30 near the groin. From here the channel continues to run superficially over the antero-lateral aspect of the upper thigh to the side of the patella and then via the anterior aspect of the lower leg and foot dorsum, terminating at the lateral side of the second toenail.

From point St 36 below the knee a branch descends via the antero-lateral aspect of the lower leg and the foot dorsum to the lateral side of the third toe. From point St 42 a branch meets with the spleen channel on the big toe.

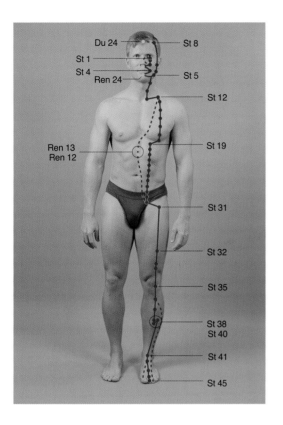

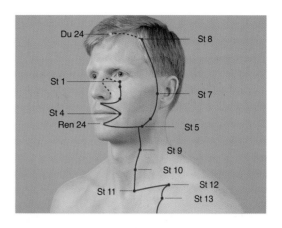

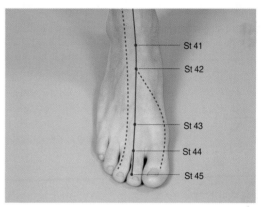

St

St 1 Cheng Qi Container of Tears

L: with the patient staring directly forward, directly below the pupil, between the eyeball and inferior infraorbital foramen

T: 0.3–0.5 cun perpendicular; no needle manipulation; no moxibustion

P: clears heat and sharpens eyesight

A: 1. diseases of the eye e.g. conjunctivitis, ceratitis, night blindness, dacryocystitis
2. tics and cramps in the facial muscles

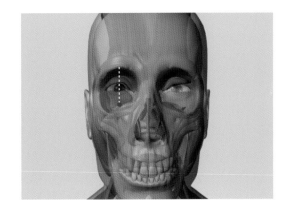

St 2 Si Bai Four Whites

L: with the patient staring directly ahead, directly below the pupil, in the depression at the infraorbital foramen

T: 0.2–0.3 cun perpendicular; no moxibustion

P: clears heat and sharpens eyesight

A: diseases of the eye e.g. conjunctivitis, ceratitis, night blindness, dacryocystitis

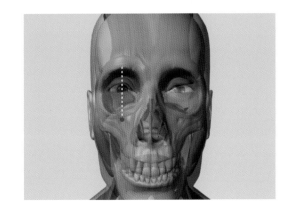

St 3 Ju Liao Great Crevice

L: with the patient staring directly ahead, directly below the pupil, on the level of the lower edge of the ala nasi

T: 0.3–0.6 cun perpendicular; moxibustion

P: clears heat and sharpens eyesight, expels wind, and activates the channel

A: 1. diseases of the eye e.g. conjunctivitis, ceratitis
2. facial paresis

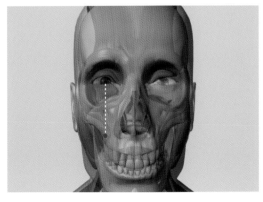

L: Location   **T:** Insertion Technique   **P:** Properties   **A:** Clinical Applications   **Pec:** Peculiarities

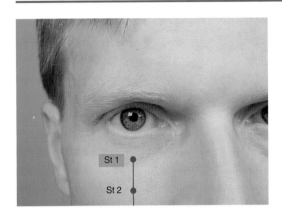

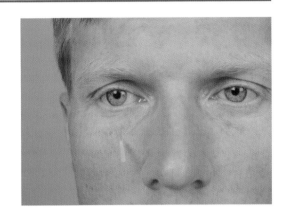

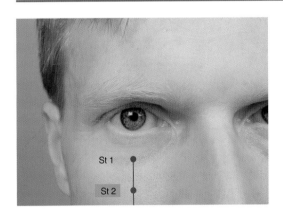

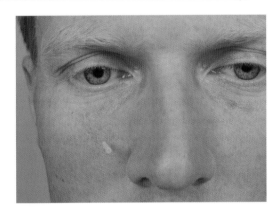

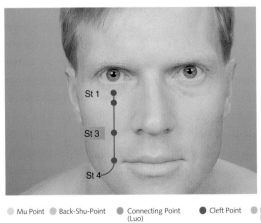

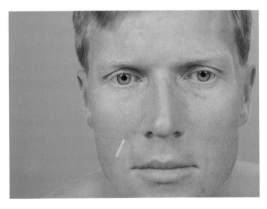

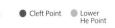

● Mu Point ● Back-Shu-Point ● Connecting Point (Luo) ● Cleft Point ● Lower He Point ● Qi-Source-Point (Yuan) ● Confluent Point ● Converging Point

St 4 Di Cang   Earth Granary

L: with the patient staring directly ahead, directly below the pupil, at 0.4 cun lateral to the corner of the mouth

T: 0.2 cun perpendicular or 0.5–0.8 cun subcutaneously towards St 6; moxibustion

P: expels wind and activates the channel

A: 1. facial paresis
2. tics and cramps in facial muscles

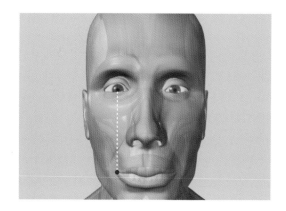

St 5 Da Ying   Great Welcome

L: on the front edge of the masseter muscle, 1.3 cun anterior and inferior to the corner of the jaw, above the palpable A. facialis

T: 0.2–0.3 cun perpendicular; moxibustion

P: expels wind and activates the channel

A: 1. facial paresis
2. toothache in the lower jaw
3. inflammation of the salivary gland

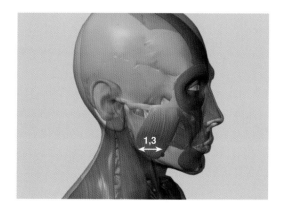

St 6 Jia Che   Jaw Bone

L: the width of a middle finger anterior and superior to the corner of the jaw; when the jaw is firmly clenched at the prominence of the masseter muscle

T: 0.3–0.4 cun perpendicular or 0.7–0.9 cun subcutaneously towards St 4; moxibustion

P: expels wind and clears heat, soothes pain and activates the channel

A: 1. acute inflammation of the bucal cavity
2. parotitis epidemica
3. facial paresis

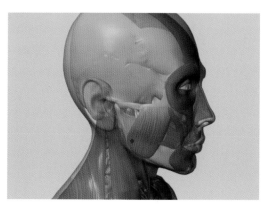

L: Location   T: Insertion Technique   P: Properties   A: Clinical Applications   Pec: Peculiarities

St

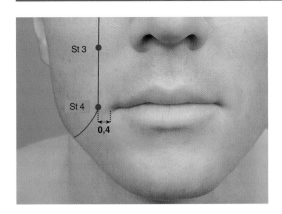

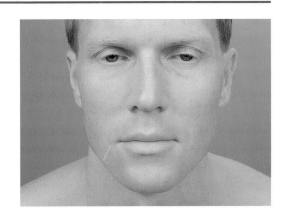

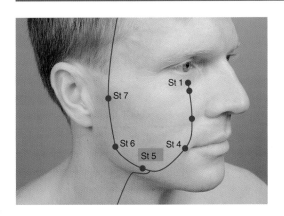

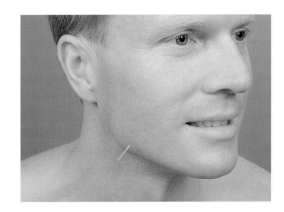

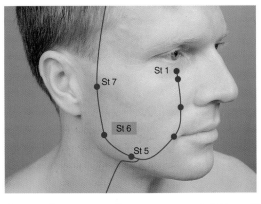

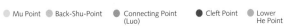

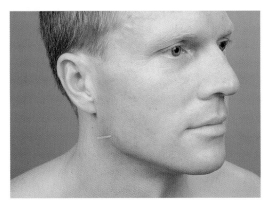

Mu Point ● Back-Shu-Point ● Connecting Point (Luo) ● Cleft Point ● Lower He Point ● Qi-Source-Point (Yuan) ● Confluent Point ● Converging Point

St 7 Xia Guan   Below the Joint

L: with closed mouth in the depression between the zygomatic arch and the incisura mandibulae

T: 0.3–0.5 cun perpendicular;
moxibustion

P: expels wind and clears heat, soothes pain and sharpens the hearing

A: 1. toothache in the upper jaw
2. trigeminus neuralgia
3. diseases of the ear e.g. deafness, tinnitus

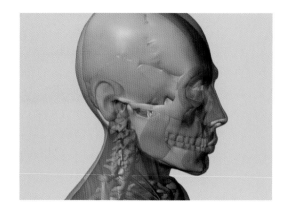

St 8 Tou Wei   Head's Binding

L: in the temple corner (in the "Head's Binding"), 0.5 cun within the ideal anterior hairline, 4.5 cun lateral to the midline

T: 0.5–0.8 subcutaneously tranvserse occipitally or caudally;
no moxibustion

P: expels wind and clears heat, soothes pain and sharpens the eyesight

A: 1. headaches on one side
2. diseases of the eye

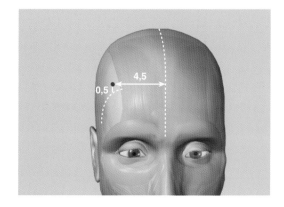

St 9 Ren Ying   Man's Welcome

L: on the front edge of the sternocleidomastoid muscle; 1.5 cun lateral to the upper edge of the laryngeal prominence, next to the carotid artery

T: 0.3–0.8 cun perpendicular, near the palpable carotid artery!;
no moxibustion

P: regulates Qi and relieves breathing difficulty, clears heat and dispels knots

A: 1. hypertension
2. bronchial asthma, spastic bronchitis
3. inflammation in the region of the pharynx and throat, tonsillitis

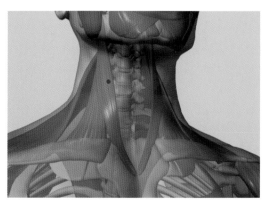

L: Location   T: Insertion Technique   P: Properties   A: Clinical Applications   Pec: Peculiarities

St

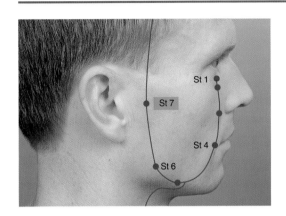

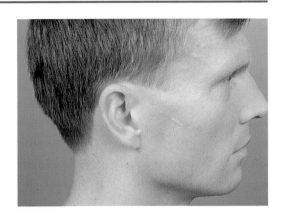

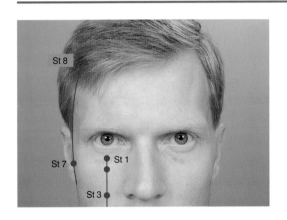

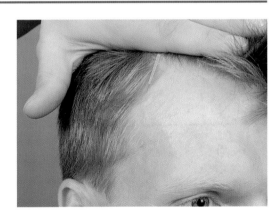

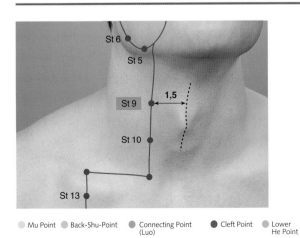

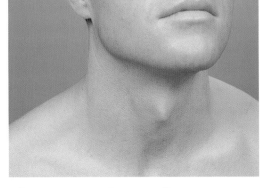

○ Mu Point ○ Back-Shu-Point ● Connecting Point (Luo) ● Cleft Point ○ Lower He Point   ● Qi-Source-Point (Yuan) ● Confluent Point ● Converging Point

St 10 Shui Tu Water Prominence

L: on the front edge of the sternocleidomastoid muscle, at the level of the lower point of the laryngeal prominence, between St 9 and St 11

T: 0.3–0.8 cun perpendicular; moxibustion

P: alleviates coughing and relieves breathing difficulty

A: 1. coughing and breathing difficulty
2. acute tonsillitis

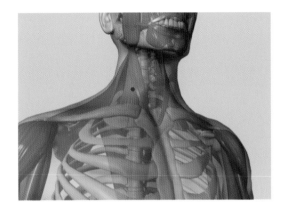

St 11 Qi She Abode of Qi

L: on the upper edge of the medial end of the clavicle, between the clavicular and sternal onset of the sternocleidomastoid muscle, directly below St 10

T: 0.3–0.4 cun perpendicular; moxibustion

P: reduces inverted Qi and relieves breathing difficulty

A: 1. acute respiratory insufficiency
2. bronchial asthma, spastic bronchitis
3. acute inflammation in the region of the pharynx and throat

Pec: CAUTION, AVOID PNEUMOTHORAX!

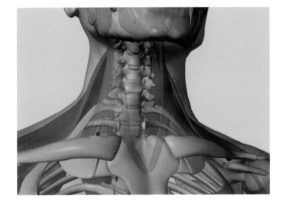

St 12 Que Pen Empty Basin

L: in the centre of the supraclavicular fossa, 4 cun lateral to the ventral midline

T: 0.2–0.4 cun perpendicular; moxibustion

P: alleviates coughing and relieves breathing difficulty, regulates Qi and soothes pain

A: 1. coughing and breathing difficulty in diseases of the trachea
2. pain in the region of the shoulder and neck
3. lymphatic drainage dysfunctions in unspecific lymphadenitis and lymphadenitis tuberculosa in the region of the neck and throat

Pec: CAUTION, AVOID PNEUMOTHORAX!

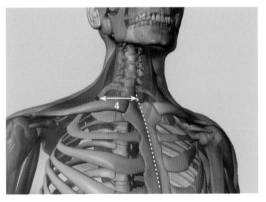

L: Location   **T:** Insertion Technique   **P:** Properties   **A:** Clinical Applications   **Pec:** Peculiarities

St

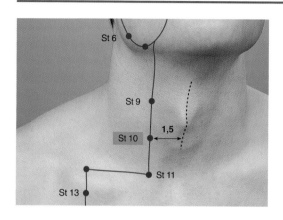

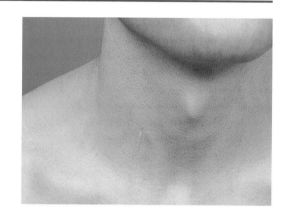

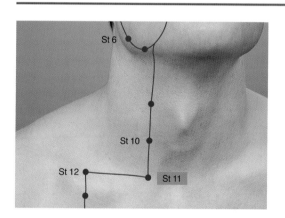

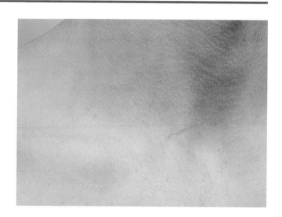

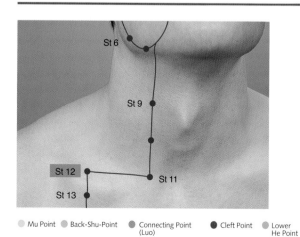

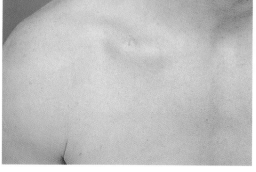

● Mu Point ● Back-Shu-Point ● Connecting Point (Luo) ● Cleft Point ● Lower He Point ● Qi-Source-Point (Yuan) ● Confluent Point ● Converging Point

St 13 Qi Hu   Qi Door

L: caudal to the centre of the lower edge of the clavicle, 4 cun lateral to the ventral midline

T: 0.3–0.5 cun oblique or subcutaneously; moxibustion

P: alleviates coughing and relieves breathing difficulty

A: coughing and breathing difficulty, spitting or coughing blood, and thoracic pain in diseases of the trachea

Pec: CAUTION, AVOID PNEUMOTHORAX!

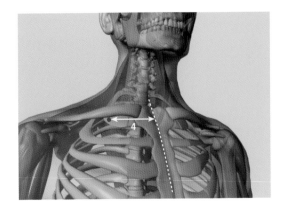

St 14 Ku Fang   Storehouse

L: in the first ICR, 4 cun lateral to the ventral midline

T: 0.3–0.5 cun oblique medially or 0.5-0.8 cun subcutaneously; moxibustion

P: clears the lung and removes heat, alleviates coughing and relieves breathing difficulty

A: infectious diseases of the trachea e.g. acute bronchitis, pneumonia, abscess of the lung

Pec: CAUTION, AVOID PNEUMOTHORAX!

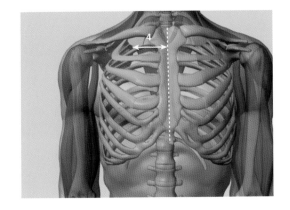

St 15 Wu Yi   Room Screen

L: in the 2nd ICR, 4 cun lateral to the ventral midline

T: 0.3–0.5 cun oblique medially or 0.5-0.8 subcutaneously; moxibustion

P: clears the lung and removes heat, alleviates coughing and transforms phlegm

A: infectious diseases of the trachea e.g. acute bronchitis, pneumonia, abscess of the lung

Pec: CAUTION, AVOID PNEUMOTHORAX!

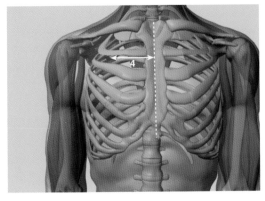

L: Location   T: Insertion Technique   P: Properties   A: Clinical Applications   Pec: Peculiarities

St

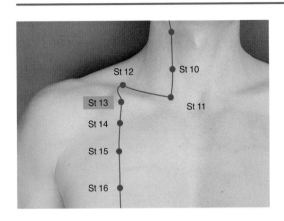
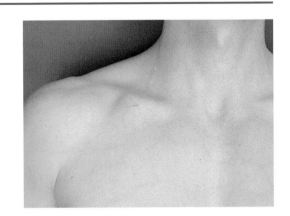

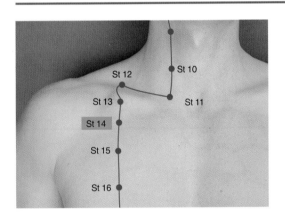
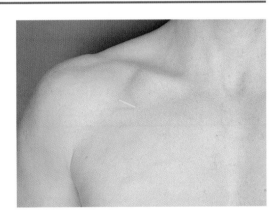

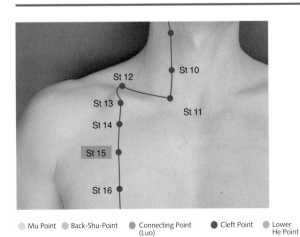
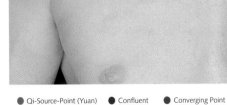

● Mu Point ● Back-Shu-Point ● Connecting Point (Luo) ● Cleft Point ● Lower He Point ● Qi-Source-Point (Yuan) ● Confluent Point ● Converging Point

St 16 Ying Chuang Breast Window

L: in the 3rd ICR, 4 cun lateral to the ventral midline

T: 0.3–0.5 cun oblique medially or 0.5–0.8 cun subcutaneously; moxibustion

P: clears the lung and relieves breathing difficulty, removes heat and suppurative sores

A: 1. coughing and respiratory insufficiency in diseases of the trachea
2. acute mastitis

Pec: CAUTION, AVOID PNEUMOTHORAX!

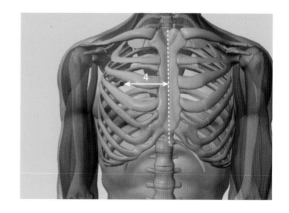

St 17 Ru Zhong Middle of the Breast

L: in the 4th ICR, 4 cun lateral to the ventral midline in the centre of the nipple

T: no acupuncture; no moxibustion; serves only to locate other points

P: none

A: none

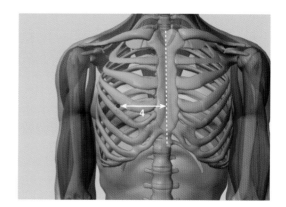

St 18 Ru Gen Root of the Breast

L: in the 5th ICR, caudal to the lower edge of the chest, 4 cun lateral to the ventral midline

T: 0.5–0.8 cun oblique or subcutaneously; moxibustion

P: stimulates lactation, removes suppurative sores, alleviates coughing and relieves breathing difficulty

A: 1. diseases of the breast e.g. insufficient postpartum lactation, acute mastitis
2. diseases of the trachea e.g. bronchitis and pneumonia

Pec: CAUTION, AVOID PNEUMOTHORAX!

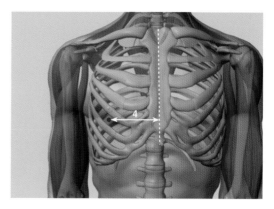

L: Location   T: Insertion Technique   P: Properties   A: Clinical Applications   Pec: Peculiarities

St

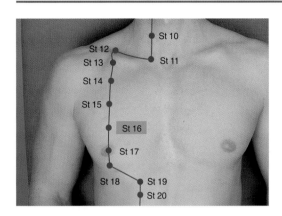

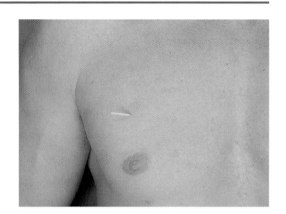

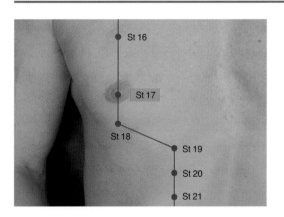

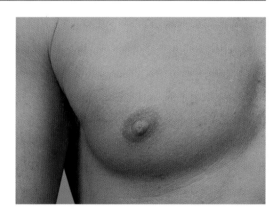

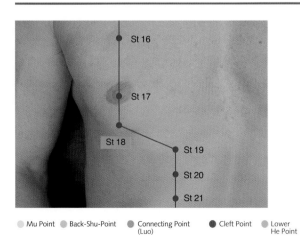

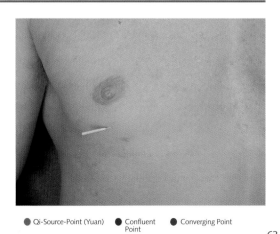

● Mu Point ● Back-Shu-Point ● Connecting Point (Luo) ● Cleft Point ● Lower He Point ● Qi-Source-Point (Yuan) ● Confluent Point ● Converging Point

St 19 Bu Rong   Not Contained

L: 6 cun superior to the umbilicus, 2 cun lateral to the ventral midline

T: 0.5–0.8 cun perpendicular; moxibustion

P: harmonizes the stomach, reduces inverted Qi, alleviates nausea and pain

A: acute gastritis, stomach pain

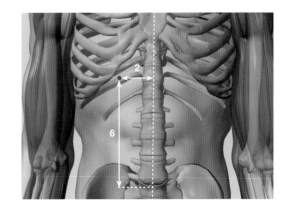

St 20 Cheng Man   Supporting Fullness

L: 5 cun superior to the umbilicus, 2 cun lateral to the ventral midline

T: 0.8–1 cun perpendicular; moxibustion

P: regulates Qi and harmonizes the stomach, reduces inverted Qi and alleviates nausea

A: 1. acute and chronic gastroenteritis
2. borborygmus, feeling of abdominal distension

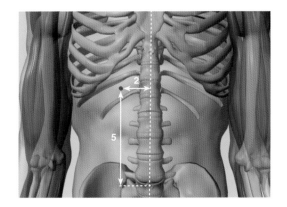

St 21 Liang Men   Beam Gate

L: 4 cun superior to the umbilicus, 2 cun lateral to the ventral midline

T: 0.8–1.2 cun perpendicular; moxibustion

P: regulates balance in stomach and intestine

A: acute and chronic gastroenteritis

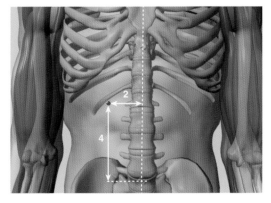

L: Location   T: Insertion Technique   P: Properties   A: Clinical Applications   Pec: Peculiarities

St

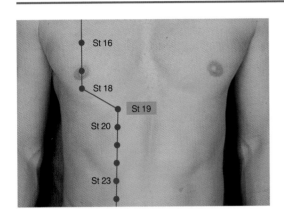

St 16
St 18
St 19
St 20
St 23

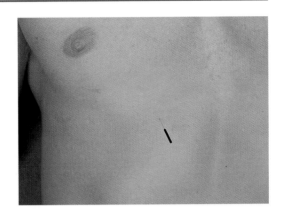

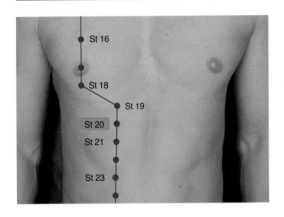

St 16
St 18
St 19
St 20
St 21
St 23

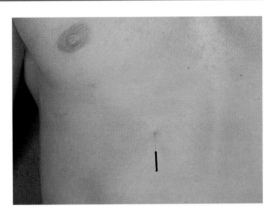

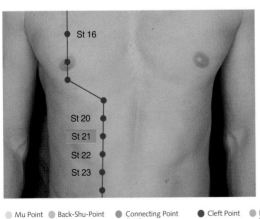

St 16
St 20
St 21
St 22
St 23

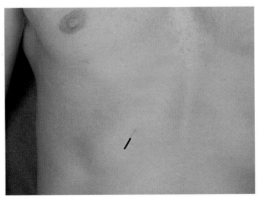

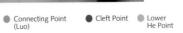

● Mu Point ● Back-Shu-Point ● Connecting Point (Luo) ● Cleft Point ● Lower He Point   ● Qi-Source-Point (Yuan) ● Confluent Point ● Converging Point

65

St 22 Guan Men   Pass Gate

L: 3 cun superior to the umbilicus, 2 cun lateral to the ventral midline

T: 0.8–1.2 cun perpendicular; moxibustion

P: regulates balance in stomach and intestine, benefits urination, reduces edema

A: 1. acute and chronic gastroenteritis
2. edema

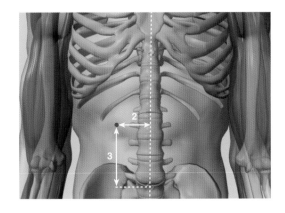

St 23 Tai Yi   Supreme Unity

L: 2 cun superior to the umbilicus, 2 cun lateral to the ventral midline

T: 0.8–1.2 cun perpendicular; moxibustion

P: pacifies spiritual strength and provides for all-round calmness, harmonizes stomach and intestine

A: 1. psychic and psychosomatic dysfunctions (sedative effect)
2. stomach pains

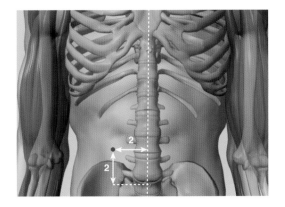

St 24 Hua Rou Men   Slippery Flesh Gate

L: 1 cun superior to the umbilicus, 2 cun lateral to the ventral midline

T: 0.8–1.2 cun perpendicular; moxibustion

P: pacifies spiritual strength and provides for all-round calmness, harmonizes stomach and intestine

A: 1. psychic and psychosomatic dysfunctions
2. acute gastritis

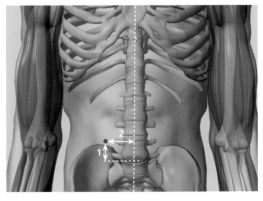

L: Location   T: Insertion Technique   P: Properties   A: Clinical Applications   Pec: Peculiarities

St

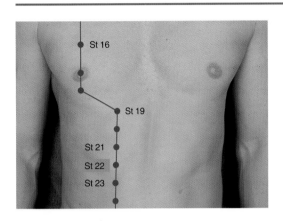

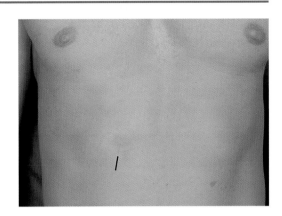

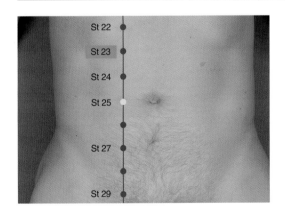

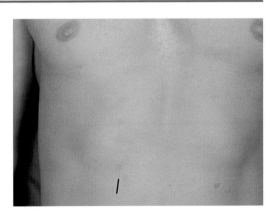

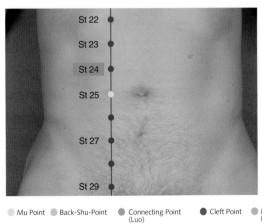

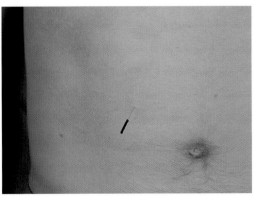

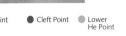

● Mu Point   ● Back-Shu-Point   ● Connecting Point (Luo)   ● Cleft Point   ● Lower He Point   ● Qi-Source-Point (Yuan)   ● Confluent Point   ● Converging Point

St 25 Tian Shu   Heaven's Pivot

L: 2 cun lateral to the umbilicus

T: 1–1.5 cun perpendicular; moxibustion

P: regulates the rise and fall of Qi, regulates the large intestine

A: 1. dysfunctions of the intestinal function in diseases of the large intestine e.g. abdominal pain, borborygmus, enteritis, dysentery, obstipation (restores balance)
2. appendicitis
3. anomalies in menstrual regularity, dysmenorrhoea

Pec: Mu (gathering) point of large intestine
CAUTION IN PREGNANCY!

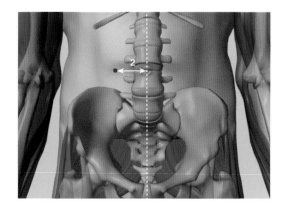

St 26 Wai Ling   Outer Mound

L: 1 cun inferior to the umbilicus, 2 cun lateral to the ventral midline

T: 1–1.5 cun perpendicular; moxibustion

P: regulates Qi and alleviates pain

A: 1. abdominal pain
2. dysmenorrhoea

Pec: CAUTION IN PREGNANCY!

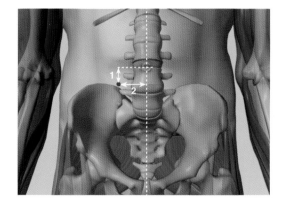

St 27 Da Ju   The Great

L: 2 cun inferior to the umbilicus, 2 cun lateral to the ventral midline

T: 1–1.5 cun perpendicular; moxibustion

P: eliminates borborygmus, benefits urination

A: 1. urinary behavior
2. external abdominal hernias

Pec: CAUTION IN PREGNANCY!

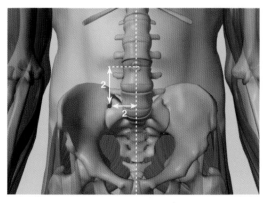

L: Location   **T:** Insertion Technique   **P:** Properties   **A:** Clinical Applications   **Pec:** Peculiarities

St

St

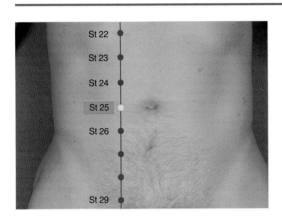
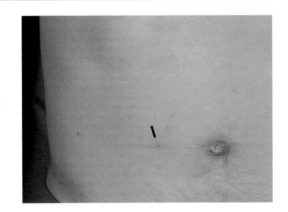

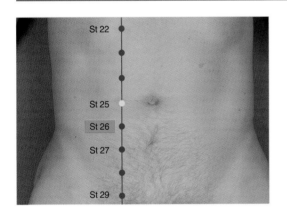
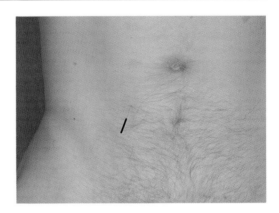

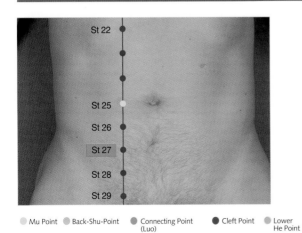
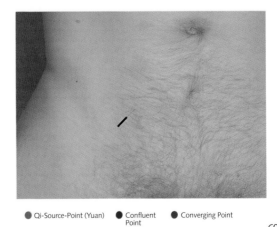

⬤ Mu Point ⬤ Back-Shu-Point ⬤ Connecting Point (Luo) ⬤ Cleft Point ⬤ Lower He Point   ⬤ Qi-Source-Point (Yuan) ⬤ Confluent Point ⬤ Converging Point

St 28 Shui Dao   Water Passage

L: 3 cun inferior to the umbilicus, 2 cun lateral to the ventral midline

T: 1–1.5 cun perpendicular; moxibustion

P: benefits the bladder, regulates menstruation, and alleviates pain

A: 1. urinary behavior
2. obstipation
3. dysmenorrhoea, female fertility dysfunctions

Pec: Caution in Pregnancy!

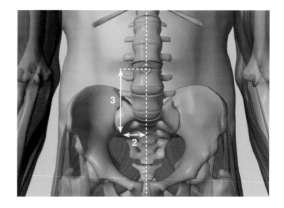

St 29 Gui Lai   Return

L: 4 cun inferior to the umbilicus, 2 cun lateral to the ventral midline

T: 1–1.5 cun perpendicular; moxibustion

P: activates Qi and alleviates pain, regulates menstruation and alleviates discharge

A: 1. external abdominal hernias

2. certain gynecological dysfunctions e.g. amenorrhoea, leucorrhoea, uterine prolapse

Pec: Caution in Pregnancy!

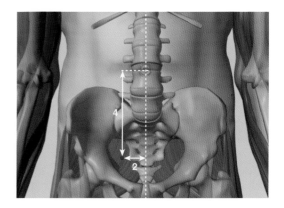

St 30 Qi Chong   Rushing Qi

L: 5 cun inferior to the umbilicus, 2 cun lateral to the ventral midline, immediately above the groin

T: 0.5–1 cun perpendicular; moxibustion

P: regulates and tonifies the chong mai, regulates menstruation and promotes fertilisation

A: 1. certain gynecological dysfunctions e.g. irregular menstruation, fertility dysfunctions, vulvitis, certain obstetric dysfunctions
2. external abdominal hernias
3. dysfunctions in male sexual function

Pec: Caution in Pregnancy!

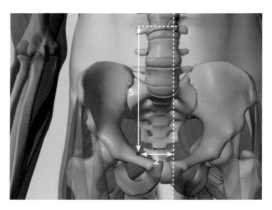

L: Location   T: Insertion Technique   P: Properties   A: Clinical Applications   Pec: Peculiarities

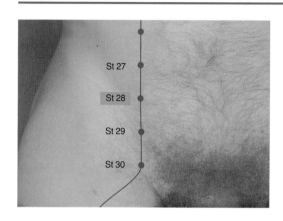

St 27
St 28
St 29
St 30

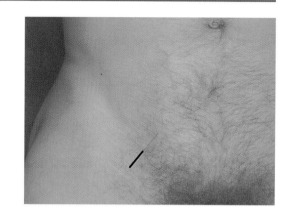

St

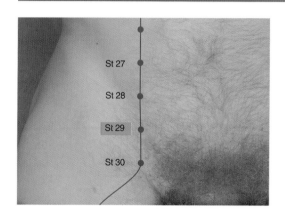

St 27
St 28
St 29
St 30

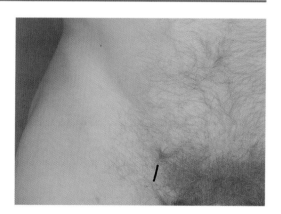

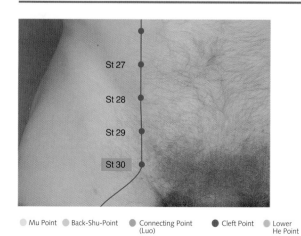

St 27
St 28
St 29
St 30

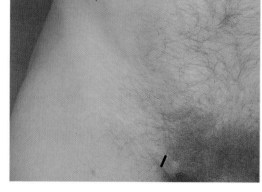

● Mu Point ● Back-Shu-Point ● Connecting Point (Luo) ● Cleft Point ● Lower He Point ● Qi-Source-Point (Yuan) ● Confluent Point ● Converging Point

St

St 31 Bi Guan   Thigh Gate

L: at the level of the inferior gluteal fold, on the connecting line between the anterior superior iliac spine and the superior lateral corner of the patella, opposite Bl 36

T: 1–2 cun perpendicular; moxibustion

P: decongests and activates the channel

A: pain, restricted movement, and numbness in the lower extremity

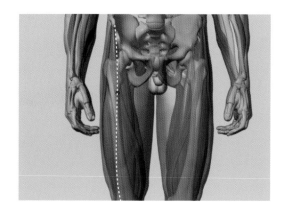

St 32 Fu Tu   Crouching Rabbit

L: on the connecting line between the anterior superior iliac spine and the superior lateral corner of the patella, at 6 cun proximal to this corner

T: 1–2 cun perpendicular; moxibustion

P: activates the channel and alleviates pain

A: pain and paraestheses in the groin area, hip, and in the lower extremity

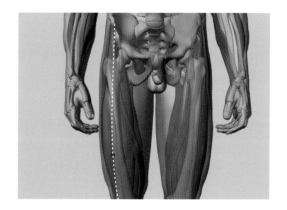

St 33 Yin Shi   Yin Market

L: on the connecting line between the anterior superior iliac spine and the superior lateral corner of the patella, at 3 cun proximal to this corner

T: 1–2 cun perpendicular; moxibustion

P: warms the channel and dispels cold

A: pain, lack of strength and cold in the regions of the groin, legs, and knees

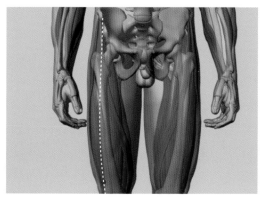

L: Location   T: Insertion Technique   P: Properties   A: Clinical Applications   Pec: Peculiarities

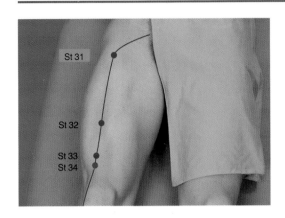

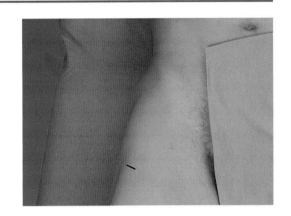

St 31

St 32

St 33
St 34

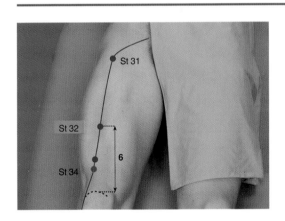

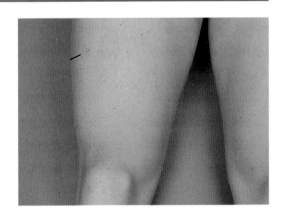

St 31

St 32

6

St 34

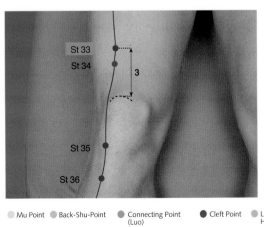

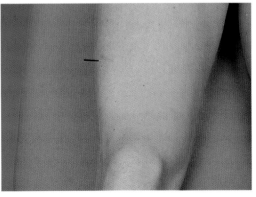

St 33

St 34

3

St 35

St 36

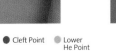

● Mu Point   ● Back-Shu-Point   ● Connecting Point (Luo)   ● Cleft Point   ● Lower He Point   ● Qi-Source-Point (Yuan)   ● Confluent Point   ● Converging Point

St 34 Liang Qiu Ridge Mound

L: when patient's knee is flexed, on the connecting line between the anterior superior iliac spine and the superior lateral corner of the patella, 2 cun proximal to this corner

T: 1–2 cun perpendicular;
moxibustion

P: harmonizes the stomach and reduces edema

A: 1. stomach pain
2. swelling and pain in the knee joint

Pec: cleft (Xi) point

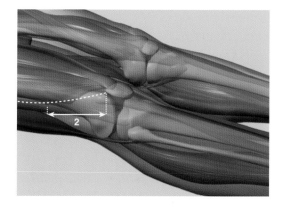

St 35 Du Bi Calf's Nose

L: when patient's knee is flexed, in the depression on the lower edge of the patella, lateral to the patellar ligament

T: 0.5–1.2 cun next to the patellar ligament, oblique proximally and medially;
moxibustion

P: activates the channel and stimulates the vessels

A: swelling and pain in the knee joint

Pec: CAUTION, AVOID SPREADING GERMS TO THE KNEE JOINT!

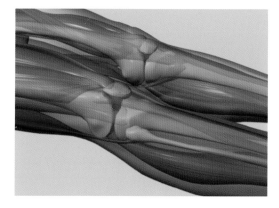

St 36 Zu San Li Leg Three Miles

L: 3 cun inferior to St 35, one middle fingerbreadth lateral to the anterior crest of the tibia, at the level of the distal edge of the tuberosity of the tibia

T: 1–2 cun perpendicular; moxibustion

P: strengthens the body and spleen, harmonizes the stomach, restores balance to Qi, decongests and activates the channel and its vessels

A: 1. strengthening of the entire body with prophylactic and immunological effects
2. dysfunctions of the digestive system
3. in all dysfunctions that can be attributed to a state of emptiness according to TCM
4. pains, restricted movement, and numbness of the lower extremity

Pec: He (sea) point (5th Shu-point)

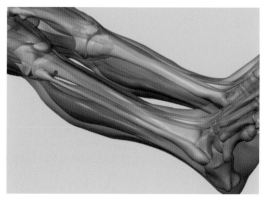

L: Location   T: Insertion Technique   P: Properties   A: Clinical Applications   Pec: Peculiarities

St

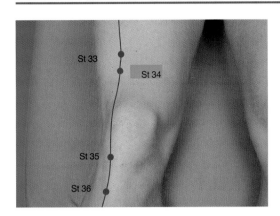

St 33
St 34
St 35
St 36

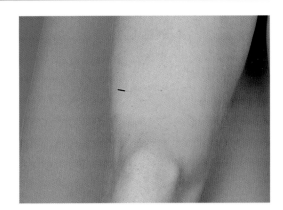

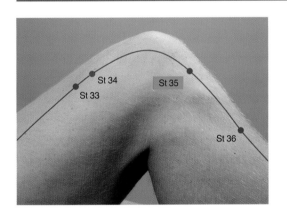

St 34
St 33
St 35
St 36

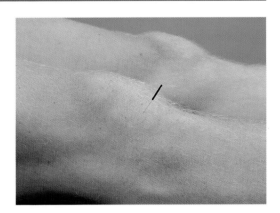

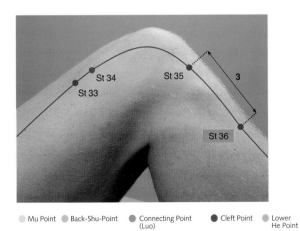

St 34
St 33
St 35
3
St 36

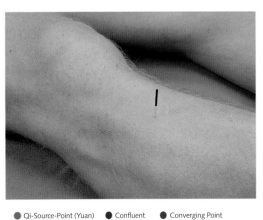

● Mu Point ● Back-Shu-Point ● Connecting Point (Luo) ● Cleft Point ● Lower He Point ● Qi-Source-Point (Yuan) ● Confluent Point ● Converging Point

75

St

St 37 Shang Ju Xu Upper Great Void

L: 6 cun inferior to St 35, one middle finger breadth
lateral to the anterior crest of the tibia

T: 1–2 cun perpendicular;
moxibustion

P: regulates and restores balance to the large intestine

A: diseases of the large intestine

Pec: lower He (sea) point of the large intestine

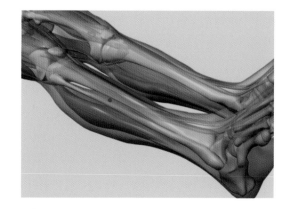

St 38 Tiao Kou Lines opening

L: 8 cun inferior to St 35, one middle finger breadth
lateral to the anterior crest of the tibia

T: 1–1.5 cun perpendicular;
moxibustion

P: decongests and activates the channel

A: 1. pains in the lower leg
2. stomach and abdominal pains
3. periarthropathia humeroscapularis

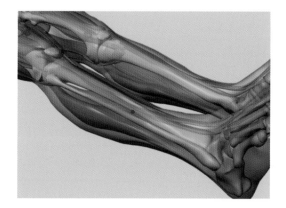

St 39 Xia Ju Xu Lower Great Void

L: 9 cun inferior to St 35 (1 cun below St 38), one
middle finger breadth lateral to the anterior crest of
the tibia

T: 1–1.5 cun perpendicular;
moxibustion

P: regulates and restores balance to the large intestine

A: 1. diseases of the small intestine (regulates and
restores balance)
2. pain and restricted movement of the lower
extremity

Pec: lower He (sea) point of the small intestine

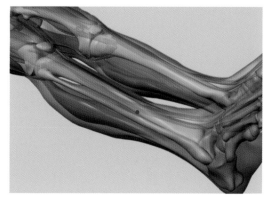

L: Location T: Insertion Technique P: Properties A: Clinical Applications Pec: Peculiarities

St

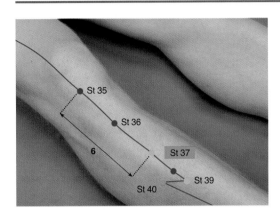

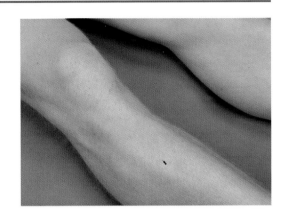

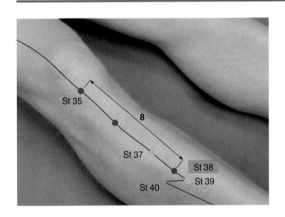

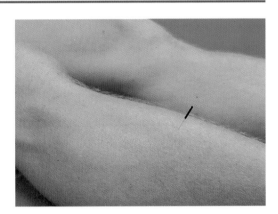

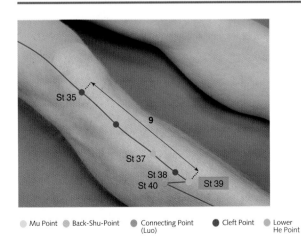

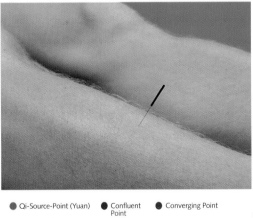

● Mu Point ● Back-Shu-Point ● Connecting Point (Luo) ● Cleft Point ● Lower He Point ● Qi-Source-Point (Yuan) ● Confluent Point ● Converging Point

St 40 Feng Long Abundant Bulge

L: 8 cun proximal to the prominence of the lateral malleolus, at the level of St 38, 2 middle finger breadths (1.5 cun) lateral to the anterior crest of the tibia

T: 1–1.5 cun perpendicular; moxibustion

P: transforms phlegm, alleviates respiratory insufficiency, provides general relaxation, and pacifies spiritual energy

A: 1. bronchial asthma, bronchitis, pneumonia, and other diseases accompanied by heavy phlegm build-up
2. psychic and psychosomatic dysfunctions, epilepsy

Pec: connecting point (Luo)

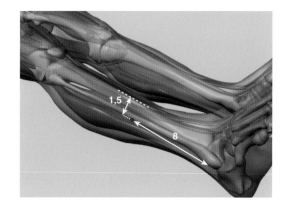

St 41 Jie Xi Stream Divide

L: in the depression of the centre of the ventral fold of the upper ankle joint, between the tendons of the extensor hallucis longus and M. extensor digitorum longus muscles

T: 0.5–1 cun perpendicular; moxibustion

P: clears the stomach and reduces inverted Qi, provides general relaxation and pacifies spiritual energy

A: 1. obstipation
2. headache; dizziness and numbness
3. fit-like psychic disease, dysfunctions in consciousness accompanied by high temperature

Pec: Jing (river) point (4th Shu-point)

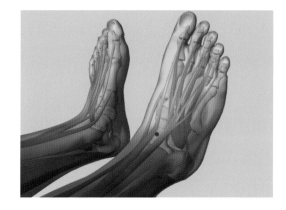

St 42 Chong Yang Rushing Yang

L: on the highest point of the foot dorsum, between the tendons of the extensor hallucis longus muscle and extensor digitorum longus muscle

T: 0.2–0.3 cun perpendicular superior to the palpable A. dorsalis pedis; moxibustion

P: harmonizes the stomach and soothes pain, decongests and activates the channel and its vessels

A: 1. stomach pain, borborygmus
2. pain on the foot dorsum, loss of foot strength
3. facial paresis

Pec: Qi-source-point (Yuan)

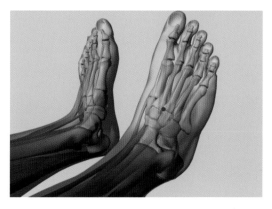

L: Location   **T:** Insertion Technique   **P:** Properties   **A:** Clinical Applications   **Pec:** Peculiarities

St

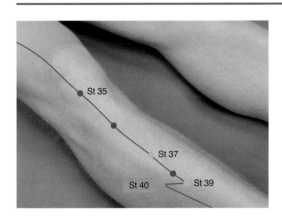

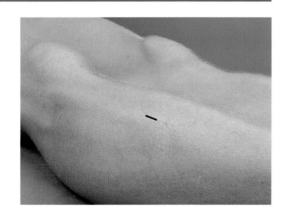

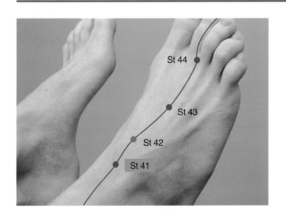

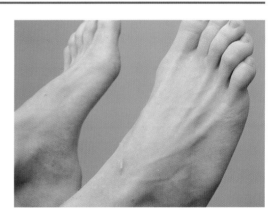

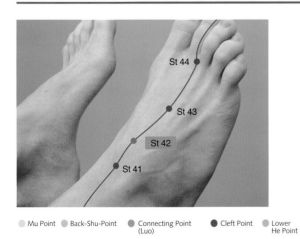

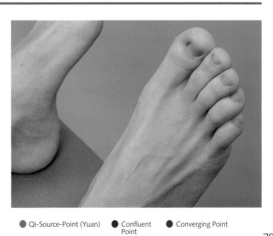

● Mu Point   ● Back-Shu-Point   ● Connecting Point (Luo)   ● Cleft Point   ● Lower He Point   ● Qi-Source-Point (Yuan)   ● Confluent Point   ● Converging Point

St 43 Xian Gu   Sunken Valley

L: in the depression in the proximal corner of the second metatarso-phalangeal joint, between the second and third metatarsal bones

T: 0.5–0.8 cun perpendicular; moxibustion

P: regulates and harmonizes the stomach and intestine, activates the channel and promotes urination

A: 1. abdominal pain
2. edemas in the lower extremity
3. pain in the foot dorsum

Pec: Shu (stream) point (3rd Shu-point)

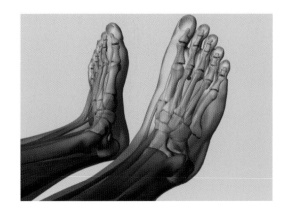

St 44 Nei Ting   Inner Courtyard

L: at the edge of the interdigital skin, between the second and third toes, at the dividing line between red and white flesh

T: 0.5–0.8 cun perpendicular or oblique; moxibustion

P: regulates and harmonizes the stomach and intestine, clears heat and reduces edemas

A: 1. certain infectious diseases of the digestive system e.g. dysentery, enteritis, gastritis
2. certain dysfunctions of the five sensory organs and in the dental or ENT regions, e.g. toothache, epistaxis, tonsillitis
3. peripheral facial paresis, frontal headache

Pec: Xing (spring) point (2nd Shu-point)

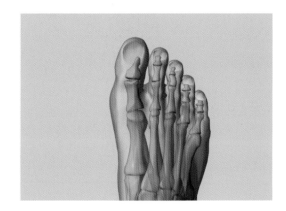

St 45 Li Dui   Strict Exchange

L: 0.1 cun proximal to the lateral border and base of the nail of the second toe

T: 0.1 cun perpendicular; prick to bleed; moxibustion

P: clears heat and expels humidity, pacifies spiritual force and secures overall relaxation

A: certain dysfunctions of the five sensory organs (ear, eye, mouth, nose, tongue) and in the dental or ENT regions e.g. toothache, rhinitis, sinusitis, epistaxis, inflammations in the region of the pharynx and throat

Pec: Jing (well) point (1st Shu-point)

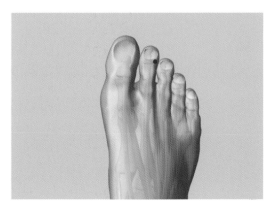

L: Location   **T:** Insertion Technique   **P:** Properties   **A:** Clinical Applications   **Pec:** Peculiarities

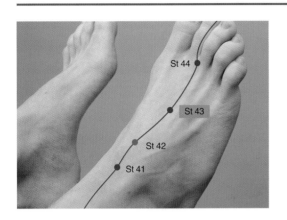

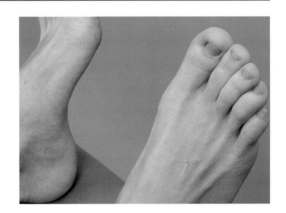

St

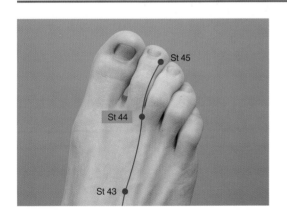

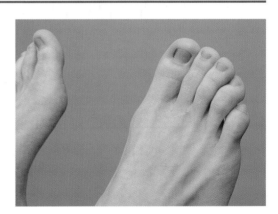

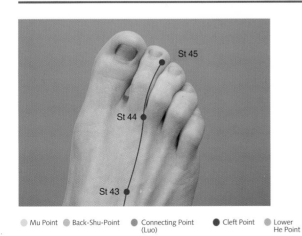

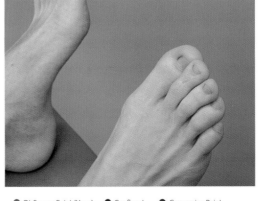

○ Mu Point ○ Back-Shu-Point ○ Connecting Point (Luo) ● Cleft Point ○ Lower He Point   ● Qi-Source-Point (Yuan) ● Confluent Point ● Converging Point

2.2.4   The spleen channel (Sp)

Synonyms

- Spleen meridian (Spleen/Pancreas Meridian)

- Foot-Taiyin-Spleen-Meridian

Channel pathway

There are 21 acupuncture points on the surface pathway of the spleen channel.

The channel begins at the inside corner of the nail of the big toe and ascends in its surface pathway from here via the instep, at the border between the sole and dorsum, in front of the medial malleolus, to the lower leg. From the lower leg the channel then runs along the posterior border of the tibia and crosses below the knee in front of the liver channel. On the upper leg it runs over the antero-medial aspect of the inner thigh.

Above the groin the channel enters in its inner pathway into the deeper layers of the points Ren 3 and Ren 4. It then reaches points Sp 14 and Sp 15 on the surface. From this stage the channel runs to the inner layers of point Ren 10 and then its inner branch runs through the abdomen to its organ, the spleen, where it connects with the stomach. It ascends further via the diaphragm to the heart and connects with the heart channel.

The surface pathway of the channel in the abdomen leads initially from the deep layers at Ren 10 back to point Sp 16, to the side of the upper abdomen. From here the channel follows, via points GB 24 and Lv 14, along the side of the chest to points Sp 17 to Sp 20.

At point Sp 20 in the 2nd ICS an inner branch leads via the deeper layers of point Lu 1 along the throat to the root of the tongue and divides in the region of the tongue base. From point Sp 20 the channel rises again into the 6th ICS, below the armpit, to point Sp 21. This is where the "Great Spleen Network Vessel" begins.

Sp

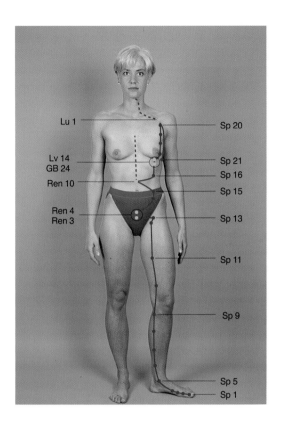

Lu 1
Sp 20
Lv 14
GB 24
Ren 10
Sp 21
Sp 16
Sp 15
Ren 4
Ren 3
Sp 13
Sp 11
Sp 9
Sp 5
Sp 1

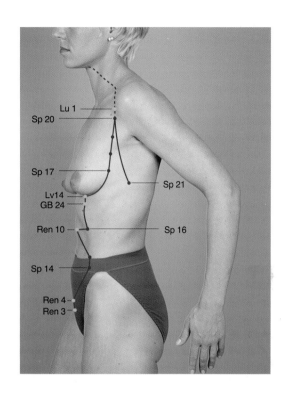

Lu 1
Sp 20
Sp 17
Sp 21
Lv14
GB 24
Ren 10
Sp 16
Sp 14
Ren 4
Ren 3

Sp

Sp 1 Yin Bai   Hidden White

L: 0.1 cun proximal to the corner of the nail of the big toe

T: 0.1 cun perpendicular;
prick to bleed; moxibustion

P: strengthens the spleen and eliminates gases, unites the blood and holds it in the veins, stops bleeding

A: 1. thoracic and abdominal sensations of tension, swelling and bloatedness
2. acute gastroenteritis
3. blood soothing

Pec: Xing (well) point (1st Shu-point)

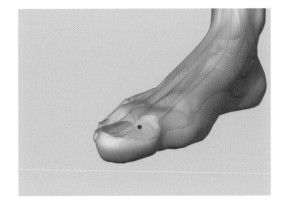

Sp 2 Da Du   Great Metropolis

L: in the depression distal and inferior to the first metatarsal-phalangeal joint at the dividing point between red and white flesh

T: 0.3–0.5 cun perpendicular;
moxibustion

P: strengthens the spleen and harmonizes the stomach

A: 1. acute and chronic gastroenteritis
2. diarrhoea in digestive dysfunctions

Pec: Xing (spring) point (2nd Shu-point)

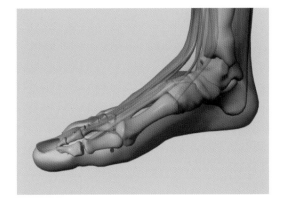

Sp 3 Tai Bai   Supreme White

L: in the depression proximal and inferior to the first metatarsal-phalangeal joint at the dividing point between red and white flesh

T: 0.5–0.8 cun perpendicular;
moxibustion

P: strengthens the spleen, resolves dampness, regulates Qi, and harmonizes the stomach

A: 1. acute and chronic gastroenteritis
2. acute and chronic dysentery
3. digestive dysfunctions

Pec: Shu (stream) point (3rd Shu-point), Qi-source-point (Yuan)

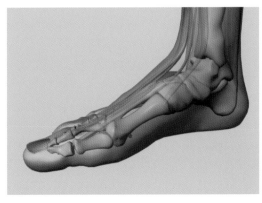

L: Location   T: Insertion Technique   P: Properties   A: Clinical Applications   Pec: Peculiarities

Sp

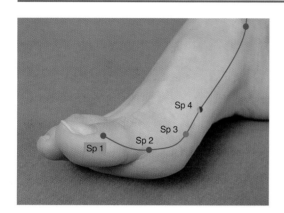
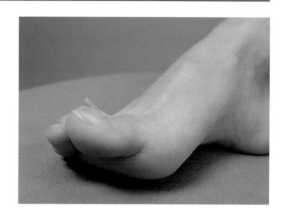

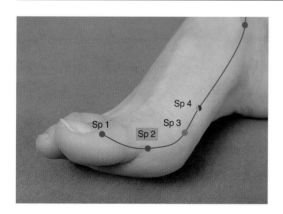
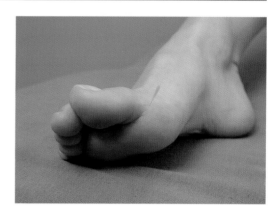

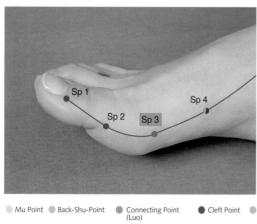
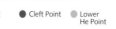
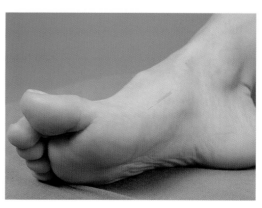

● Mu Point ● Back-Shu-Point ● Connecting Point (Luo) ● Cleft Point ● Lower He Point ● Qi-Source-Point (Yuan) ● Confluent Point ● Converging Point

Sp

Sp 4 Gong Sun   Grandfather–Grandson

L: in the depression, distal and inferior to the basis of the first metatarsal bone, at the dividing line between red and white flesh

T: 0.6–1.2 cun perpendicular; moxibustion

P: strengthens the spleen, resolves dampness, harmonizes the stomach, and regulates the middle Jiao

A: 1. acute and chronic gastritis, acute and chronic enteritis
2. chronic dysentery
3. gases and abdominal pain of various sources

Pec: connecting point (Luo), confluent point (Ba Mai Jiao Hui) of the Chong Mai

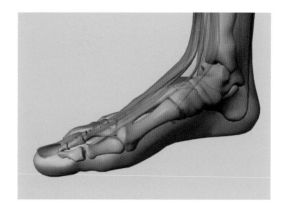

Sp 5 Shang Qiu   Shang Mound

L: in the depression ventral and distal to the medial malleolus, in the middle between the tuberosity of the navicular and the prominence of the medial malleolus

T: 0.5–0.8 cun perpendicular; moxibustion

P: strengthens the spleen and calms diarrhoea

A: 1. chronic enteritis
2. digestive dysfunctions

Pec: Jing (river) point (4th Shu-point)

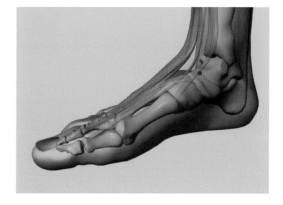

Sp 6 San Yin Jiao   Three Yin Intersection

L: 3 cun proximal to the prominence of the medial malleolus, dorsal to the medial crest of the tibia

T: 1–1.5 cun perpendicular; moxibustion

P: strengthens the spleen, resolves and expels dampness; it restores balance to the Yin and blood, liver, and kidneys

A: 1. many gynecological and obstetric dysfunctions
2. chronic enteritis, chronic diarrhoea
3. dysfunctions to the male sexual function
4. dysfunctions in bladder function, e.g. urinary retention
5. dysfunctions in movement in the lower extremity

Pec: CAUTION, CAN INDUCE LABOUR IF STRONG MANIPULATION APPLIED!

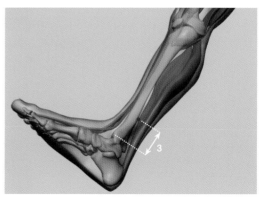

L: Location   **T:** Insertion Technique   **P:** Properties   **A:** Clinical Applications   **Pec:** Peculiarities

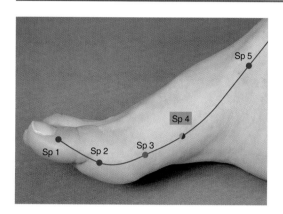

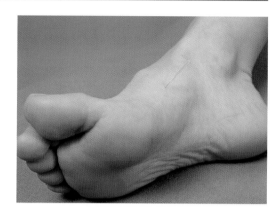

Sp

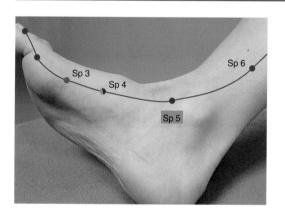

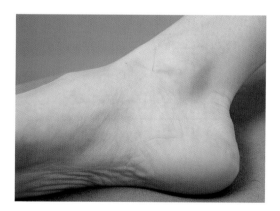

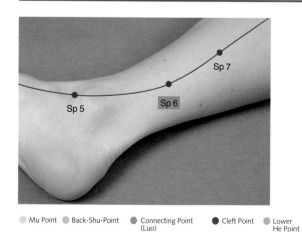

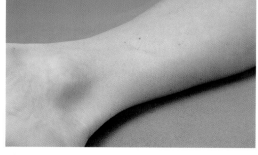

○ Mu Point ○ Back-Shu-Point ● Connecting Point (Luo) ● Cleft Point ○ Lower He Point ● Qi-Source-Point (Yuan) ● Confluent Point ● Converging Point

Sp 7 Lou Gu   Leaking Valley

L: 6 cun proximal to the prominence of the medial
malleolus, dorsal to the medial crest of the tibia

T: 1–1.5 cun perpendicular;
moxibustion

P: strengthens the spleen and expels dampness

A: 1. intestinal gases, sensation of abdominal tension,
swelling, and fullness
2. urinary retention, difficult urination

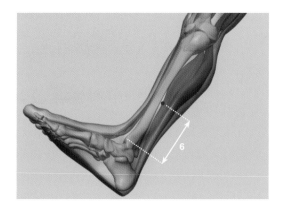

Sp 8 Di Ji   Earth Pivot

L: 3 cun inferior to Sp 9, on the connection line
between the prominence of the medial malleolus
and Sp 9

T: 1–1.5 cun perpendicular;
moxibustion

P: strengthens the spleen and expels dampness,
regulates menstruation and invigorates blood

A: 1. chronic diarrhoea, chronic dysentery
2. some gynecological dysfunctions e.g. irregular
menstruation, dysmenorrhoea, myoma of the
uterus, ovarian cysts

Pec: cleft (Xi) point

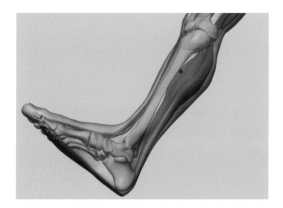

Sp 9 Yin Ling Quan   Yin Mound Spring

L: in the depression, distal and dorsal to the medial
condyle of the tibia

T: 1–2 cun perpendicular;
moxibustion

P: strengthens the spleen and expels dampness,
restores balance to body fluids

A: 1. acute and chronic enteritis
2 edema propensity
3. dysfunctions in the bladder function e.g. urinary
retention, urinary incontinence (restores balance)
4. pain in the region of the knee joint

Pec: He (sea) point (5th Shu-point)

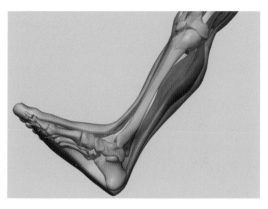

L: Location   **T:** Insertion Technique   **P:** Properties   **A:** Clinical Applications   **Pec:** Peculiarities

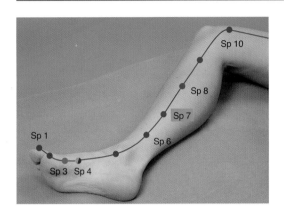
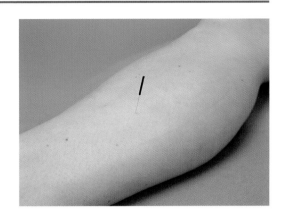

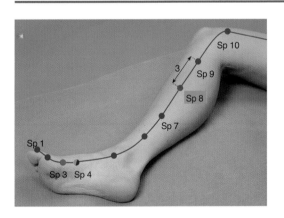
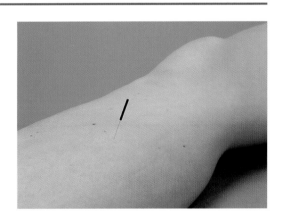

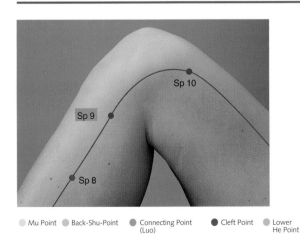
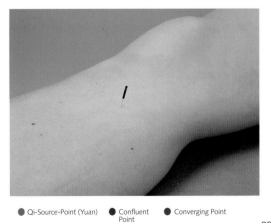

● Mu Point ● Back-Shu-Point ● Connecting Point (Luo) ● Cleft Point ● Lower He Point   ● Qi-Source-Point (Yuan) ● Confluent Point ● Converging Point

Sp 10 Xue Hai   Sea of Blood

L: with the patient's knee flexed, 2 cun proximal to the medial superior border of the patella on the bulge of the vastus medialis muscle

T: 1–1.5 cun perpendicular; moxibustion

P: regulates menstruation and invigorates the blood, expels dampness and alleviates nausea

A: 1. some gynecological dysfunctions e.g. irregular menstruation, dysmenorrhoea, amenorrhoea, anovulatory dysfunctional uterine hemorrhages
2. pain on the inner aspect of the upper thigh
3. urticaria, eczema

Pec: symptomatic point in allergies

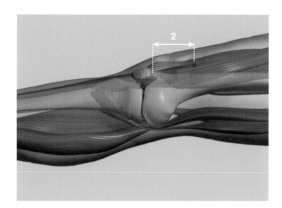

Sp 11 Ji Men   Winnowing Gate

L: 6 cun proximal to Sp 10 on the connecting line between Sp 10 and Sp 12

T: 0.5–1 cun perpendicular above the A. femoralis; moxibustion

P: clears heat, mobilises the urinary tract, and expels urine

A: 1. urinary retention and urinary incontinence
2. infections of the urinary tract

Pec: deep needling may puncture the femoral artery

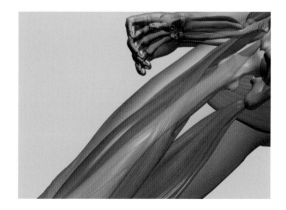

Sp 12 Chong Men   Rushing Gate

L: on the lateral end of the groin, 3.5 cun lateral to the central point of the upper edge of the symphyses, lateral to the A. iliaca externa

T: 0.5–1 cun perpendicular above the A. iliaca externa; moxibustion

P: regulates Qi, resolves and expels dampness

A: 1. external abdominal hernias
2. urinary retention

Pec: CAUTION IN PREGNANCY!

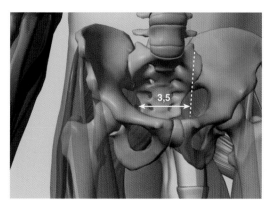

L: Location   T: Insertion Technique   P: Properties   A: Clinical Applications   Pec: Peculiarities

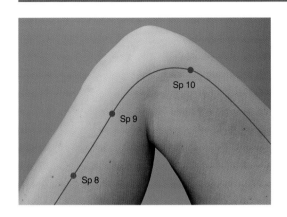

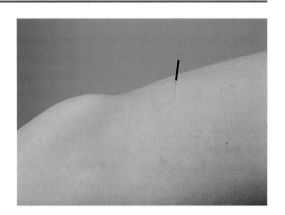

Sp

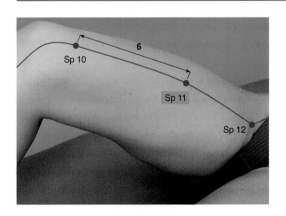

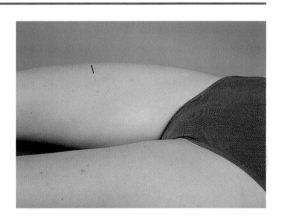

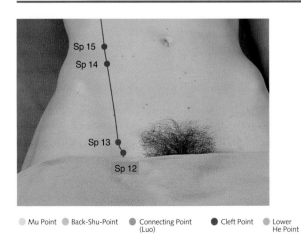

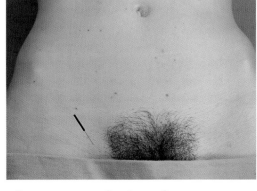

⚪ Mu Point ⚪ Back-Shu-Point ⚪ Connecting Point (Luo) ⚫ Cleft Point ⚪ Lower He Point ⚫ Qi-Source-Point (Yuan) ⚫ Confluent Point ⚫ Converging Point

Sp 13 Fu She   Abode of the Fu

L: 4 cun lateral to the ventral midline, 0.7 cun superior and lateral to Sp 12, 4 cun inferior to the umbilical centre

T: 1–1.5 cun perpendicular; moxibustion

P: regulates intestine and stomach

A: 1. abdominal sensation of tension, swelling, and borborygmus
    2. external abdominal hernias

Pec: CAUTION IN PREGNANCY!

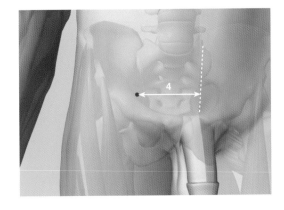

Sp 14 Fu Jie   Abdomen Knot

L: 1.3 cun inferior to Sp 15, 4 cun lateral to the ventral midline

T: 1–2 cun perpendicular; moxibustion

P: warms spleen and alleviates diarrhoea

A: chronic diarrhoea

Pec: CAUTION IN PREGNANCY!

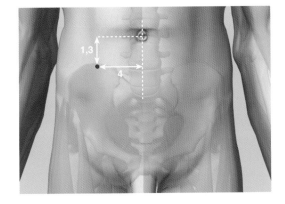

Sp 15 Da Heng   Great Horizontal

L: 4 cun lateral to the centre of the umbilicus

T: 1–2 cun perpendicular; moxibustion

P: regulates Qi and alleviates pain, restores balance to the large intestine

A: 1. pain in the lower abdomen
    2. chronic diarrhoeas, chronic dysenteries
    3. obstipation

Pec: CAUTION IN PREGNANCY!

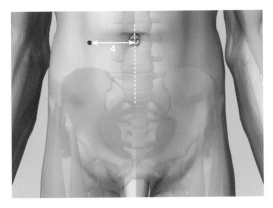

L: Location   **T:** Insertion Technique   **P:** Properties   **A:** Clinical Applications   **Pec:** Peculiarities

Sp

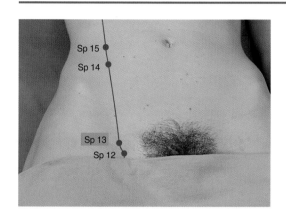

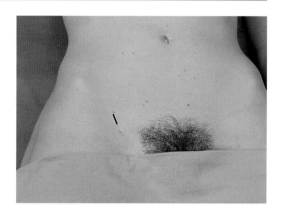

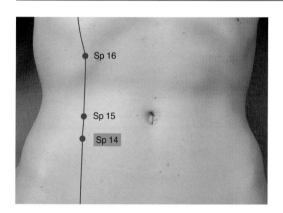

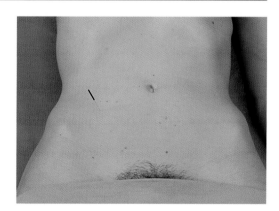

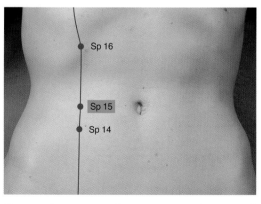

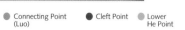

● Mu Point ● Back-Shu-Point ● Connecting Point (Luo) ● Cleft Point ● Lower He Point ● Qi-Source-Point (Yuan) ● Confluent Point ● Converging Point

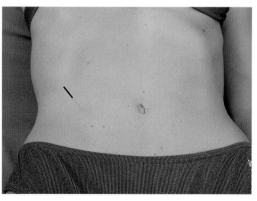

93

Sp 16 Fu Ai Abdomen Sorrow

L: 3 cun superior to the centre of the umbilicus, 4 cun lateral to the ventral midline

T: 1–1.5 cun perpendicular; moxibustion

P: strengthens the spleen and eliminates nutrition congestion, activates and descends Fu (palace) organ Qi

A: 1. periumbilical pain
2. acute and chronic dysenteries
3. obstipation

Pec: CAUTION, AVOID PNEUMOTHORAX!

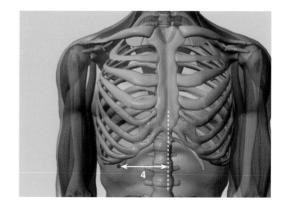

Sp 17 Shi Dou Food Cavity

L: in the 5th ICR, 6 cun lateral to the ventral midline

T: 0.5–0.8 cun oblique or laterally subcutaneous; moxibustion

P: regulates Qi and alleviates pain, harmonizes the stomach and descends inverted Qi

A: 1. intercostal neuralgia
2. esophagitis, swallowing difficulties

Pec: CAUTION, AVOID PNEUMOTHORAX!

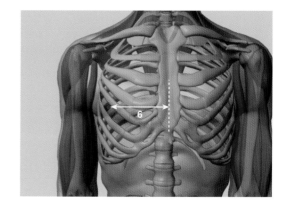

Sp 18 Tian Xi Heavenly Stream

L: in the 4th ICR, 6 cun lateral to the ventral midline

T: 0.5–0.8 cun oblique or laterally subcutaneous; moxibustion

P: unbinds the chest and stimulates lactation

A: 1. thoracic pain

2. disease of the breast, e.g. mastodynia, insufficient post-partum milk

Pec: CAUTION, AVOID PNEUMOTHORAX!

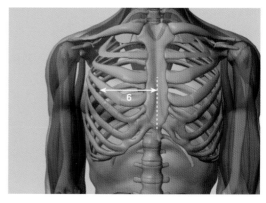

L: Location   **T:** Insertion Technique   **P:** Properties   **A:** Clinical Applications   **Pec:** Peculiarities

Sp

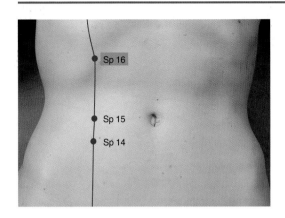

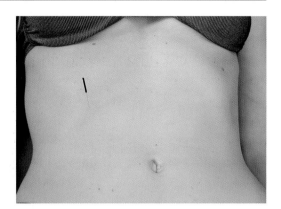

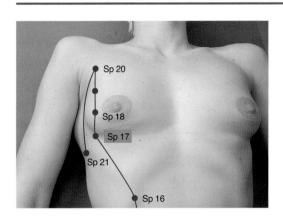

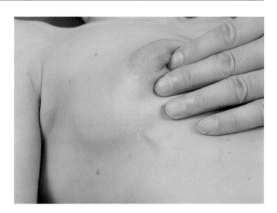

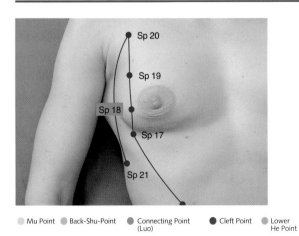

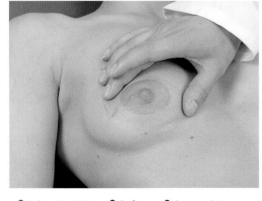

⬤ Mu Point ⬤ Back-Shu-Point ⬤ Connecting Point (Luo) ⬤ Cleft Point ⬤ Lower He Point   ⬤ Qi-Source-Point (Yuan) ⬤ Confluent Point ⬤ Converging Point

95

Sp 19 Xiong Xiang Chest Village

L: in the 3rd ICR, 6 cun lateral to the ventral midline

T: 0.5–0.8 cun oblique or laterally subcutaneous; moxibustion

P: unbinds the chest and alleviates pain

A: thoracic pain, e.g. intercostal neuralgia

Pec: CAUTION, AVOID PNEUMOTHORAX!

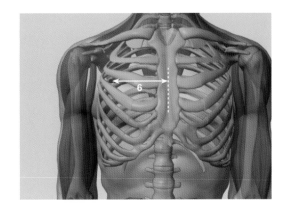

Sp 20 Zhou Rong Encircling Glory

L: in the 2nd ICR, 6 cun lateral to the ventral midline

T: 0.5–0.8 cun oblique or laterally subcutaneous; moxibustion

P: unbinds the chest, regulates Qi, alleviates coughing, and eliminates phlegm

A: 1. intercostal neuralgia
2. pneumonia, abscess of the lung

Pec: CAUTION, AVOID PNEUMOTHORAX!

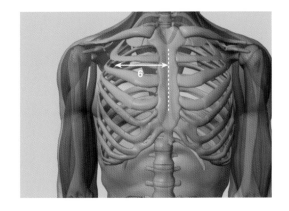

Sp 21 Da Bao Great Enveloping

L: in the 6th ICR, in the mid-axillary line

T: 0.5–0.8 cun oblique or laterally subcutaneous; moxibustion

P: encircles the blood and holds it in the veins, harmonizes the blood, unbinds the chest, and alleviates pain

A: 1. chest or side pain
2. joint pains in general

Pec: Departure point of the "Great Luo-connecting point of the Spleen"
CAUTION, AVOID PNEUMOTHORAX!

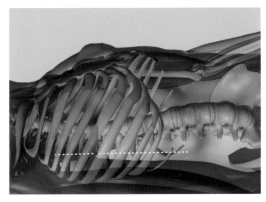

L: Location   T: Insertion Technique   P: Properties   A: Clinical Applications   Pec: Peculiarities

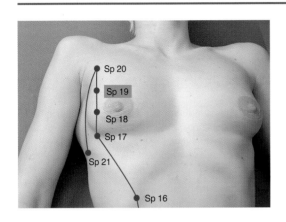
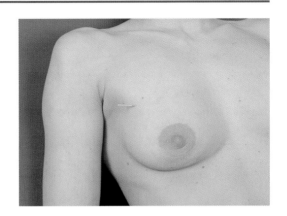

Sp

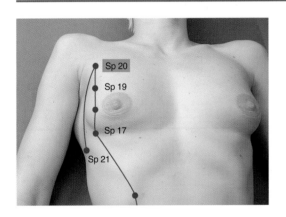
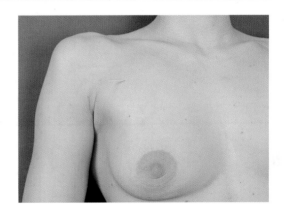

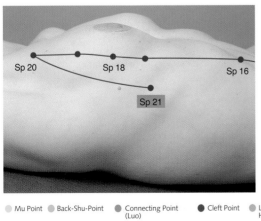
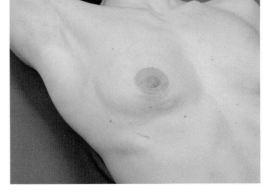

● Mu Point ● Back-Shu-Point ● Connecting Point (Luo) ● Cleft Point ● Lower He Point ● Qi-Source-Point (Yuan) ● Confluent Point ● Converging Point

2.2.5   The heart channel (He)

Synonyms

- Heart meridian
- Hand-Shaoyin-Heart-Channel

Channel pathway

There are 9 acupuncture points in the surface pathway of the heart channel.

The inner channel pathway originates at the heart and the "heart-system," with all its connections to the other organs. The descending part of the channel traverses the diaphragm to connect with the small intestine. The ascending part ascends alongside the esophagus, connects with the root of the tongue, and to the "eye system," i.e. the eyeball and accompanying tissues. The main pathway of the channel runs through the lung and leaves the chest cavity from the side in the axilla, at point He 1.

The surface pathway comes from the axilla and runs, firstly, to the medial aspect of the inner upper arm, the inside of the elbow joint and finally to the antero-medial aspect of the inside of the lower arm. In the region of the wrist joint the channel runs radially past the pisiform bone, then via the palm of the hand to the radial corner of the nail of the little finger.

He

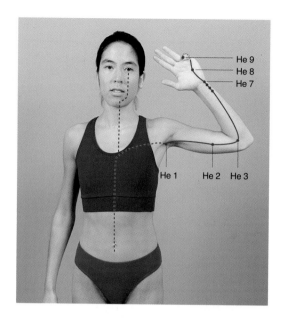

He 9
He 8
He 7

He 1   He 2   He 3

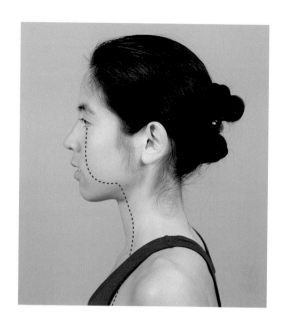

He

He 1 Ji Quan Summit Spring

L: at the tip of the axilla above the palpable A. axiliaris

T: 0.3–0.5 cun perpendicular or oblique above the palpable A. axiliaris; moxibustion

P: regulates Qi and unbinds the chest, decongests and activates the channel

A: 1. palpitations, pains in the heart region, thoracic feeling of bloatedness, other functional diseases of the heart

2. paralyses and haemorrhagic dysfunctions of the upper extremity

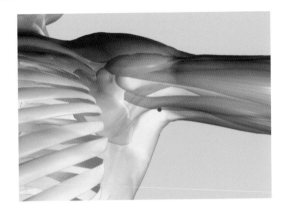

He 2 Qing Ling Green Spirit

L: 3 cun proximal to the cubital crease on the inner side of the upper arm, on the connecting line between He 1 and He 3, in the channel medial to M. biceps brachii

T: 0.5–1 cun perpendicular; moxibustion

P: relaxes tendons and alleviates pain

A: pain in the upper arm

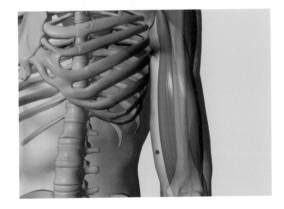

He 3 Shao Hai Lesser Sea

L: (with the patient's elbow flexed) midway between the medial end of the cubital crease and the medial epicondyle of the humerus

T: 0.5–1 cun perpendicular; moxibustion

P: calms the heart and pacifies the spirit

A: 1. manic-depressive dysfunctions, amnesic dysfunctions and forgetfulness

2. pain in the heart region

Pec: He (sea) point (5th Shu-point)

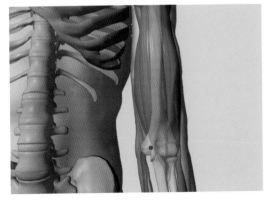

L: Location   T: Insertion Technique   P: Properties   A: Clinical Applications   Pec: Peculiarities

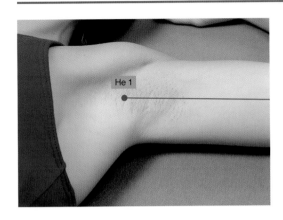

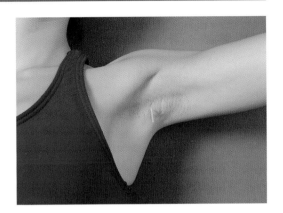

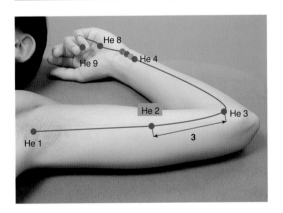

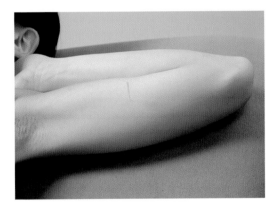

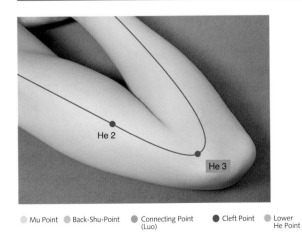

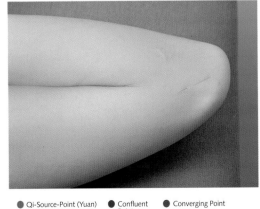

● Mu Point ● Back-Shu-Point ● Connecting Point (Luo) ● Cleft Point ● Lower He Point   ● Qi-Source-Point (Yuan) ● Confluent Point ● Converging Point

He

He 4 Ling Dao Spirit Path

L: 1.5 cun proximal to the distal wrist crease, on the radial side of the tendon of flexor carpi ulnaris

T: 0.3–0.5 cun perpendicular; moxibustion

P: calms the heart and pacifies strength of spirit

A: 1. pain in the heart region

2. psychogenic restlessness

Pec: Jing (river) point (4th Shu-point)

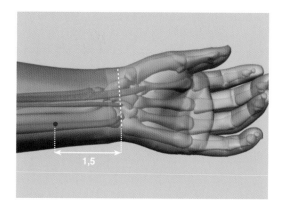

He 5 Tong Li Penetrating the Interior

L: 1 cun proximal to the distal wrist crease on the radial side of the tendon of flexor carpi ulnaris

T: 0.3–0.5 cun perpendicular; moxibustion

P: calms the heart and pacifies strength of spirit, opens the senses and benefits the tongue

A: 1. pain in the heart region, palpitations, and other functional diseases of the heart

2. psycho-emotional instability

3. sudden loss of voice

Pec: connecting point (Luo)

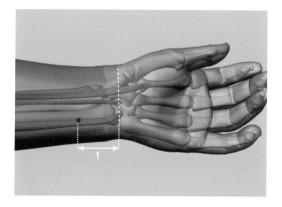

He 6 Yin Xi Yin Cleft

L: 0.5 cun proximal to the distal wrist crease on the radial side of the tendon of flexor carpi ulnaris

T: 0.3–0.5 cun perpendicular; moxibustion

P: calms the heart, clears heat, and cools the blood

A: 1. pectoral angina

2. epistaxis, coughing or spitting of blood, hemotemesis and other forms of blood loss from superior orifices

Pec: cleft (Xi) point

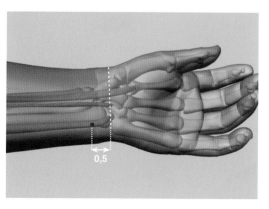

L: Location   **T:** Insertion Technique   **P:** Properties   **A:** Clinical Applications   **Pec:** Peculiarities

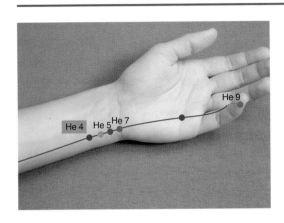

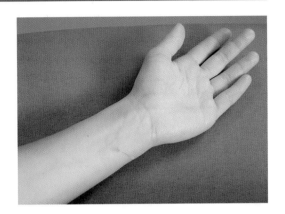

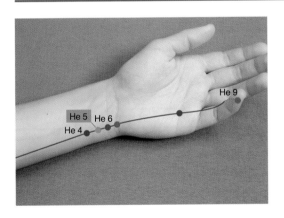

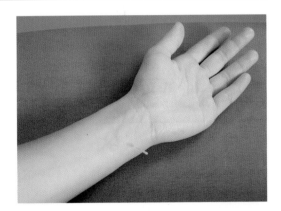

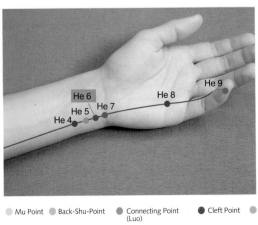

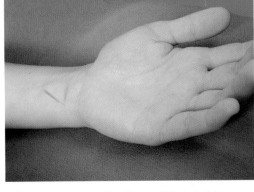

⬤ Mu Point   ⬤ Back-Shu-Point   ⬤ Connecting Point (Luo)   ⬤ Cleft Point   ⬤ Lower He Point   ⬤ Qi-Source-Point (Yuan)   ⬤ Confluent Point   ⬤ Converging Point

He 7 Shen Men Spirit Gate

L: at the ulnar end of the distal wrist crease, in the depression between the radial side of the tendon of flexor carpi ulnaris, at the proximal border of the pisiform bone

T: 0.3–0.5 cun perpendicular; moxibustion

P: supports and calms the heart, pacifies the spirit, and resolves depressions

A: 1. pains in the heart region, palpitations, and other functional disorders of the heart
  2. psychic and psychosomatic dysfunctions, stage fright, exam fright

Pec: Shu (stream) point (3rd Shu-point), Qi-source-point (Yuan)

He

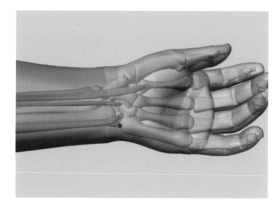

He 8 Shao Fu Lesser Palace

L: on the palm between the fourth and fifth metacarpal bones, where the tip of the little finger lies when a fist is clenched

T: 0.3–0.5 cun perpendicular; moxibustion

P: clears the heart and pacifies the spirit

A: 1. pains in the heart region
  2. psycho-emotional instability
  3. dysfunctions in the region of the uterus and vulva e.g. colpitis and uterine prolapse

Pec: Xing (spring) point (2nd Shu-point)

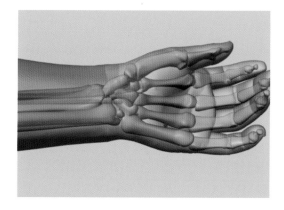

He 9 Shao Chong Lesser Rushing

L: 0.1 cun proximal and lateral to the radial corner of the nail of the little finger

T: 0.1 cun perpendicular; prick to bleed; moxibustion

P: clears heat and pacifies the spirit, opens the senses and revives consciousness

A: 1. pains in the heart region, sensation of thoracic fullness, and other functional disorders of the heart
  2. psychic and psychosomatic dysfunctions
  3. loss of consciousness accompanied by fever

Pec: Jing (well) point (1st Shu-point)

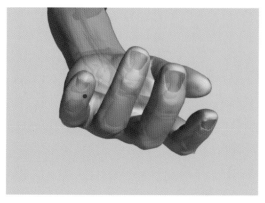

L: Location   **T:** Insertion Technique   **P:** Properties   **A:** Clinical Applications   **Pec:** Peculiarities

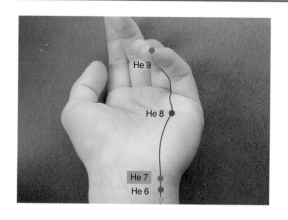

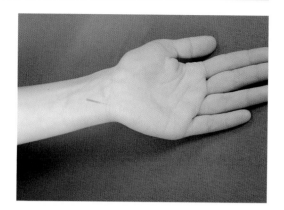

He

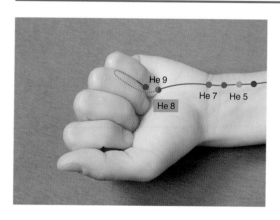

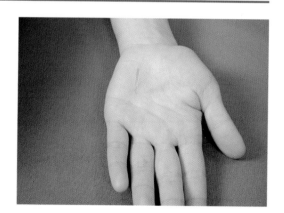

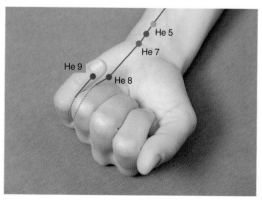

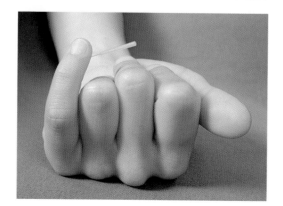

- Mu Point
- Back-Shu-Point
- Connecting Point (Luo)
- Cleft Point
- Lower He Point
- Qi-Source-Point (Yuan)
- Confluent Point
- Converging Point

2.2.6   The small intestine channel (SI)

Synonyms

• Small intestine meridian

• Hand-Taiyang Small Intestine Channel

Channel pathway

There are 19 acupuncture points in the surface pathway of the small intestine channel.

The small intestine primary channel originates at the ulnar corner of the nail of the little finger. It ascends in its surface pathway, over the outside aspect of the little finger and the hand at the dividing line between the skin of the dorsum and the palm, to the region of the wrist. The channel then ascends, via the ulnar region of the outside of the lower arm, the Canalis nervi ulnaris, and the posterior aspect of the outside of the upper arm, to the posterior aspect of the shoulder joint. It zigzags over the scapula and branches to connect with the seventh cervical vertebra (Du 14).

From here the inner pathway of the channel descends through the superior fossa of the clavicle and connects with the heart. It further descends alongside the esophagus through the diaphragm, reaching the stomach, and finally connects with its organ, the small intestine.

The surface pathway runs from the superior clavicular fossa, alongside the neck and over the lower jaw to the cheekbone (SI 18), branching to the inner corner of the eye (Bl 1) and then connecting with the bladder channel. Before reaching point SI 18, a branch runs from the cheek to the outer corner of the eye (GB 1), before finally entering the ear at point SI 19.

SI

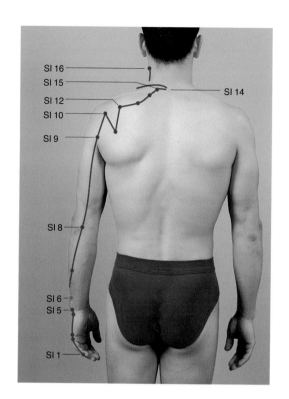

SI 16
SI 15
SI 14
SI 12
SI 10
SI 9
SI 8
SI 6
SI 5
SI 1

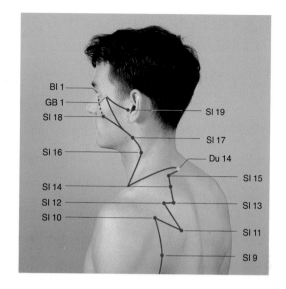

BI 1
GB 1
SI 18
SI 19
SI 17
SI 16
Du 14
SI 15
SI 14
SI 12
SI 13
SI 10
SI 11
SI 9

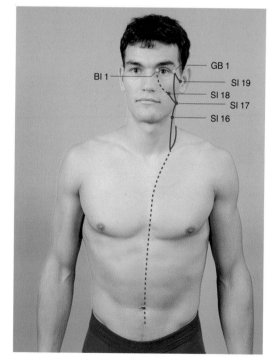

GB 1
BI 1
SI 19
SI 18
SI 17
SI 16

SI

SI 1 Shao Ze Lesser Marsh

L: 0.1 cun proximal and lateral to the ulnar corner of the nail of the little finger

T: 0.1 cun perpendicular; prick to bleed; moxibustion

P: promotes body fluids and lactation, clears heat and opens the senses

A: 1. diseases of the breast e.g. insufficient post-partum lactation, acute mastitis
2. fever, absence of sweating, pain in the pharynx and throat in the first phase of a "cold"
3. loss of consciousness, coma (complementary or emergency measure)

Pec: Jing (well) point (1st Shu-point)

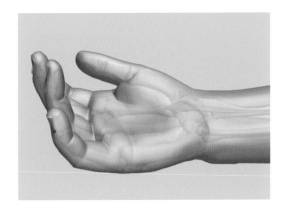

SI

SI 2 Qian Gu Front Valley

L: with the patient's fist loosely clenched, at the ulnar end of the distal crease of the fifth metacarpo-phalangeal joint, on the dividing line between red and white flesh

T: 0.3–0.5 cun perpendicular; moxibustion

P: clears the heart and promotes general calmness, sharpens hearing and eyesight

A: 1. epilepsy, psychic and psychosomatic dysfunctions (sedative effect)
2. certain diseases of the five sensory organs e.g. tinnitus, rhinitis, laryngitis, pharyngitis, inflammation of the eye
3. pain and paraestheses of the little finger

Pec: Xing (spring) point (2nd Shu-point)

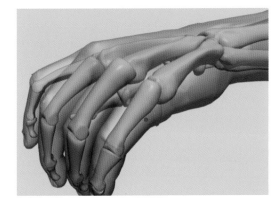

SI 3 Hou Xi Back Stream

L: with the patient's fist loosely clenched, at the ulnar end of the proximal crease of the fifth metacarpo-phalangeal joint, on the dividing line between red and white flesh

T: 0.3–0.5 cun perpendicular; moxibustion

P: clears the heart and promotes general calmness, eliminates inflammation and sharpens eyesight

A: 1. inflammation of the eye
2. epilepsy, psychic and psychosomatic dysfunctions
3. pains on the lower arm, wrist, and fingers
4. disorders of the cervical-spinal column, lumbar pain

Pec: Shu (stream) point (3rd Shu-point), confluent point (Ba Mai Jiao Hui) of the Du Mai

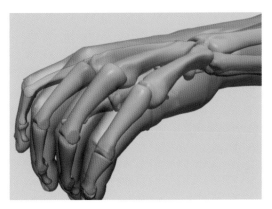

L: Location   **T:** Insertion Technique   **P:** Properties   **A:** Clinical Applications   **Pec:** Peculiarities

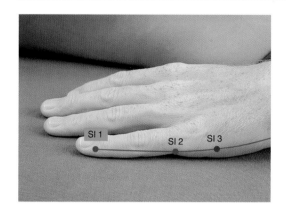

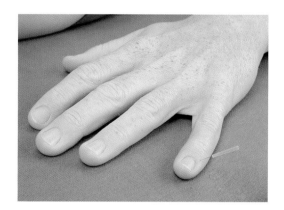

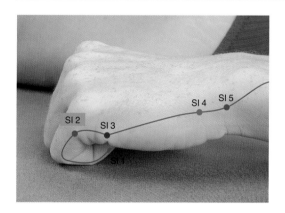

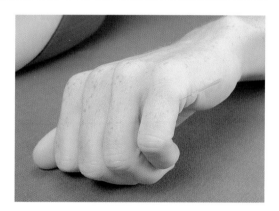

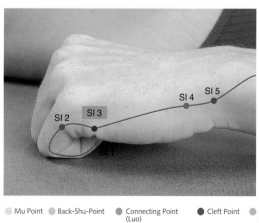

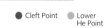

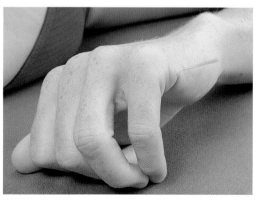

○ Mu Point ○ Back-Shu-Point ○ Connecting Point (Luo) ● Cleft Point ○ Lower He Point   ● Qi-Source-Point (Yuan) ● Confluent Point ● Converging Point

SI 4 Wan Gu Wrist Bone

L: in the depression between the base of the fifth metacarpal bone and the triquetral bone, on the dividing line between red and white flesh

T: 0.3–0.5 cun perpendicular; moxibustion

P: activates the channel and alleviates pain, promotes bile and reduces jaundice

A: 1. wrist pains

2. jaundice

Pec: Qi-source-point (Yuan)

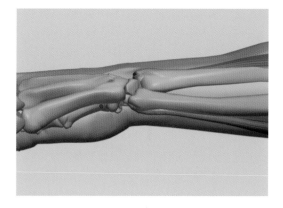

SI 5 Yang Gu Yang Valley

L: in the depression distal to the styloid process of the ulna, at the level of the ulnar end of the distal wrist crease

T: 0.3–0.5 cun perpendicular; moxibustion

P: clears heat and liberates the surface, activates the channel and alleviates pain

A: 1. fever, absence of sweating, headaches and dizziness in "colds"

2. wrist pains

Pec: Jing (river) point (4th Shu-point)

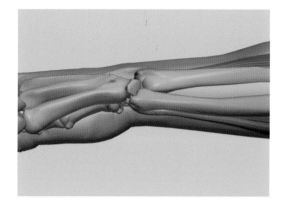

SI 6 Yang Lao Nourishing the Old

L: with the patient's palm placed on the chest, on the outer aspect of the lower arm, in the depression proximal and radial to the styloid process of the ulna

T: 0.5–0.8 cun oblique or perpendicular; moxibustion

P: activates the channel and alleviates pain

A: 1. pains in the upper extremity

2. lumbago

Pec: cleft (Xi) point

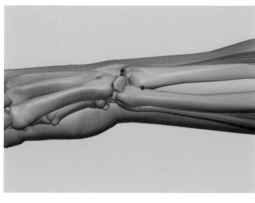

L: Location   T: Insertion Technique   P: Properties   A: Clinical Applications   Pec: Peculiarities

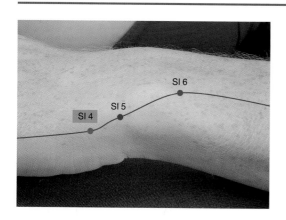

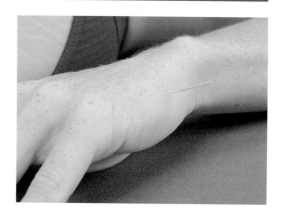

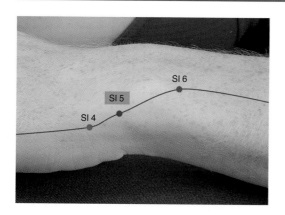

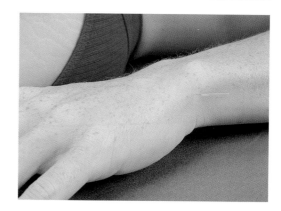

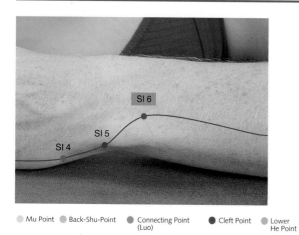

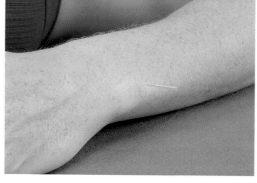

SI

○ Mu Point   ○ Back-Shu-Point   ● Connecting Point (Luo)   ● Cleft Point   ○ Lower He Point   ● Qi-Source-Point (Yuan)   ● Confluent Point   ● Converging Point

SI 7 Zhi Zheng Branch of the Upright

L: on the outside aspect of the lower arm, 5 cun proximal to the dorsal wrist crease, on the connecting line between SI 5 and SI 8

T: 0.5–0.8 cun oblique or perpendicular; moxibustion

P: promotes general calmness and pacifies the spirit, decongests and activates the channel

A: 1. psychic and psychosomatic dysfunctions, psycho-emotional change

2. pain in the lower arm

Pec: connecting point (Luo)

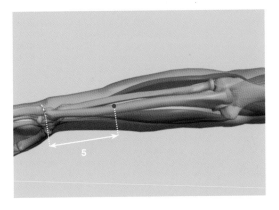

SI 8 Xiao Hai Small Sea

L: in the depression between the olecranon process and the epicondyle of the humerus

T: 0.3–0.5 cun perpendicular; moxibustion

P: pacifies the spirit and releases cramp, relaxes the tendons and alleviates pain

A: 1. epilepsy, psychic and psychosomatic dysfunctions (sedative and cramp-releasing)

2. pains radiating from the small intestine channel

Pec: He (sea) point (5th Shu-point)

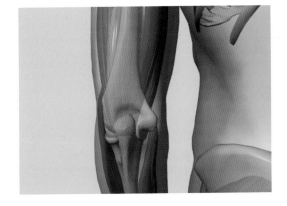

SI 9 Jian Zhen True Shoulder

L: with the arm in adducted position, 1 cun superior to the dorsal end of the axillary crease

T: 1–1.5 cun perpendicular; moxibustion

P: eliminates inflammation and reduces swelling, activates the channel

A: 1. dysfunctions of lymphatic discharge in unspecific lymphadenitis and lymphadenitis tuberculosa in the region of the neck, throat, and axilla

2. pain in the region of the shoulder joint and upper arm

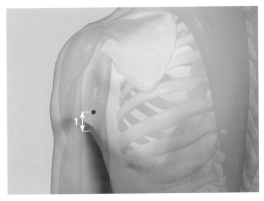

L: Location   **T:** Insertion Technique   **P:** Properties   **A:** Clinical Applications   **Pec:** Peculiarities

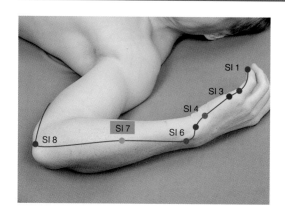

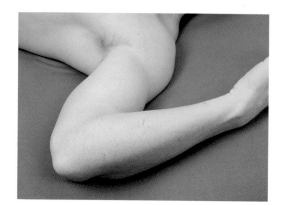

SI

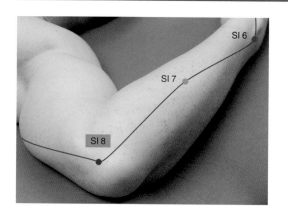

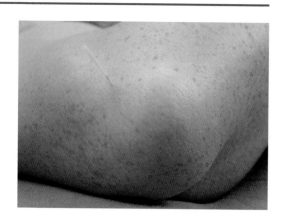

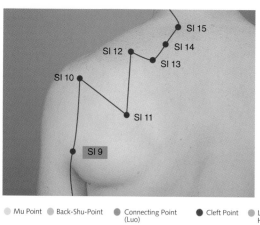

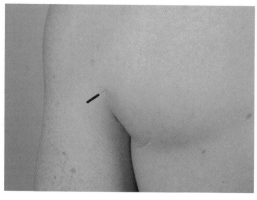

● Mu Point   ● Back-Shu-Point   ● Connecting Point (Luo)   ● Cleft Point   ● Lower He Point   ● Qi-Source-Point (Yuan)   ● Confluent Point   ● Converging Point

SI 10 Nao Shu Upper Arm Shu

L: with the arm in adducted position, superior to the dorsal end of the axillary crease, in the depression inferior to the inferior edge of the scapular spine

T: 0.5–1.5 cun perpendicular; moxibustion

P: eliminates inflammation and reduces swelling, relaxes the tendons and activates the vessels

A: 1. dysfunctions of lymphatic discharge in unspecific lymphadenitis and lymphadenitis tuberculosa in the region of the neck, throat, and axilla
2. pain in the region of the shoulder joint and upper arm

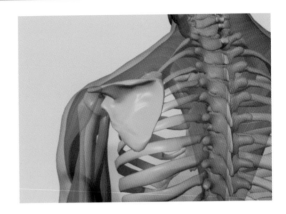

SI 11 Tian Zong Heavenly Gathering

L: in the centre of the fossa infraspinata, at the dividing line from the upper to middle third of the connecting line, between the lower border of the scapular spine and the inferior angle of the scapula

T: 0.5–1 cun perpendicular or oblique; moxibustion

P: descends Qi and alleviates breathing difficulty, relaxes the tendons and alleviates pain

A: 1. spastic bronchitis, bronchial asthma
2. pains in the region of the neck; shoulder joint and upper arm

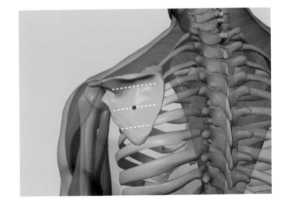

SI 12 Bing Feng Grasping the Wind

L: superior to SI 11, in the depression in the midpoint of the fossa supraspinata

T: 0.5–1 cun perpendicular or oblique; moxibustion

P: activates the channel and alleviates pain

A: pain and paraestheses in the region of the neck, shoulder, and upper arm

Pec: CAUTION, AVOID PNEUMOTHORAX!

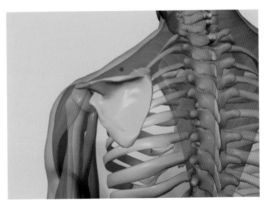

L: Location   T: Insertion Technique   P: Properties   A: Clinical Applications   Pec: Peculiarities

SI

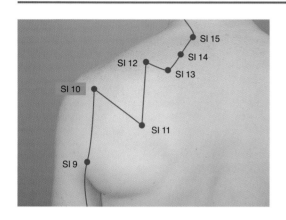

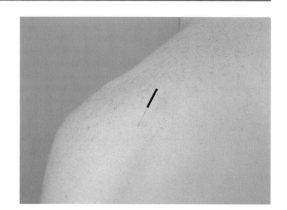

SI

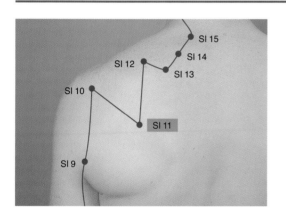

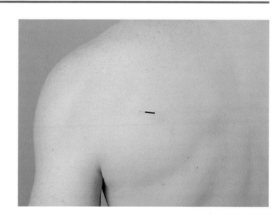

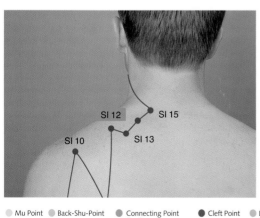

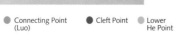

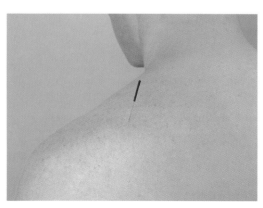

Mu Point   Back-Shu-Point   Connecting Point (Luo)   Cleft Point   Lower He Point   Qi-Source-Point (Yuan)   Confluent Point   Converging Point

115

SI 13 Qu Yuan   Crooked Wall

L: at the medial end of the fossa supraspinata, at the midpoint between SI 10 and the spinous process Th2

T: 0.5–1 cun perpendicular or oblique; moxibustion

P: relaxes the tendons and alleviates pain

A: pain in the region of the neck and shoulder

Pec: CAUTION, AVOID PNEUMOTHORAX!

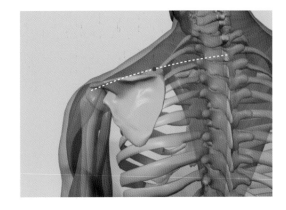

SI 14 Jian Wai Shu   Outer Shoulder Shu

L: at the level of the depression below the spinous process Th1, 3 cun lateral to the dorsal midline

T: 0.5–0.8 cun oblique; moxibustion

P: relaxes the tendons and alleviates pain

A: pain in the region of the neck and shoulder

Pec: CAUTION, AVOID PNEUMOTHORAX!

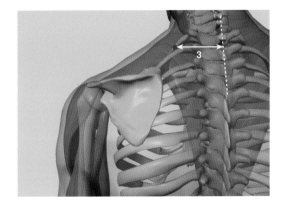

SI 15 Jian Zhong Zhu   Middle Shoulder Shu

L: at the level of the depression below the spinous process C7, 2 cun lateral to the dorsal midline

T: 0.5–0.8 cun oblique; moxibustion

P: descends lung Qi and liberates the surface

A: fever, absence of sweating and coughing in infectious diseases of the superior respiratory tract

Pec: CAUTION, AVOID PNEUMOTHORAX!

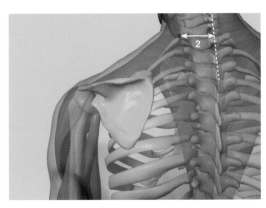

L: Location   **T:** Insertion Technique   **P:** Properties   **A:** Clinical Applications   **Pec:** Peculiarities

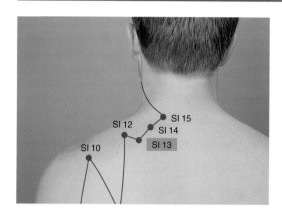

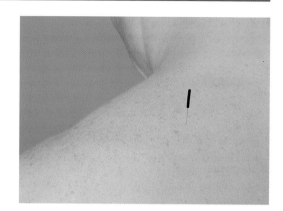

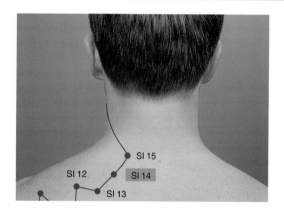

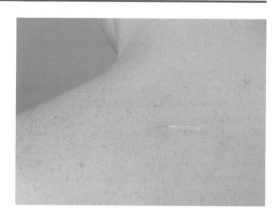

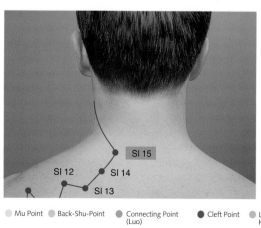

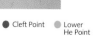

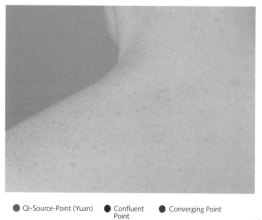

● Mu Point ● Back-Shu-Point ● Connecting Point (Luo) ● Cleft Point ● Lower He Point ● Qi-Source-Point (Yuan) ● Confluent Point ● Converging Point

SI 16 Tian Chuang Heavenly Window

L: on the posterior border of the sternocleidomastoid muscle lateral to the laryngeal prominence, dorsal LI 18

T: 0.5–1 cun perpendicular; moxibustion

P: sharpens hearing and relieves upper body orifices

A: 1. diseases of the ear e.g. tinnitus, deafness
2. pain and swelling in the region of the pharynx and throat

Pec: CAUTION, AVOID NEEDLING OF THE CAROTID ARTERY!

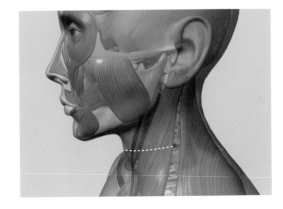

SI 17 Tian Rong Heavenly Appearance

L: dorsal to the angle of the jaw, in the depression at the anterior border of the sternocleidomastoid muscle

T: 0.5–1 cun perpendicular; moxibustion

P: relieves the pharynx and reduces edema, sharpens hearing and relieves the upper body orifices

A: 1. acute inflammation in the region of the pharynx and the throat
2. tinnitus, deafness

Pec: CAUTION, AVOID NEEDLING OF CAROTID ARTERY AND JUGULAR VEIN!

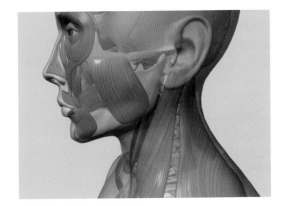

SI 18 Quan Liao Cheek Bone Crevice

L: directly below the outer canthus in the depression below the zygomatic bone

T: 0.3–0.5 cun perpendicular or 0.5–1 cun oblique; moxibustion

P: returns to correct position and relieves cramp, activates the channel and alleviates pain

A: 1. facial paresis, tics, and facial cramps
2. trigeminal neuralgia

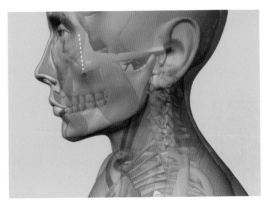

L: Location   T: Insertion Technique   P: Properties   A: Clinical Applications   Pec: Peculiarities

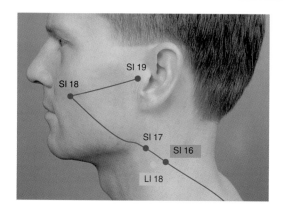

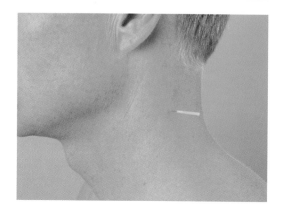

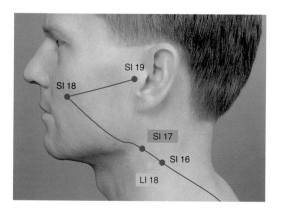

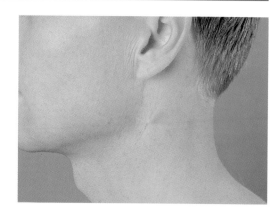

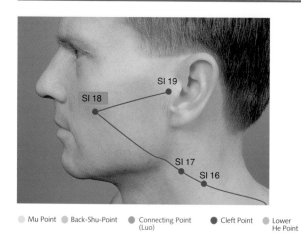

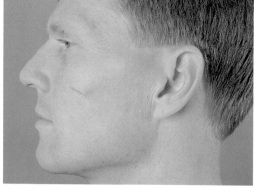

SI

● Mu Point　● Back-Shu-Point　● Connecting Point (Luo)　● Cleft Point　● Lower He Point　　● Qi-Source-Point (Yuan)　● Confluent Point　● Converging Point

119

SI 19 Ting Gong   Listening Palace

L: with the patient's mouth slightly opened, in the depression ventral to the tragus and dorsal to the caput manibulae

T: 1–1.5 cun perpendicular; moxibustion

P: sharpens hearing and relieves the upper body orifices

A: 1. diseases of the ear
2. trigeminal neuralgia (especially of the first branch), dysfunctions of the jaw

Pec: CAUTION, AVOID SPREADING GERMS TO THE JAW!

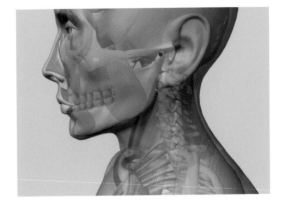

SI

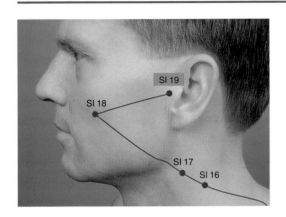
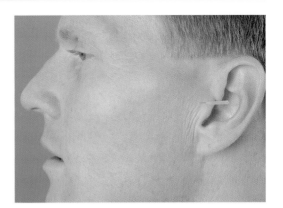

⬤ Mu Point ⬤ Back-Shu-Point ⬤ Connecting Point (Luo) ⬤ Cleft Point ⬤ Lower He Point ⬤ Qi-Source-Point (Yuan) ⬤ Confluent Point ⬤ Converging Point

2.2.7 The bladder channel (Bl)

Synonyms

• Bladder-Meridian

• Foot-Taiyang Bladder Channel

Channel pathway

There are 67 acupuncture points on the surface pathway of the Bladder channel.

In its surface pathway the channel originates at the inner canthus of the eye and ascends along the forehead to the Du Mai on the anterior hairline (Du 24). From here the channel runs laterally to points Bl 3 and Bl 4 and further over the skull. At the vertex the channel runs from Bl 7 to the Du Mai (Du 20) and then to Bl 8. From the vertex branches enter the brain, in the direction of the tip of the ear at point GB 8. From point Bl 9 the channel returns to the Du Mai (Du 16) and then descends to point Bl 10. After crossing the skull the channel separates at point Bl 10 into its two principal branches along the spine. These run almost parallel to the midline.

The first branch first runs over the seventh cervical vertebra (Du 14) and first thoracic vertebra (Du 13), from where it descends along the spine at 1.5 cun lateral to the midline to the region of the sacrum, at the level of the fourth sacral foramen. The channel then returns cranially toward the midline where it descends from the first sacral vertebra, via the sacral foramen, to the centre of the buttocks and finally, via the centre of the posterior aspect of the thigh, to the popliteal fossa at Bl 40.

In the lumbar region (Bl 23 and Bl 52) the inner channel pathway branches via the lumbar muscles into the interior, where it connects with the kidney and its organ, the bladder.

The surface pathway of the second branch descends from point Bl 10 and paravertebrally from the second thoracic vertebra, but more distant from the midline, along the inner border of the scapula to the lumbar-sacral region (Bl 54). From here it descends further over the buttocks (GB 30) and the posterior aspect of the thigh to the popliteal fossa (Bl 40).

Both channel branches meet at point Bl 40 in the popliteal fossa and descend via the middle of the calf along the Achilles tendon to the heel. The channel circles the outer bones from behind and follows the fifth metatarsal bone on the border between dorsum and sole, to end at the outer nail corner of the little toe.

Bl

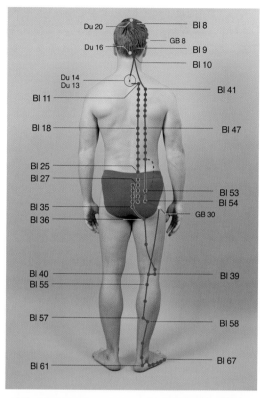

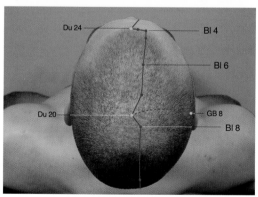

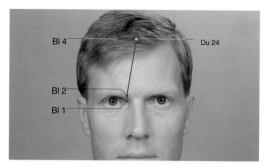

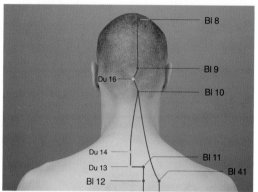

Bl

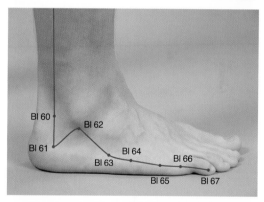

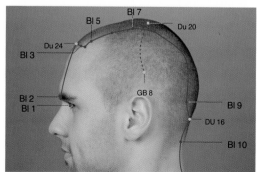

Bl 1 Jing Ming Bright Eyes

L: in the depression 0.1 cun medial and superior to the inner canthus of the eye

T: eyeball to be pushed firmly downwards and sidewards, 0.5–1 cun perpendicular directly alongside the inner border of the orbit, no needle manipulation! No moxibustion!

P: clears heat and sharpens eyesight

A: diseases of the eye e.g. conjunctivitis, ceratitis, dim vision, irregular refraction

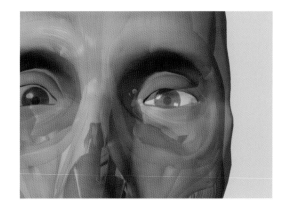

Bl 2 Zuan Zhu Gathered Bamboo

L: in the depression at the medial end of the eyebrow in the incisura frontalis

T: 0.5–0.8 cun subcutaneously; no moxibustion

P: expels wind and alleviates pain, clears heat and sharpens eyesight

A: 1. frontal headache, frontal sinusitis
2. diseases of the eye

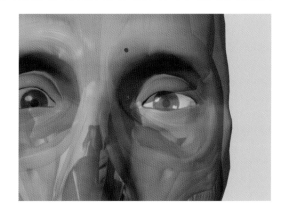

Bl 3 Mei Chong Eyebrows' Pouring

L: directly superior to Bl 2, 0.5 cun within the ideal anterior hairline

T: 0.3–0.5 cun subcutaneously; moxibustion

P: expels wind and alleviates pain, clears heat and calms the spirit

A: 1. headache
2. epilepsy

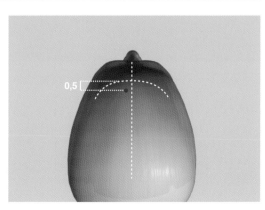

L: Location   T: Insertion Technique   P: Properties   A: Clinical Applications   Pec: Peculiarities

Bl

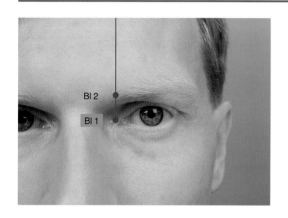

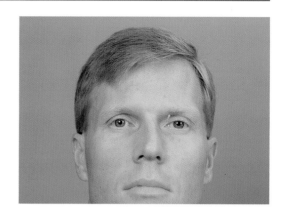

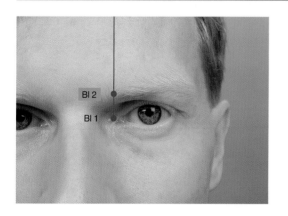

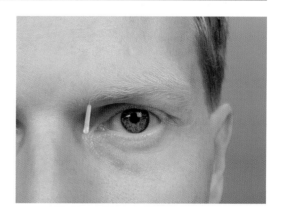

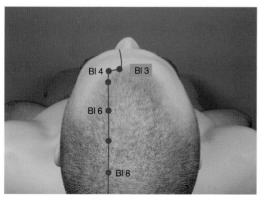

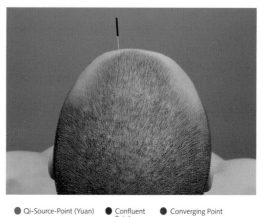

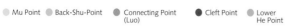

● Mu Point ● Back-Shu-Point ● Connecting Point (Luo) ● Cleft Point ● Lower He Point ● Qi-Source-Point (Yuan) ● Confluent Point ● Converging Point

Bl 4 Qu Cha(i) Crooked Curve

L: 0.5 cun within the ideal anterior hairline, 1.5 cun lateral to the midline, at the crossing from the medial to the central third of the connecting line, between Du 24 and St 8

T: 0.5-0.8 cun subcutaneously; moxibustion

P: clears heat and sharpens eyesight, expels wind and activates the upper orifices

A: 1. headache
2. diseases of the eye e.g. dim vision
3. diseases of the nose e.g. "congested nose," epistaxis

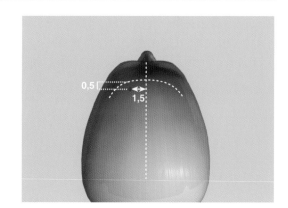

Bl 5 Wu Chu Fifth Place

L: 1 cun within the ideal anterior hairline, 1.5 cun lateral to the midline

T: 0.5–0.8 cun subcutaneously; moxibustion

P: expels wind and clears heat, sharpens eyesight and releases cramp

A: 1. headache
2. dim vision
3. epilepsy

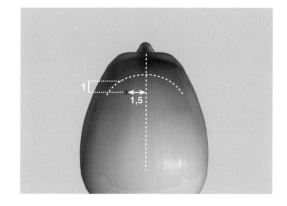

Bl 6 Cheng Guang Receiving Light

L: 2.5 cun within the ideal anterior hairline, 1.5 cun lateral to the midline

T: 0.3–0.5 cun subcutaneously; moxibustion

P: expels wind and clears heat, sharpens eyesight and alleviates pain

A: 1. headache
2. glaucoma

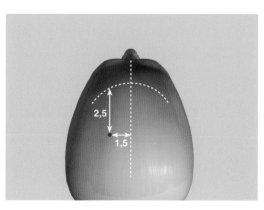

L: Location T: Insertion Technique P: Properties A: Clinical Applications Pec: Peculiarities

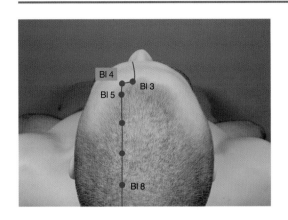

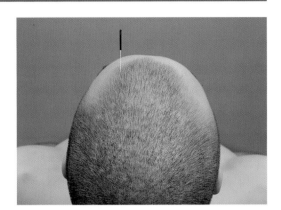

Bl

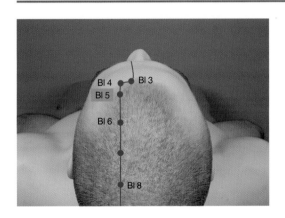

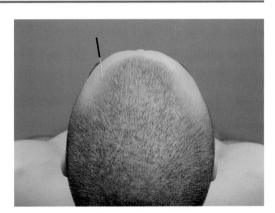

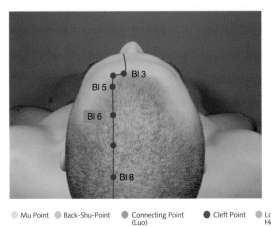

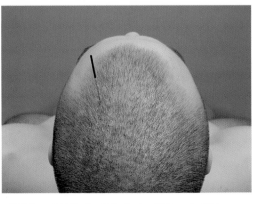

⬤ Mu Point ⬤ Back-Shu-Point ⬤ Connecting Point (Luo) ⬤ Cleft Point ⬤ Lower He Point ⬤ Qi-Source-Point (Yuan) ⬤ Confluent Point ⬤ Converging Point

Bl 7 Tong Tian   Heavenly Connection

L: 4 cun within the ideal anterior hairline, 1.5 cun
lateral to the midline

T: 0.3–0.5 cun subcutaneously;
moxibustion

P: clears heat and expels wind, alleviates pain and
relieves the upper orifices

A: 1. diseases of the nose
2. headache
3. hypertension

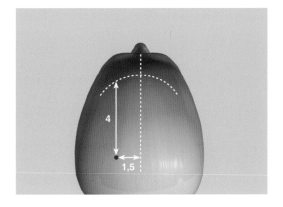

Bl 8 Luo Que   Declining Connection

L: 5.5 cun within the ideal anterior hairline, 1.5 cun
lateral to the midline

T: 0.3–0.5 cun subcutaneously;
moxibustion

P: pacifies the liver and expels wind, clears the heart
and pacifies the spirit

A: 1. hypertension
2. psychic and psychosomatic dysfunctions, epilepsy

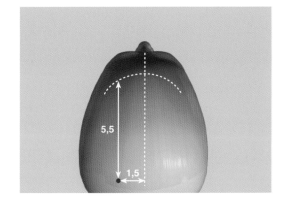

Bl 9 Yu Zhen   Jade Pillow

L: 2.5 cun within the ideal posterior hairline, at the
level of the upper ridge of the external occipital
protuberance, 1.5 cun lateral to the midline

T: 0.3–0.5 cun subcutaneously;
moxibustion

P: clears heat and expels wind, sharpens eyesight and
descends inverted Qi

A: 1. headache
2. diseases of the eye, e.g. glaucoma

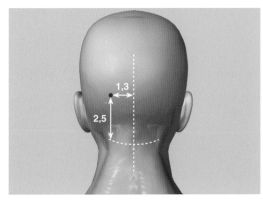

L: Location   T: Insertion Technique   P: Properties   A: Clinical Applications   Pec: Peculiarities

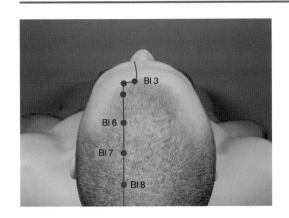

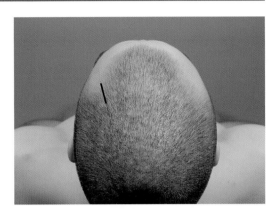

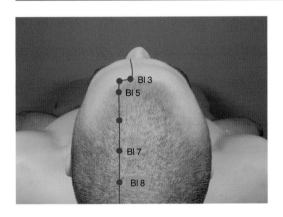

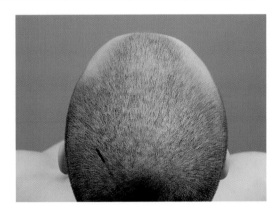

Bl

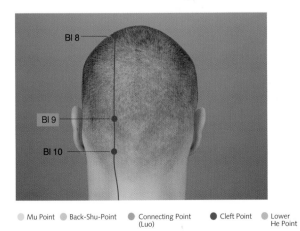

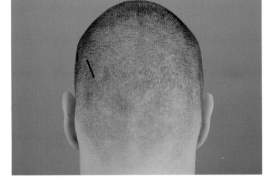

⬤ Mu Point ⬤ Back-Shu-Point ⬤ Connecting Point (Luo) ⬤ Cleft Point ⬤ Lower He Point ⬤ Qi-Source-Point (Yuan) ⬤ Confluent Point ⬤ Converging Point

Bl 10 Tian Zhu   Celestial Pillar

L: 0.5 cun within the ideal anterior hairline, 1.3 cun lateral to the midline in the depression at the lateral edge of the trapezius muscle

T: 0.5–0.8 cun perpendicular or oblique medially; moxibustion

P: opens the senses and restores consciousness, clears heat and expels wind

A: 1. headache
2. vertebro-basiliar insufficiency
3. cervicobrachial syndrome

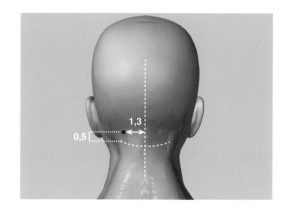

Bl 11 Da Zhu   Great Shuttle

L: at the level of the depression inferior to the spinous process Th1, 1.5 cun lateral to the dorsal midline

T: 0.5–0.8 cun oblique medially; moxibustion

P: clears heat and liberates the surface, strengthens the bones and alleviates pain

A: 1. infections of the superior respiratory tract
2. cervicobrachial syndrome

Pec: meeting (master) point (Hui) of the bones
CAUTION, AVOID PNEUMOTHORAX!

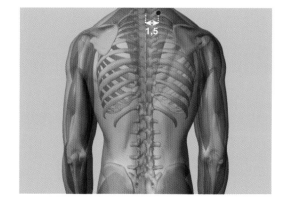

Bl 12 Feng Men   Wind Gate

L: at the level of the depression inferior to the spinous process Th2, 1.5 cun lateral to the dorsal midline

T: 0.5–0.8 cun oblique medially; moxibustion

P: expels wind and liberates the surface, clears the lungs and alleviates coughing

A: 1. infections of the superior trachea
2. acute and chronic bronchitis

Pec: CAUTION, AVOID PNEUMOTHORAX!

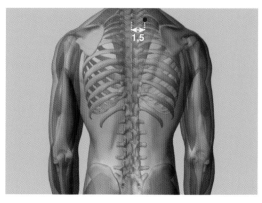

L: Location   T: Insertion Technique   P: Properties   A: Clinical Applications   Pec: Peculiarities

Bl

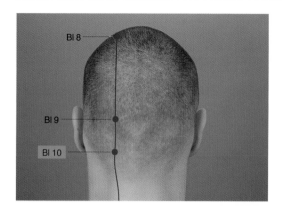

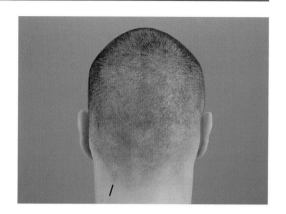

Bl

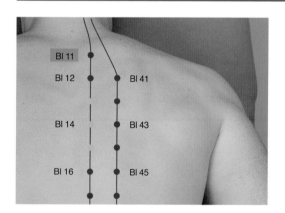

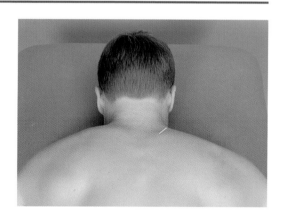

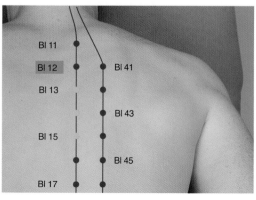

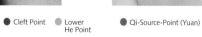

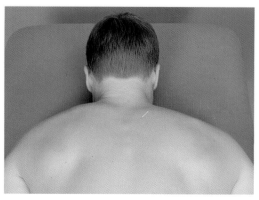

⬤ Mu Point   ⬤ Back-Shu-Point   ⬤ Connecting Point (Luo)   ● Cleft Point   ⬤ Lower He Point   ⬤ Qi-Source-Point (Yuan)   ● Confluent Point   ⬤ Converging Point

131

Bl 13 Fei Shu   Lung Shu

L: at the level of the depression inferior to the spinous process Th3, 1.5 cun lateral to the dorsal midline

T: 0.5–0.8 cun oblique medially; moxibustion

P: liberates the surface and disseminates lung Qi, descends Qi and alleviates breathing difficulty

A: 1. infections of the superior trachea
2. bronchial asthma
3. diseases of the lung, e.g. pneumonia

Pec: back-Shu-point of the lung
CAUTION, AVOID PNEUMOTHORAX!

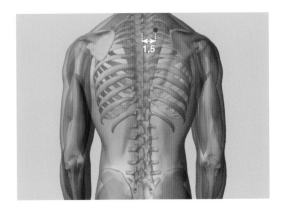

Bl

Bl 14 Jue Yin Shu   Jue Yin Shu

L: at the level of the depression inferior to the spinous process Th4, 1.5 cun lateral to the dorsal midline

T: 0.5–0.8 cun oblique medially; moxibustion

P: unbinds the chest and descends inverted Qi, calms the heart and alleviates pain

A: 1. coronary diseases, e.g. dysfunctions of the heartbeat
2. coughing

Pec: back-Shu-point of the Pericardium
CAUTION, AVOID PNEUMOTHORAX!

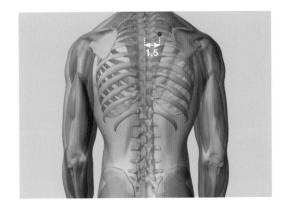

Bl 15 Xin Shu   Heart Shu

L: at the level of the depression inferior to the spinous process Th5, 1.5 cun lateral to the dorsal midline

T: 0.5–0.8 cun oblique medially; moxibustion

P: unbinds the chest and descends Qi, calms the heart and pacifies the spirit

A: 1. diseases of the heart
2. psychic and psychosomatic dysfunctions

Pec: back-Shu-point of the heart
CAUTION, AVOID PNEUMOTHORAX!

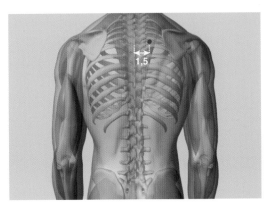

L: Location   **T:** Insertion Technique   **P:** Properties   **A:** Clinical Applications   **Pec:** Peculiarities

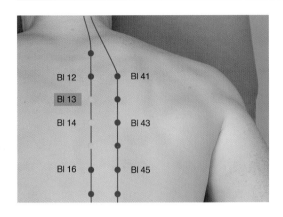

Bl 12
Bl 13
Bl 14
Bl 16

Bl 41
Bl 43
Bl 45

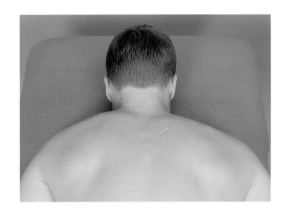

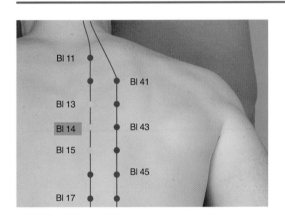

Bl 11
Bl 13
Bl 14
Bl 15
Bl 17

Bl 41
Bl 43
Bl 45

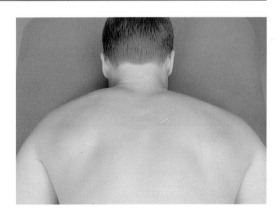

BI

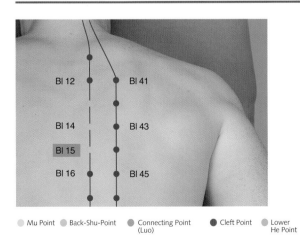

Bl 12
Bl 14
Bl 15
Bl 16

Bl 41
Bl 43
Bl 45

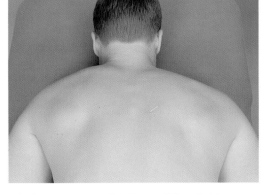

| ● Mu Point | ● Back-Shu-Point | ● Connecting Point (Luo) | ● Cleft Point | ● Lower He Point | ● Qi-Source-Point (Yuan) | ● Confluent Point | ● Converging Point |

Bl 16 Du Shu   Governor Shu

L: at the level of the depression inferior to the spinous process Th6, 1.5 cun lateral to the dorsal midline

T: 0.5–0.8 cun oblique medially; moxibustion

P: unbinds the chest and alleviates pain, regulates Qi and eliminates tension

A: 1. pectoral angina
2. stomach pains, abdominal pain

Pec: CAUTION, AVOID PNEUMOTHORAX!

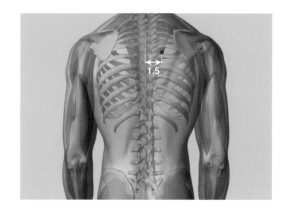

Bl 17 Ge Shu   Diaphragm Shu

L: at the level of the depression inferior to the spinous process Th7, 1.5 cun lateral to the dorsal midline

T: 0.5–0.8 cun oblique medially; moxibustion

P: replenishes and soothes the blood, unbinds the chest and alleviates pain, descend inverted Qi

A: 1. anemia
2. stopping the bleeding from superior orifices e.g. epistaxis, coughing or spitting blood
3. bronchial asthma, spastic bronchitis
4. hiccups

Pec: meeting (master) point (Hui) of the blood
CAUTION, AVOID PNEUMOTHORAX!

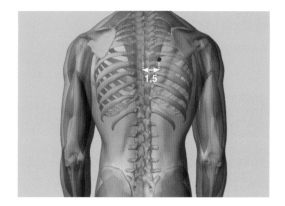

Bl 18 Gan Shu   Liver Shu

L: at the level of the depression inferior to the spinous process Th9, 1.5 cun lateral to the dorsal midline

T: 0.5–0.8 cun oblique medially; moxibustion

P: decongests the liver and benefits bile, promotes all-round calmness and releases cramp

A: 1. certain liver and gall bladder dysfunctions e.g. hepatitis, cholecystitis
2. psychic and psychosomatic dysfunctions e.g. epilepsy
3. diseases of the eye e.g. glaucoma, night blindness, diseases of the eye nerve

Pec: back-Shu-point of the liver
CAUTION, AVOID PNEUMOTHORAX!

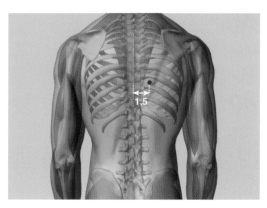

Bl

L: Location   T: Insertion Technique   P: Properties   A: Clinical Applications   Pec: Peculiarities

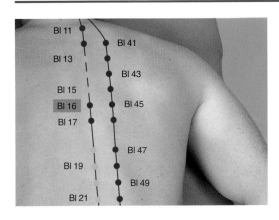

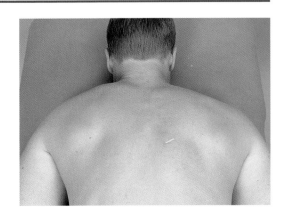

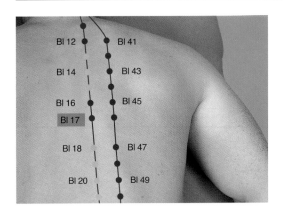

BI

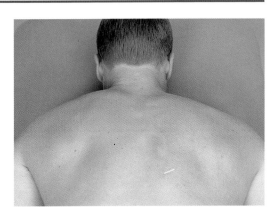

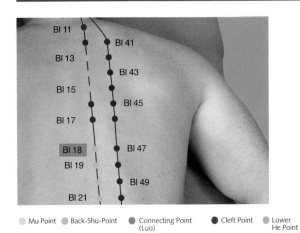

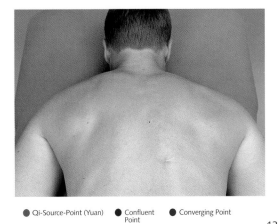

● Mu Point ● Back-Shu-Point ● Connecting Point (Luo) ● Cleft Point ● Lower He Point   ● Qi-Source-Point (Yuan) ● Confluent Point ● Converging Point

BI 19 Dan Shu Gall Bladder Shu

L: at the level of the depression inferior to the spinous process Th10, 1.5 cun lateral to the dorsal midline

T: 0.5–0.8 cun oblique medially; moxibustion

P: clears heat and transforms phlegm, benefits bile, and alleviates pain

A: diseases of the gall bladder, e.g. cholecystitis, cholelithiasis

Pec: back-Shu-point of the gall bladder
CAUTION, AVOID PNEUMOTHORAX!

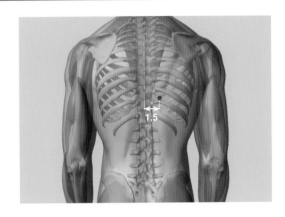

BI 20 Pi Shu Spleen Shu

L: at the level of the depression inferior to the spinous process Th11, 1.5 cun lateral to the dorsal midline

T: 0.5–0.8 cun oblique medially; moxibustion

P: strengthens the spleen, promotes urination, increases clarity, and alleviates diarrhoea

A: 1. chronic gastritis, chronic enteritis, digestive dysfunctions
2. dyspeptic diarrhoea in children
3. edemas

Pec: back-Shu-point of the spleen
CAUTION, AVOID PNEUMOTHORAX!

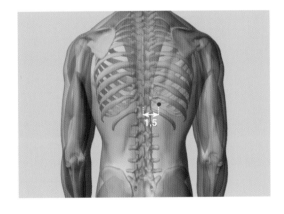

BI 21 Wei Shu Stomach Shu

L: at the level of the depression inferior to the spinous process Th12, 1.5 cun lateral to the dorsal midline

T: 0.5–0.8 cun oblique medially; moxibustion

P: harmonizes the stomach and alleviates pain, regulates the centre and descends inverted Qi

A: acute and chronic gastritis, stomach pains

Pec: back-Shu-point of the stomach
CAUTION, AVOID PNEUMOTHORAX!

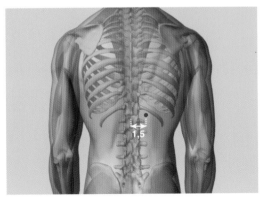

L: Location   **T:** Insertion Technique   **P:** Properties   **A:** Clinical Applications   **Pec:** Peculiarities

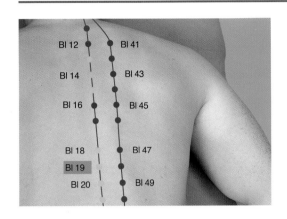

Bl 12   Bl 41
Bl 14   Bl 43
Bl 16   Bl 45
Bl 18   Bl 47
Bl 19
Bl 20   Bl 49

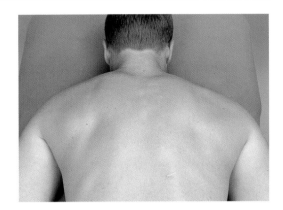

Bl

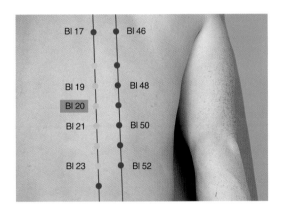

Bl 17   Bl 46
Bl 19   Bl 48
Bl 20
Bl 21   Bl 50
Bl 23   Bl 52

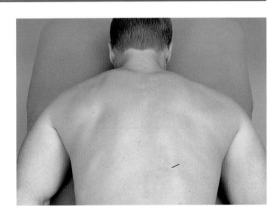

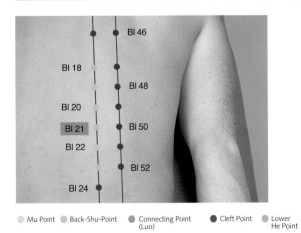

Bl 46
Bl 18
Bl 48
Bl 20
Bl 21   Bl 50
Bl 22
Bl 52
Bl 24

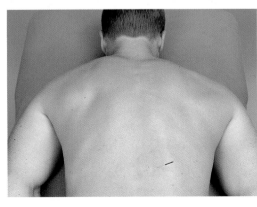

○ Mu Point   ○ Back-Shu-Point   ● Connecting Point (Luo)   ● Cleft Point   ○ Lower He Point   ● Qi-Source-Point (Yuan)   ● Confluent Point   ● Converging Point

137

Bl 22 San Jiao Shu   San Jiao Shu

L: at the level of the depression inferior to the spinous process L1, 1.5 cun lateral to the dorsal midline

T: 0.5–1 cun perpendicular; moxibustion

P: regulates the Sanjiao, strengthens the spleen, and promotes urination

A: 1. acute and chronic gastritis, acute and chronic enteritis, digestive dysfunctions
2. edema

Pec: back-Shu-point of the San Jiao

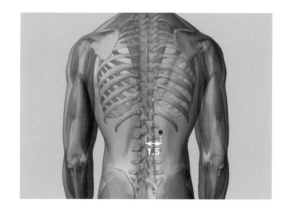

Bl 23 Shen Shu   Kidney Shu

Bl

L: at the level of the depression inferior to the spinous process L2, 1.5 cun lateral to the dorsal midline

T: 0.5–1 cun perpendicular; moxibustion

P: supports the kidney and enriches the yin, regulates menstruation, and promotes urination

A: 1. dysfunctions in male sexual function
2. certain gynecological dysfunctions, e.g. irregular menstruation, leucorrhoea
3. urinary incontinence
4. lumbalgia

Pec: back-Shu-point of the kidney

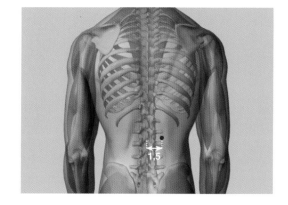

Bl 24 Qi Hai Shu   Sea of Qi Shu

L: at the level of the depression inferior to the spinous process L3, 1.5 cun lateral to the dorsal midline

T: 0.5–1 cun perpendicular; moxibustion

P: replenishes the kidney and increases Qi, regulates menstruation and alleviates pain

A: 1. dysmenorrhoea
2. lumbalgia

Pec: CAUTION IN PREGNANCY!

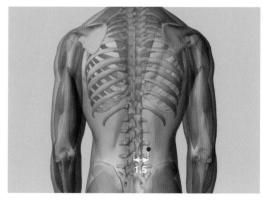

L: Location   **T:** Insertion Technique   **P:** Properties   **A:** Clinical Applications   **Pec:** Peculiarities

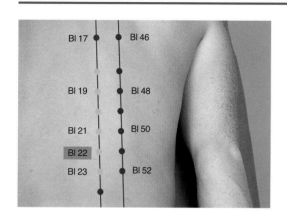

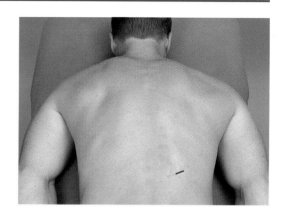

Bl

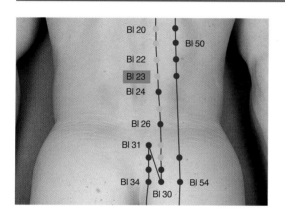

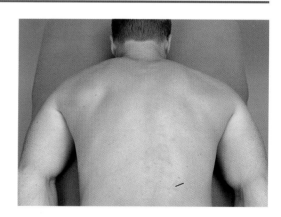

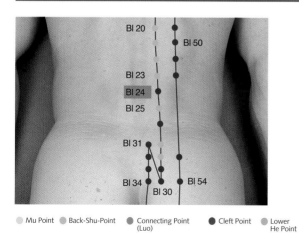

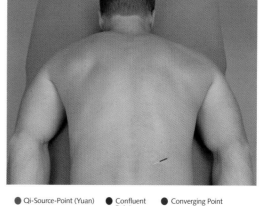

○ Mu Point ○ Back-Shu-Point ● Connecting Point (Luo) ● Cleft Point ○ Lower He Point ● Qi-Source-Point (Yuan) ● Confluent Point ● Converging Point

Bl 25 Da Chang Shu Large Intestine Shu

L: at the level of the depression inferior to the spinous process L4, 1.5 cun lateral to the dorsal midline

T: 0.8–1.2 cun perpendicular; moxibustion

P: restores balance to the large intestine, regulates Qi and alleviates pain

A: 1. dysfunctions in the urinary function in diseases of the large intestine (regulatory effect)
2. lumbalgia, ischialgia

Pec: back-Shu-point of the large intestine
CAUTION IN PREGNANCY!

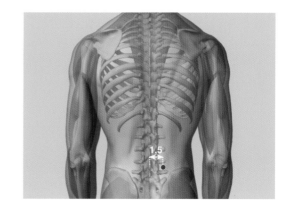

Bl 26 Guan Yuan Shu Gate of Origin Shu

L: at the level of the depression inferior to the spinous process L5, 1.5 cun lateral to the dorsal midline

T: 0.8–1.2 cun perpendicular or oblique laterally; moxibustion

P: expands and replenishes source Qi, regulates the stools, and passage of water

A: 1. dysfunctions in the function of the intestine
2. dysfunctions in the function of the bladder e.g. urinary incontinence, urinary retention
3. lumbalgia

Pec: CAUTION IN PREGNANCY!

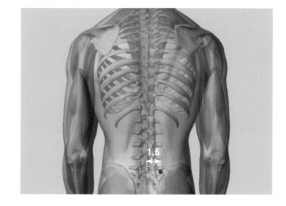

Bl 27 Xiao Chang Shu Small Intestine Shu

L: at the level of the first dorsal sacral foramen, 1.5 cun lateral to the dorsal midline

T: 0.8–1.2 cun perpendicular or oblique laterally; moxibustion

P: regulates defecation and urination

A: 1. infections of the urinary tract
2. infectious diseases of the intestine, e.g. enteritis, dysentery
3. lumbalgia

Pec: back-Shu-point of the small intestine
CAUTION IN PREGNANCY!

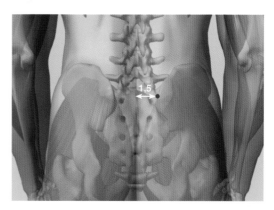

L: Location   **T:** Insertion Technique   **P:** Properties   **A:** Clinical Applications   **Pec:** Peculiarities

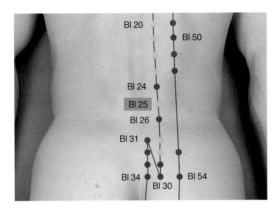

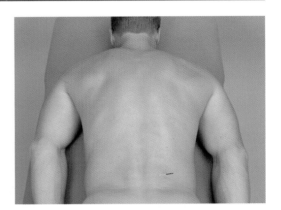

Bl

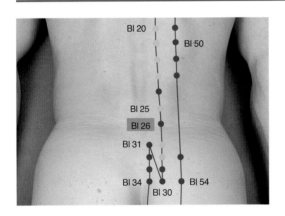

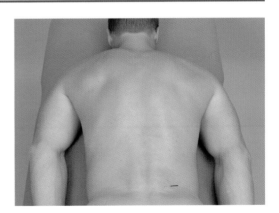

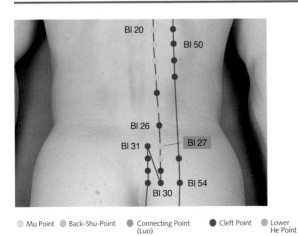

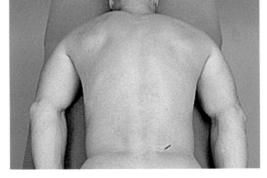

● Mu Point   ● Back-Shu-Point   ● Connecting Point (Luo)   ● Cleft Point   ● Lower He Point   ● Qi-Source-Point (Yuan)   ● Confluent Point   ● Converging Point

Bl 28 Pang Guang Shu   Bladder Shu

L: at the level of the second posterior sacral foramen, 1.5 cun lateral to the dorsal midline

T: 0.8–1.2 cun perpendicular or oblique laterally; moxibustion

P: clears heat, promotes urination, decongests and activates the primary channel and its vessels

A: 1. infections of the urinary tract
2. vulvitis, colpitis
3. pains in the lumbo-sacral region

Pec: back-Shu-point of the bladder
CAUTION IN PREGNANCY!

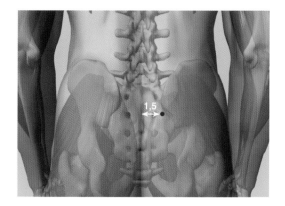

Bl 29 Zhong Lu Shu   Mid-Spine Shu

L: at the level of the third posterior sacral foramen, 1.5 cun lateral to the dorsal midline

T: 1–1.5 cun perpendicular; moxibustion

P: restores balance to the large intestine, regulates Qi and alleviates pain

A: 1. dysentery
2. pains in the lumbo-sacral region

Pec: CAUTION IN PREGNANCY!

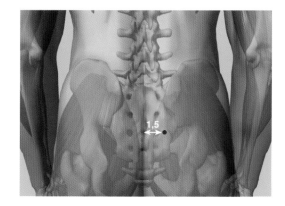

Bl 30 Bai Huan Shu   White Ring Shu

L: at the level of the fourth posterior sacral foramen, 1.5 cun lateral to the dorsal midline

T: 1–1.5 cun perpendicular; moxibustion

P: supports the kidneys and promotes menstruation

A: 1. certain gynecological dysfunctions, e.g. irregular menstruation, leucorrhoea
2. pains in the lumbo-sacral region

Pec: CAUTION IN PREGNANCY!

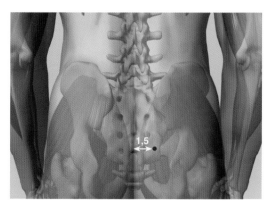

L: Location   **T:** Insertion Technique   **P:** Properties   **A:** Clinical Applications   **Pec:** Peculiarities

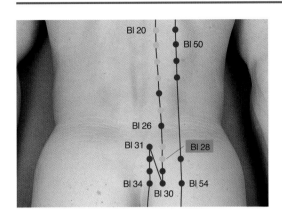

BI 20
BI 50
BI 26
BI 31
BI 28
BI 34
BI 54
BI 30

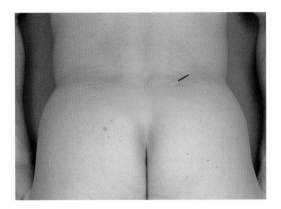

Bl

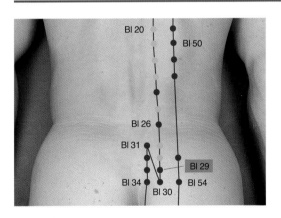

BI 20
BI 50
BI 26
BI 31
BI 29
BI 34
BI 54
BI 30

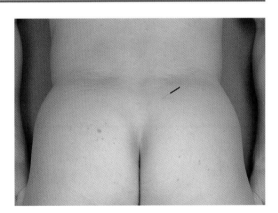

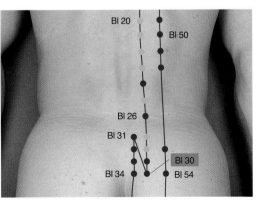

BI 20
BI 50
BI 26
BI 31
BI 30
BI 34
BI 54

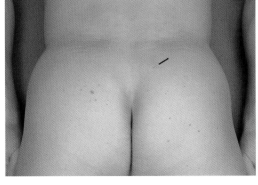

● Mu Point ● Back-Shu-Point ● Connecting Point (Luo) ● Cleft Point ● Lower He Point ● Qi-Source-Point (Yuan) ● Confluent Point ● Converging Point

Bl 31 Shang Liao   Upper Crevice

L: at the midpoint between the posterior superior iliac spine and the dorsal midline in the first posterior sacral foramen

T: 1–1.5 cun perpendicular; moxibustion

P: promotes menstruation and replenishes Qi, assists the yang and increases essence

A: 1. certain gynecological dysfunctions, e.g. irregular menstruation, uterine prolapse, leucorrhoea
       2. male sexual dysfunction

Pec: CAUTION IN PREGNANCY!

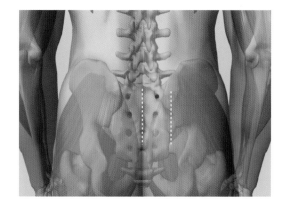

Bl 32 Ci Liao   Second Crevice

L: medial and inferior to the posterior superior iliac spine in the second posterior sacral foramen

T: 1–1.5 cun perpendicular; moxibustion

P: clears and facilitates urination and clears heat, regulates Qi and promotes menstruation

A: 1. certain gynecological dysfunctions, e.g. inflammation in the small pelvis, irregular menstruation, dysmenorrhoea
       2. paraestheses in the lower extremity

Pec: CAUTION IN PREGNANCY!

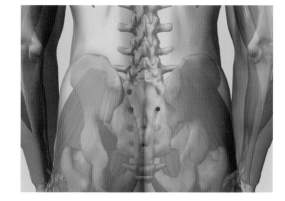

Bl 33 Zhong Liao   Middle Crevice

L: medial and inferior to Bl 32, in the third posterior sacral foramen

T: 1–1.5 cun perpendicular; moxibustion

P: promotes menstruation and regulates flow

A: 1. certain gynecological dysfunctions, e.g. irregular menstruation, endo-/myometritis, adnexitis
       2. pain in the lumbo-sacral region

Pec: CAUTION IN PREGNANCY!

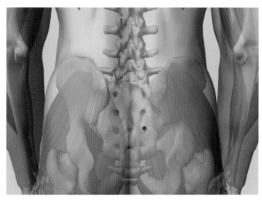

Bl

L: Location   T: Insertion Technique   P: Properties   A: Clinical Applications   Pec: Peculiarities

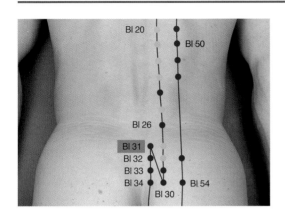

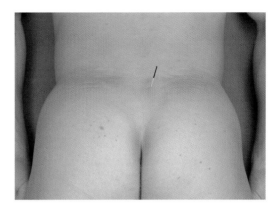

Bl

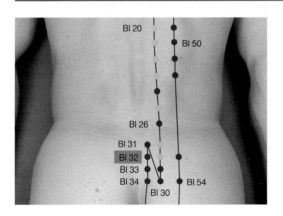

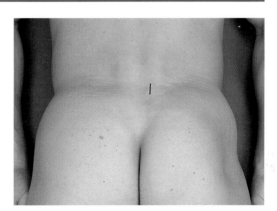

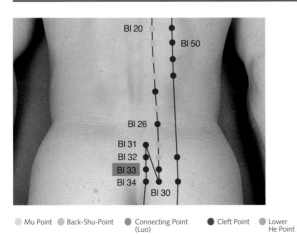

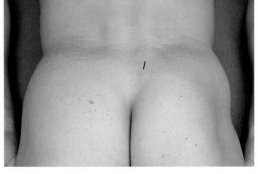

● Mu Point   ● Back-Shu-Point   ● Connecting Point (Luo)   ● Cleft Point   ● Lower He Point   ● Qi-Source-Point (Yuan)   ● Confluent Point   ● Converging Point

Bl 34 Xia Liao   Lower Crevice

L: medial and inferior to Bl 33, in the fourth posterior sacral foramen

T: 1–1.5 cun perpendicular; moxibustion

P: clears heat and transforms dampness, restores balance to defecation and urination

A: 1. acute and chronic enteritis
2. urinary retention

Pec: CAUTION IN PREGNANCY!

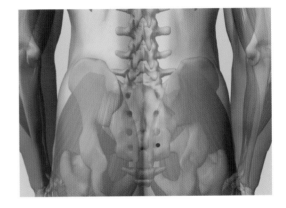

Bl 35 Hui Yang   Meeting of Yang

L: 0.5 cun lateral to the tip of the coccyx

T: 1–1.5 cun perpendicular; moxibustion

P: alleviates discharge and cures hemorrhoids

A: 1. acute and chronic endometritis, acute and chronic adnexitis
2. hemorrhoids

Pec: CAUTION IN PREGNANCY!

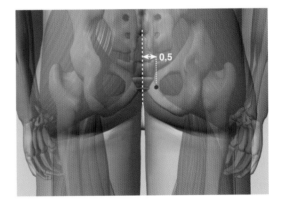

Bl 36 Cheng Fu   Hold and Support

L: in the centre of the inferior gluteal crease

T: 1–2 cun perpendicular; moxibustion

P: eliminates hemorrhoids and alleviates pain, decongests and activates the channel and its vessels

A: 1. hemorrhoids
2. pains in the buttocks, sacrum, and upper thigh

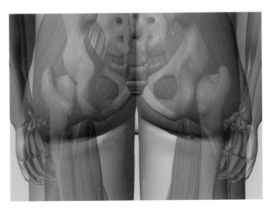

Bl

L: Location   **T:** Insertion Technique   **P:** Properties   **A:** Clinical Applications   **Pec:** Peculiarities

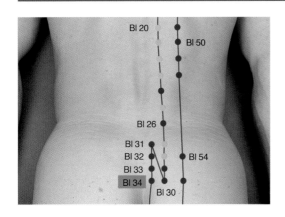

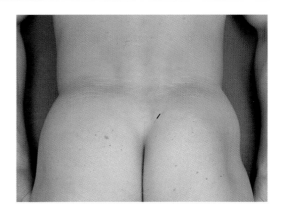

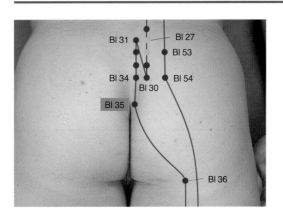

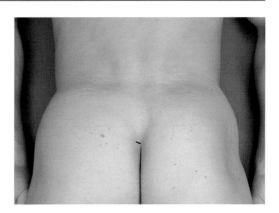

Bl

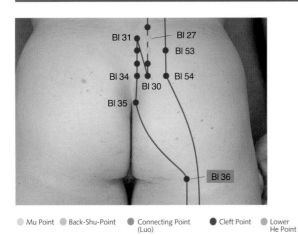

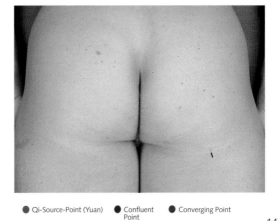

● Mu Point　● Back-Shu-Point　● Connecting Point (Luo)　● Cleft Point　● Lower He Point　● Qi-Source-Point (Yuan)　● Confluent Point　● Converging Point

147

Bl 37 Yin Men   Gate of Abundance

L: 6 cun distal to the inferior gluteal crease (Bl 36), on the connecting line between Bl 36 and Bl 40, about 8 cun proximal to Bl 39

T: 1–2 cun perpendicular; moxibustion

P: decongests and activates the channel and its vessels

A: 1. pain in the back and lumbar region
2. ischialgia

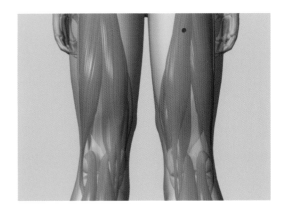

Bl 38 Fu Xi   Floating Cleft

Bl

L: 1 cun proximal to Bl 39, on the medial side of the tendon of the M. biceps femoris

T: 1–1.5 cun perpendicular; moxibustion

P: relaxes the tendons and activates the vessels

A: local pain, paraestheses

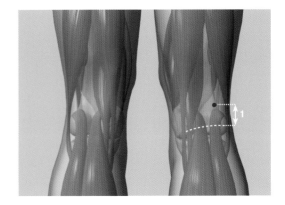

Bl 39 Wei Yang   Outside of the Crook

L: at the lateral end of the popliteal crease, on the medial side of the M. biceps femoris

T: 1–1.5 cun perpendicular; moxibustion

P: promotes urination and facilitates water discharge, regulates the sanjiao

A: 1. dysfunctions in the distribution of body fluids in urine e.g. urinary retention, urinary incontinence, edema (restores balance)
2. sensations of abdominal swelling and tension

Pec: lower He (sea) point of the sanjiao

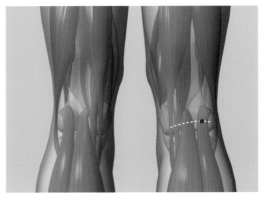

L: Location   T: Insertion Technique   P: Properties   A: Clinical Applications   Pec: Peculiarities

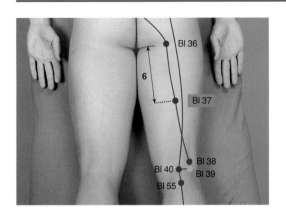
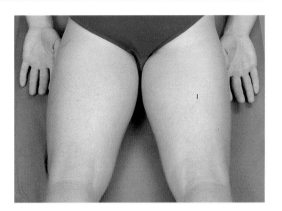
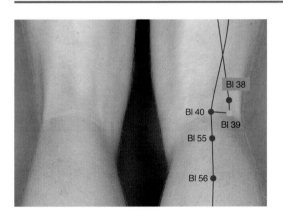
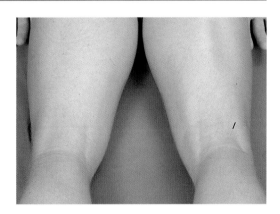
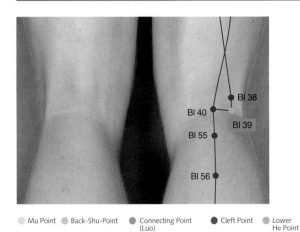
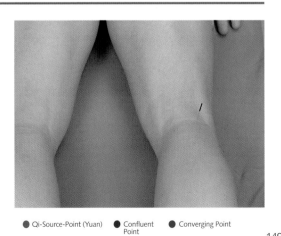

Bl

○ Mu Point ○ Back-Shu-Point ○ Connecting Point (Luo) ● Cleft Point ○ Lower He Point   ● Qi-Source-Point (Yuan) ● Confluent Point ● Converging Point

149

Bl 40 Wei Zhong Middle of the Crook

L: in the middle of the popliteal crease

T: 1–1.5 cun perpendicular; prick superficial popliteal veins to bleed; moxibustion

P: clears heat and restores clarity to the senses, decongests and activates the channel and its vessels

A: 1. sudden loss of consciousness in cerebro-vascular and cerebral diseases
2. loss of movement, pains and cramp in the lower extremity
3. lumbago
4. acute and chronic gastroenteritis

Pec: He (sea) point (5th Shu-point)

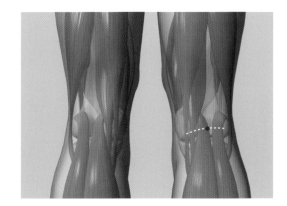

Bl 41 Fu Fen Attached Branch

L: at the level of the depression inferior to the spinous process Th2, 3 cun lateral to the dorsal midline at the level of Bl 12

T: 0.5–0.8 cun oblique medially; moxibustion

P: disseminates and expels wind and cold, activates the vessels and alleviates pain

A: pain in the region of the shoulder and back

Pec: Caution, avoid Pneumothorax!

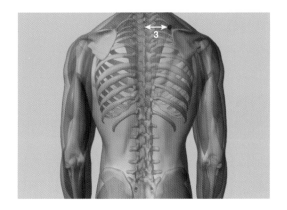

Bl 42 Po Hu Door of the Corporeal Soul

L: at the level of the depression inferior to the spinous process Th3, 3 cun lateral to the dorsal midline

T: 0.5–0.8 cun oblique medially; moxibustion

P: purifies and descends lung Qi, loosens the tendons and activates the vessels

A: 1. diseases of the lung such as bronchitis, bronchial asthma
2. pains in the region of the shoulder, neck, and back

Pec: Caution, avoid Pneumothorax!

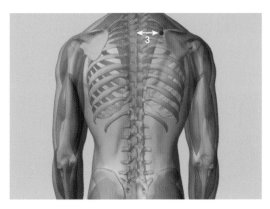

L: Location   T: Insertion Technique   P: Properties   A: Clinical Applications   Pec: Peculiarities

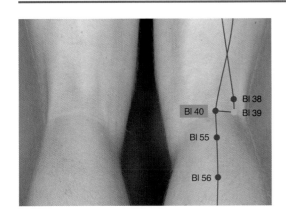

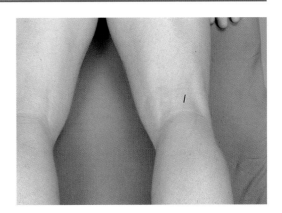

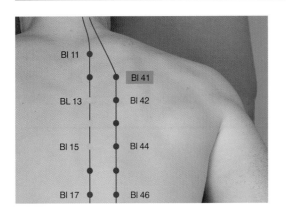

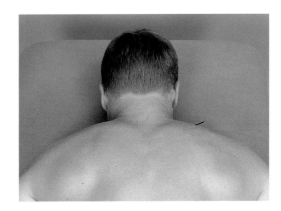

BI

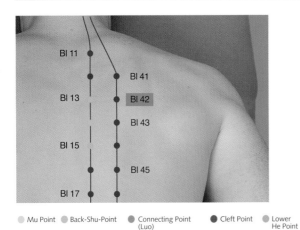

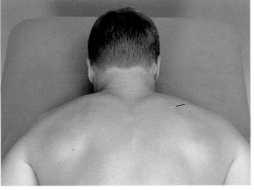

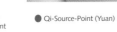

● Mu Point   ● Back-Shu-Point   ● Connecting Point (Luo)   ● Cleft Point   ● Lower He Point   ● Qi-Source-Point (Yuan)   ● Confluent Point   ● Converging Point

Bl 43 Gao Huang Vital Region

L: at the level of the depression inferior to the spinous process Th4, 3 cun lateral to the dorsal midline

T: 0.5–0.8 cun oblique medially; moxibustion

P: alleviates coughing and breathing difficulty, loosens the tendons, and activates the vessels

A: 1. infections of the lung, chronic bronchitis, emphysema of the lung
2. pain in the region of the shoulder, neck, and back

Pec: CAUTION, AVOID PNEUMOTHORAX!

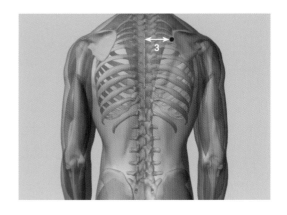

Bl 44 Sheng Tang Hall of the Spirit

L: at the level of the depression inferior to the spinous process Th5, 3 cun lateral to the dorsal midline

T: 0.5–0.8 cun oblique medially; moxibustion

P: alleviates coughing and breathing difficulty

A: acute and chronic bronchitis, bronchial asthma

Pec: CAUTION, AVOID PNEUMOTHORAX!

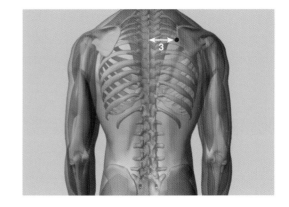

Bl 45 Yi Xi That hurts!

L: at the level of the depression inferior to the spinous process Th6, 3 cun lateral to the dorsal midline

T: 0.5–0.8 cun oblique medially; moxibustion

P: alleviates coughing and breathing difficulty, activates the channel and alleviates pain

A: 1. acute and chronic bronchitis
2. pains in the region of the shoulder, back, and ribs

Pec: CAUTION, AVOID PNEUMOTHORAX!

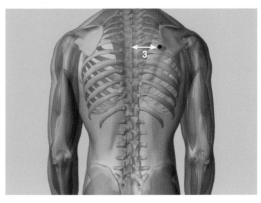

L: Location   **T:** Insertion Technique   **P:** Properties   **A:** Clinical Applications   **Pec:** Peculiarities

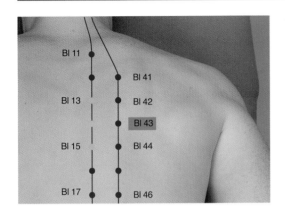

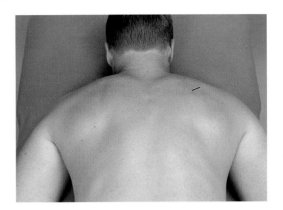

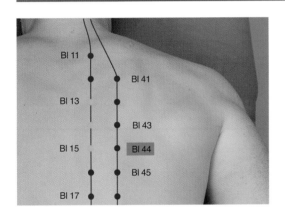

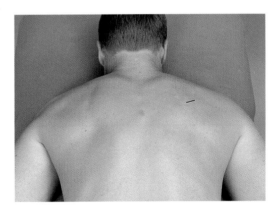

Bl

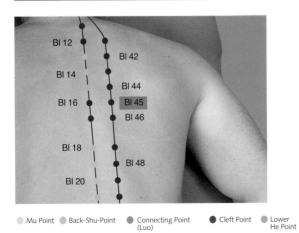

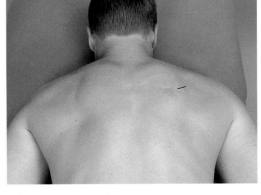

● Mu Point ● Back-Shu-Point ● Connecting Point (Luo) ● Cleft Point ● Lower He Point ● Qi-Source-Point (Yuan) ● Confluent Point ● Converging Point

Bl 46 Ge Guan Diaphragm Gate

L: at the level of the depression inferior to the spinous process Th7, 3 cun lateral to the dorsal midline

T: 0.5–0.8 cun oblique medially; moxibustion

P: descends inverted Qi and harmonizes the stomach

A: esophagitis, gastritis

Pec: CAUTION, AVOID PNEUMOTHORAX!

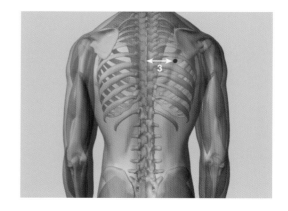

Bl 47 Hun Men Gate of the Ethereal Soul

L: at the level of the depression inferior to the spinous process Th9, 3 cun lateral to the dorsal midline

T: 0.5–0.8 cun oblique medially; moxibustion

P: decongests the liver and strengthens the spleen, descends inverted Qi and harmonizes the stomach

A: 1. hepatitis
2. acute and chronic gastroenteritis

Pec: CAUTION, AVOID PNEUMOTHORAX!

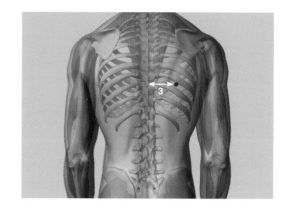

Bl 48 Yang Gang Yang's Key Link

L: at the level of the depression inferior to the spinous process Th10, 3 cun lateral to the dorsal midline

T: 0.5–0.8 cun oblique medially; moxibustion

P: strengthens the spleen and transforms dampness, decongests the liver and promotes the gall bladder

A: 1. acute and chronic gastroenteritis
2. cholecystitis

Pec: CAUTION, AVOID PNEUMOTHORAX!

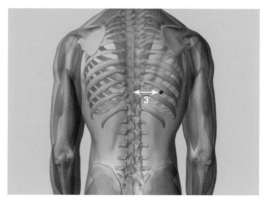

L: Location **T:** Insertion Technique **P:** Properties **A:** Clinical Applications **Pec:** Peculiarities

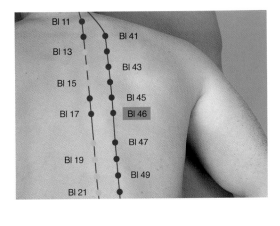

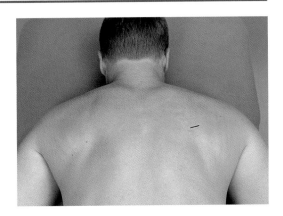

BI

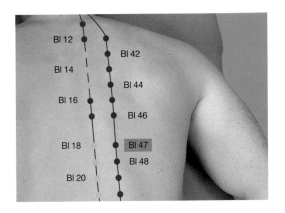

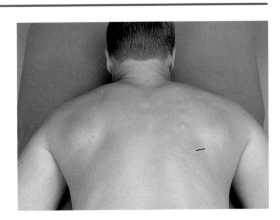

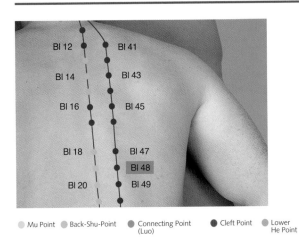

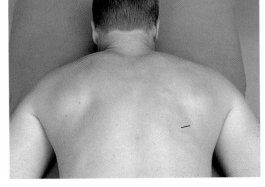

Mu Point Back-Shu-Point Connecting Point (Luo) Cleft Point Lower He Point Qi-Source-Point (Yuan) Confluent Point Converging Point

155

Bl 49 Yi She   Abode of Thought

L: at the level of the depression inferior to the spinous process Th11, 3 cun lateral to the dorsal midline

T: 0.5–0.8 cun oblique medially; moxibustion

P: strengthens the spleen and harmonizes the stomach

A: acute and chronic gastroenteritis

Pec: CAUTION, AVOID PNEUMOTHORAX!

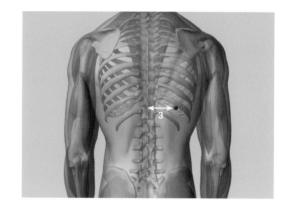

Bl 50 Wei Cang   Stomach Granary

L: at the level of the depression inferior to the spinous process Th12, 3 cun lateral to the dorsal midline

T: 0.5–0.8 cun oblique medially; moxibustion

P: harmonizes the stomach and promotes digestion

A: 1. acute and chronic gastroenteritis
2. digestive dysfunctions in children

Pec: CAUTION, AVOID PNEUMOTHORAX!

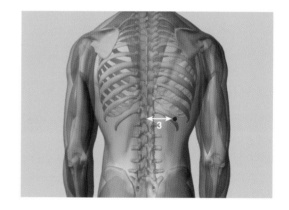

Bl 51 Huang Men   Vitals Gate

L: at the level of the depression inferior to the spinous process L1, 3 cun lateral to the dorsal midline

T: 0.5–0.8 cun oblique medially; moxibustion

P: regulates Qi and reduces edema

A: 1. swelling of the liver and spleen
2. habitual constipation

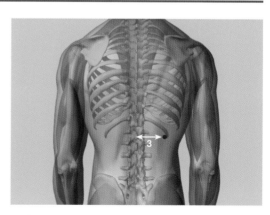

L: Location   T: Insertion Technique   P: Properties   A: Clinical Applications   Pec: Peculiarities

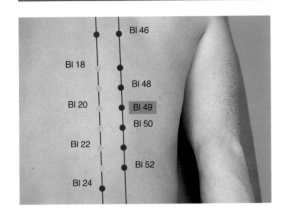

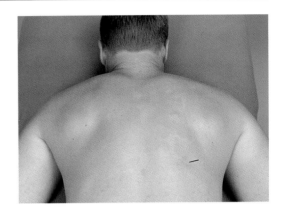

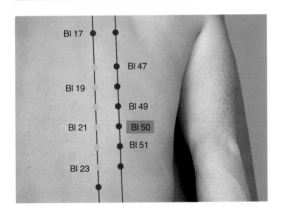

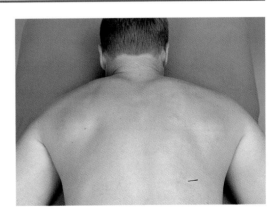

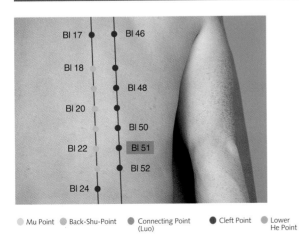

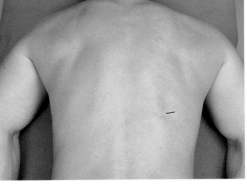

● Mu Point   ● Back-Shu-Point   ● Connecting Point (Luo)   ● Cleft Point   ● Lower He Point   ● Qi-Source-Point (Yuan)   ● Confluent Point   ● Converging Point

Bl 52 Zhi Shi   Residence of the Will

L: at the level of the depression inferior to the spinous process L2, 3 cun lateral to the dorsal midline

T: 0.5–0.8 cun oblique medially; moxibustion

P: supports the kidneys and firms the essence, clears and expels dampness and heat

A: 1. male sexual dysfunction
2. urinary infections
3. lumbalgia

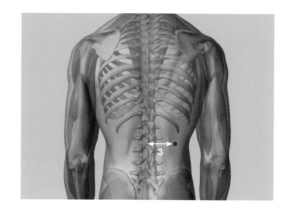

Bl 53 Bao Huang   Bladder's Vitals

L: at the level of the second sacral foramen, 3 cun lateral to the dorsal midline (at the same level as Bl 28 and Bl 32)

T: 1–1.5 cun perpendicular; moxibustion

P: clears heat, expels dampness, promotes defecation, and urination

A: 1. urinary retention
2. constipation
3. pain in the lumbo-sacral region

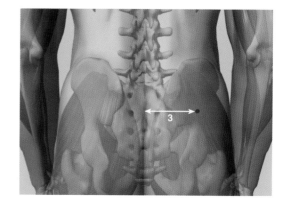

Bl 54 Zhi Bian   Order's Limit

L: at the level of the fourth sacral foramen, 3 cun lateral to the dorsal midline

T: 1.5–2 cun perpendicular; moxibustion

P: clears heat and cures hemorrhoids, activates the channel and alleviates pain

A: 1. hemorrhoids
2. prostatis, prostate adenoma
3. ischialgia

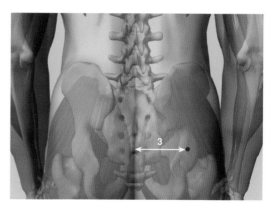

L: Location   T: Insertion Technique   P: Properties   A: Clinical Applications   **Pec:** Peculiarities

Bl

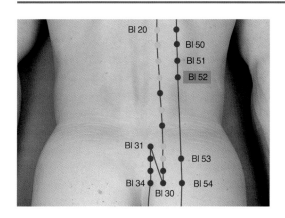

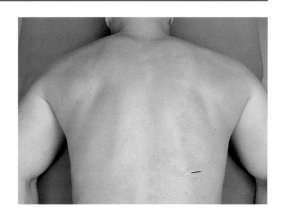

BI

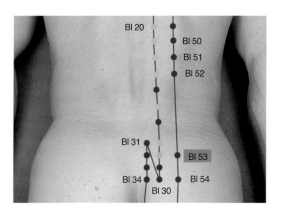

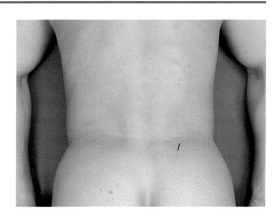

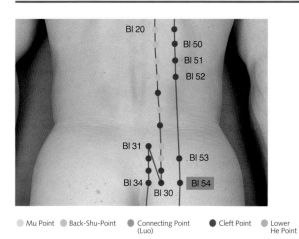

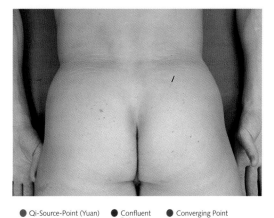

● Mu Point　● Back-Shu-Point　● Connecting Point (Luo)　● Cleft Point　● Lower He Point　● Qi-Source-Point (Yuan)　● Confluent Point　● Converging Point

159

Bl 55 He Yang   Confluence of Yang

L: 2 cun distal to Bl 40 on the connecting line between Bl 40 and Bl 57

T: 1–2 cun perpendicular;
moxibustion

P: promotes Qi and alleviates pain, regulates menstruation and alleviates uterine bleeding

A: 1. external abdominal hernias
2. anovulatory dysfunctional uterine bleeding
3. pains in the region of the LWS and the lower extremity

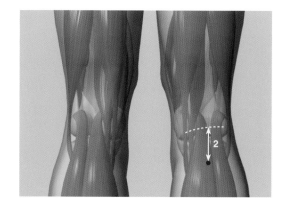

Bl 56 Cheng Jin   Support the Sinews

L: 5 cun distal to Bl 40 at the centre of the belly of the gastrocnemius muscle, on the connecting line between Bl 40 and Bl 57

T: 1–1.5 cun perpendicular;
moxibustion

P: clears heat and cures hemorrhoids, relaxes the tendons and alleviates pain

A: 1. hemorrhoids
2. cramps of the calf, pains in the lower leg

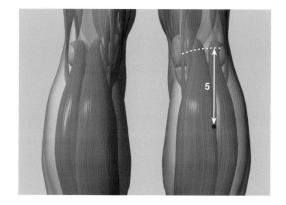

Bl 57 Cheng Shan   Support the Mountain

L: at the tip of the depression formed between the twin bellies of the gastrocnemius muscle, in the centre between Bl 40 and Bl 60

T: 1–2 cun perpendicular;
moxibustion

P: clears heat and eliminates hemorrhoids, relaxes the tendons and alleviates pain

A: 1. hemorrhoids
2. constipation
3. cramps of the calf, pains in the lower leg

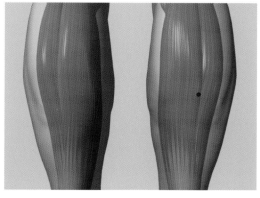

Bl

L: Location   T: Insertion Technique   P: Properties   A: Clinical Applications   Pec: Peculiarities

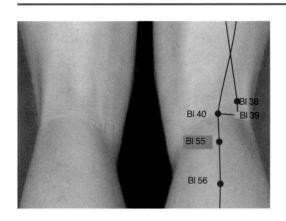

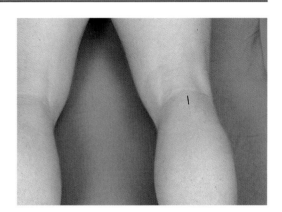

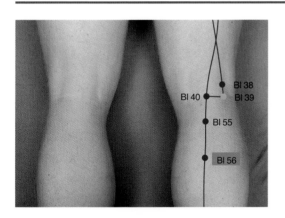

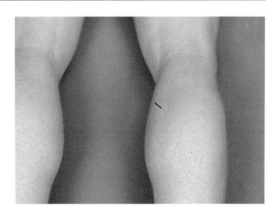

Bl

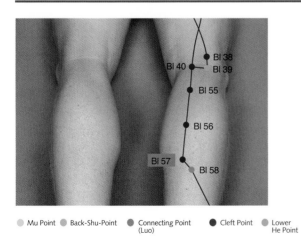

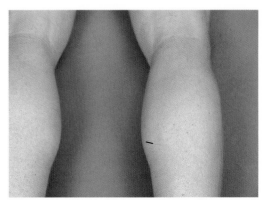

● Mu Point ● Back-Shu-Point ● Connecting Point (Luo) ● Cleft Point ● Lower He Point   ● Qi-Source-Point (Yuan) ● Confluent Point ● Converging Point

Bl 58 Fei Yang Soaring Upwards

L: 7 cun proximal to Bl 60, 1 cun lateral and distal to Bl 57, between the gastrocnemius muscle and the soleus muscle

T: 1–1.5 cun perpendicular; moxibustion

P: clears heat and eliminates hemorrhoids, expels wind, and alleviates pain

A: 1. hemorrhoids
2. neck headache
3. rhinitis, epistaxis

Pec: connecting point (Luo)

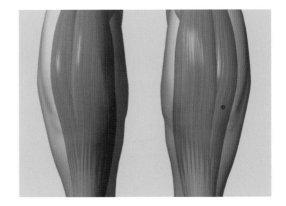

Bl 59 Fu Yang Instep Yang

L: 3 cun directly proximal to Bl 60

T: 0.8–1.2 cun perpendicular; moxibustion

P: expels wind and alleviates pain, decongests and activates the channel and its vessels

A: 1. headache
2. pain and numbness of the lower leg

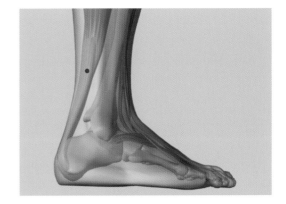

Bl 60 Kun Lun Kunlun Mountains

L: at the midpoint between the prominence of the lateral malleolus and the Achilles tendon

T: 0.5–0.8 cun perpendicular; moxibustion

P: expels wind and clears heat, activates the channel and alleviates pain

A: 1. neck headache
2. lumbalgia
3. pains in the heel
4. protracted labour

Pec: Jing (river) point (4th Shu-point)
CAUTION IN PREGNANCY (WHEN STRONG MANIPULATION APPLIED)!

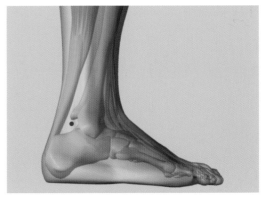

L: Location   T: Insertion Technique   P: Properties   A: Clinical Applications   Pec: Peculiarities

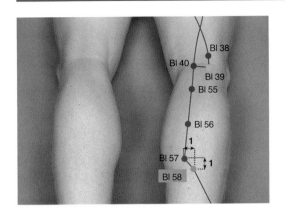

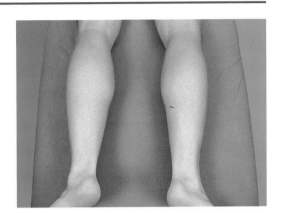

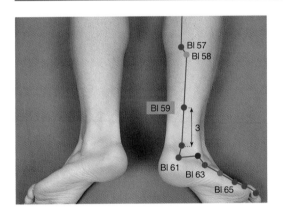

BI

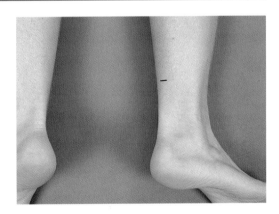

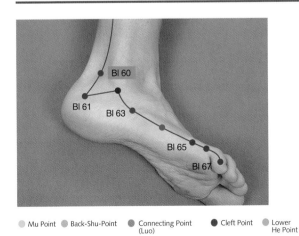

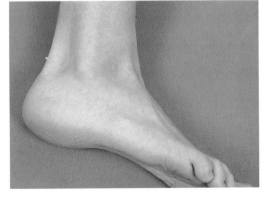

● Mu Point ● Back-Shu-Point ● Connecting Point (Luo) ● Cleft Point ● Lower He Point   ● Qi-Source-Point (Yuan) ● Confluent Point ● Converging Point

Bl 61 Pu Can Servant's Respect

L: dorsal and distal to the lateral malleolus, distal to Bl 60 on the side of the calcaneus, between red and white flesh

T: 0.3–0.5 cun perpendicular; moxibustion

P: relaxes the tendons and alleviates pain

A: 1. cramps and loss of strength in the calf muscles
2. pains in the heel

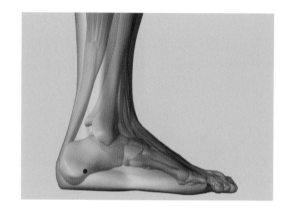

Bl 62 Shen Mai Extending Vessel

L: in the depression distal to the lateral malleolus

T: 0.3–0.5 cun perpendicular; moxibustion

P: promotes general calmness and alleviates cramps, expels wind and alleviates pain

A: 1. headache, dizziness, dazed state
2. sleeping disorders, epilepsy, psychic and psychosomatic dysfunctions (sedative and cramp-releasing function)
3. pains in the heel

Pec: confluent point (Ba Mai Jiao Hui) of the Yang Qiao Mai

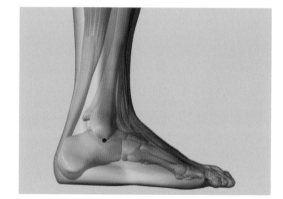

Bl 63 Jin Men Golden Gate

L: distal to the anterior border of the lateral malleolus, distal to the cuboid bone

T: 0.3–0.5 cun perpendicular; moxibustion

P: promotes general calmness and relaxes cramps, decongests and activates the channel and its vessels

A: 1. epileptic fits
2. lumbalgia
3. pains in region of the lateral malleolus

Pec: cleft (Xi) point

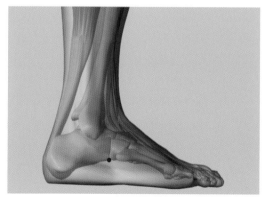

L: Location   T: Insertion Technique   P: Properties   A: Clinical Applications   Pec: Peculiarities

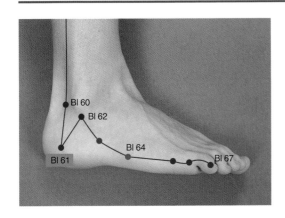

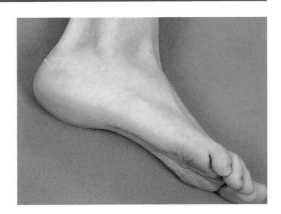

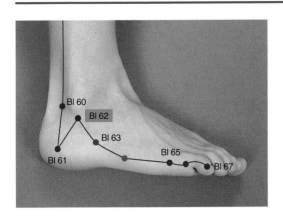

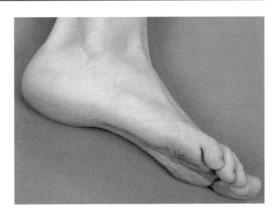

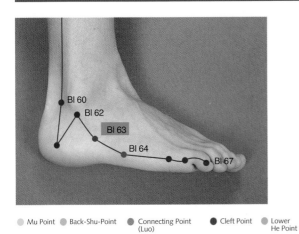

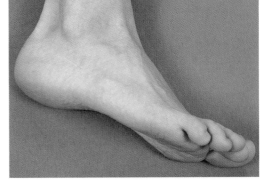

🔘 Mu Point   🔘 Back-Shu-Point   🔘 Connecting Point (Luo)   ⚫ Cleft Point   🔘 Lower He Point   🔘 Qi-Source-Point (Yuan)   ⚫ Confluent Point   ⚫ Converging Point

Bl 64 Jing Gu Capital Bone

L: inferior to the tuberosity of the fifth metatarsal bone, at the dividing line between red and white flesh

T: 0.3–0.5 cun perpendicular; moxibustion

P: suppresses cramps and alleviates falling sickness, sharpens eyesight and relaxes the tendons

A: 1. epileptic fits
2. lumbo-ischialgia
3. ceratitis

Pec: Qi-source-point (Yuan)

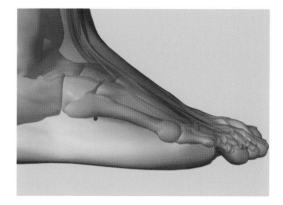

Bl 65 Shu Gu Restraining Bone

L: proximal to the fifth metatarso-phalangeal joint at the dividing line between red and white flesh

T: 0.3–0.5 cun perpendicular; moxibustion

P: pacifies and strengthens the spirit, clears heat, and alleviates pain

A: 1. psychic and psychosomatic disorders
2. neck headache
3. local pain, pain at the posterior side of the lower leg

Pec: Shu (stream) point (3rd Shu-point)

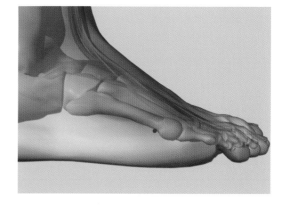

Bl 66 Zu Tong Gu Foot Connecting Valley

L: inferior to the fifth metatarso-phalangeal joint, at the dividing line between red and white flesh

T: 0.2–0.3 cun perpendicular; moxibustion

P: pacifies the spirit and alleviates pain

A: 1. psychic and psychosomatic disorders
2. neck headache

Pec: Xing (spring) point (2nd Shu-point)

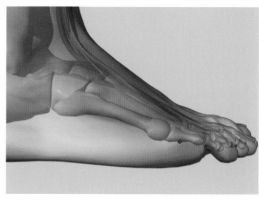

L: Location   **T:** Insertion Technique   **P:** Properties   **A:** Clinical Applications   **Pec:** Peculiarities

Bl

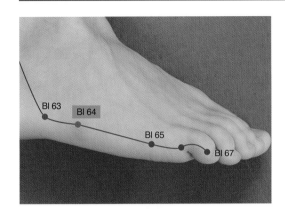

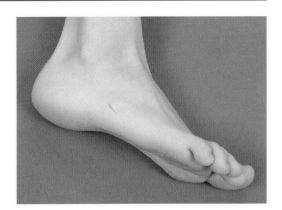

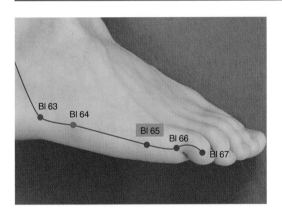

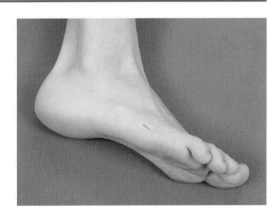

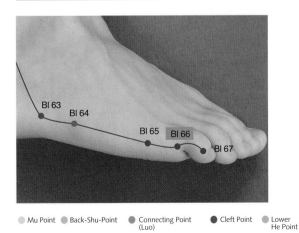

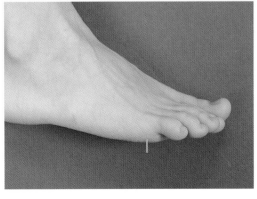

● Mu Point ● Back-Shu-Point ● Connecting Point (Luo) ● Cleft Point ● Lower He Point ● Qi-Source-Point (Yuan) ● Confluent Point ● Converging Point

Bl 67 Zhi Yin Reaching Yin

L: 0.1 cun proximal and lateral to the lateral border and base of the nail of the little toe

T: 0.1 cun perpendicular; moxibustion

P: expels wind and clears heat, turns the fetus and removes stases

A: 1. headache
2. rhinitis, epistaxis
3. malposition of fetus
4. additional obstetric dysfunctions, e.g. protracted labour, retention of placenta

Pec: Jing (well) point (1st Shu-point)
CAUTION IN PREGNANCY (IF STRONG MANIPULATION APPLIED)!

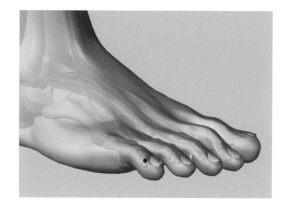

Bl

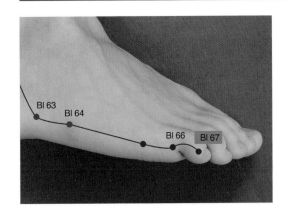

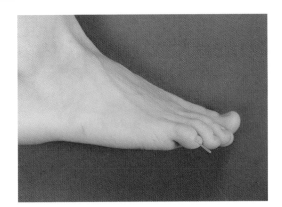

BI

● Mu Point ● Back-Shu-Point ● Connecting Point (Luo) ● Cleft Point ● Lower He Point ● Qi-Source-Point (Yuan) ● Confluent Point ● Converging Point

2.2.8   The kidney channel (Ki)

Synonyms

- The kidney-meridian

- The Foot-Shaoyin Kidney Channel

Channel pathway

There are 27 acupuncture points on the surface pathway of the kidney channel.

The surface pathway of the channel originates at the underside of the little toe and ascends to point Ki 1 on the sole of the foot. From here, the channel traverses the arch of the foot to the navicular bone and the region inferior to the bone on the instep of the foot. The channel then performs a loop, which reaches under the inner bone and ascends again to the posterior part of the inner side of the lower leg in front of the Achilles tendon. However, point Ki 8 is located at the posterior border of the tibia, distal to point Sp 6, which is also traversed by the kidney channel. The channel then continues to ascend the leg to the medial side of the popliteal fossa and traverses the posterior aspect of the inner thigh to the region of the pubic symphisis.

The inner pathway of the channel begins at point Ki 11, ascending over the spine before branching off to connect with its organ, the kidney, and connecting with the bladder. Another branch runs from the kidney via the liver and diaphragm to the lung, where it connects with the heart and where other branches in the centre of the chest lead to the pericardium channel. From the lung the channel ascends lateral to the larynx and pharynx to terminate at the root of the tongue.

The surface pathway ascends from the pubic symphisis to the lower and upper abdomen, where the channel runs strictly parallel to the midline. It then traverses the chest alongside the midline at a slightly greater distance from the midline to the angle at the chest and clavicle joint. From about point Ki 25 a branch runs to the heart and lungs.

Ki

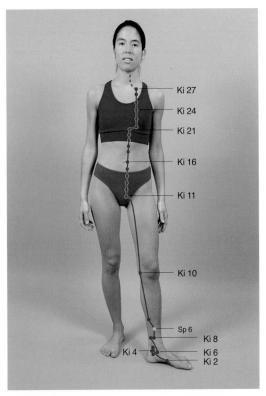

Ki 27
Ki 24
Ki 21
Ki 16
Ki 11
Ki 10
Sp 6
Ki 8
Ki 4
Ki 6
Ki 2

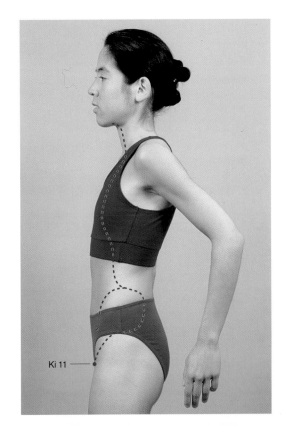

Ki 11

Ki

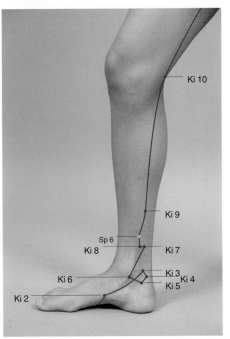

Ki 10
Ki 9
Sp 6
Ki 8
Ki 7
Ki 6
Ki 3
Ki 4
Ki 5
Ki 2

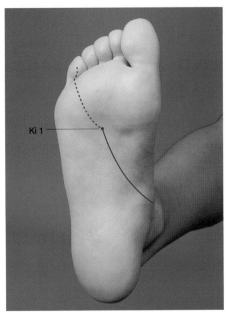

Ki 1

171

Ki 1 Yong Quan Gushing Spring

L: with the patient's foot plantar flexed, in the depression formed in the anterior part of the sole, approximately one third of the distance from the anterior and posterior aspect of the sole

T: 0.5–1 cun perpendicular; moxibustion

P: enriches Yin and replenishes the kidneys, soothes the liver, and dissipates wind

A: 1. chronic laryngitis, chronic pharyngitis
2. loss of voice with psychosomatic background
3. urinary retention
4. headache; dizziness and dazed state

Pec: Jing (well) point (1st Shu-point)

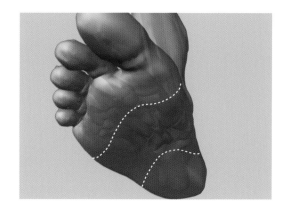

Ki 2 Ran Gu Blazing Valley

L: on the medial side of the foot plantar to the navicular tuberosity, on the dividing line between red and white flesh

T: 0.5–1 cun perpendicular; moxibustion

P: supports the kidney and strengthens essence, regulates menstruation and activates the vessels

A: 1. certain gynecological disorders, e.g. irregular menstruation, uterine prolapse, colpitis
2. male sexual dysfunctions
3. pain and restricted movement of the foot and lower extremity

Pec: Xing (spring) point (2nd Shu-point)

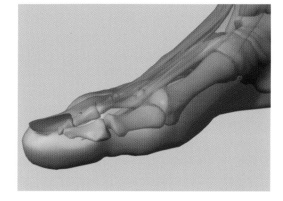

Ki 3 Tai Xi Supreme Stream

L: in the depression between the prominence of the medial malleolus and the Achilles tendon

T: 0.5–1 cun perpendicular; moxibustion

P: enriches the Yin and replenishes the kidney, soothes the liver and descends Yang, decongests and activates the channel and its vessels

A: 1. hypertension; dizziness and dazed state
2. chronic laryngitis, chronic pharyngitis
3. tinnitus, deafness
4. male sexual dysfunction
5. restricted movement in the lower extremity

Pec: Shu (stream) point (3rd Shu-point), Qi-source-point (Yuan)

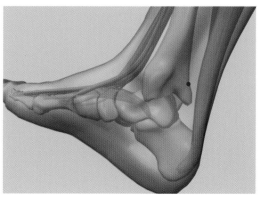

Ki

L: Location   T: Insertion Technique   P: Properties   A: Clinical Applications   Pec: Peculiarities

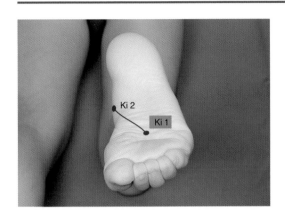

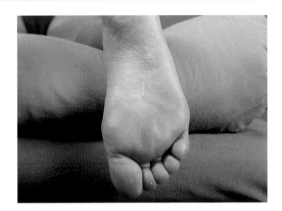

Ki

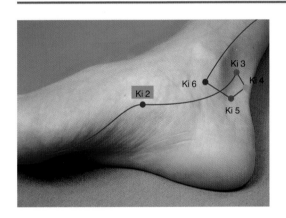

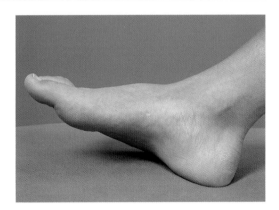

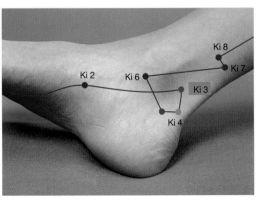

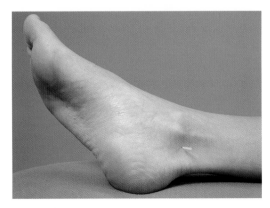

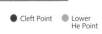

○ Mu Point ○ Back-Shu-Point ● Connecting Point (Luo) ● Cleft Point ○ Lower He Point ● Qi-Source-Point (Yuan) ● Confluent Point ● Converging Point

Ki 4 Da Zhong Great Cup

L: 0.5 cun distal and dorsal to Ki 3, on the inner aspect of the Achilles tendon

T: 0.3–0.5 cun perpendicular; moxibustion

P: supports the kidney and alleviates breathing difficulty, regulates defecation and urination

A: 1. chronic bronchitis
2. constipation
3. urinary retention
4. pain in the heel

Pec: connecting point (Luo)

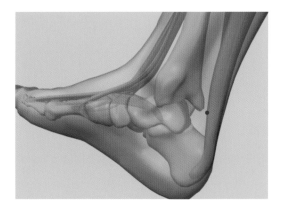

Ki 5 Shui Quan Water Spring

L: distal and dorsal to the medial malleolus, 1 cun inferior to Ki 3, in the depression medial to the calcaneal tuberosity

T: 0.3–0.5 cun perpendicular; moxibustion

P: activates the blood and stimulates menstruation

A: certain gynecological disorders, e.g. irregular menstruation, amenorrhoea, uterine prolapse

Pec: cleft (Xi) point

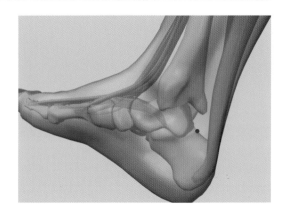

Ki 6 Zhao Hai Shining Sea

L: in the depression inferior to the inferior border of the medial malleolus

T: 0.3–0.5 cun perpendicular; moxibustion

P: enriches the Yin and pacifies the spirit, regulates menstruation and alleviates discharge

A: 1. numbness, narcolepsy, fatigue
2. certain gynecological disorders, e.g. irregular menstruation, dysmenorrhoea, leucorrhoea, acute inflammation of the small pelvis, uterine prolapse
3. chronic pharyngitis

Pec: confluent point (Ba Mai Jiao Hui) of the Yin Qiao Mai

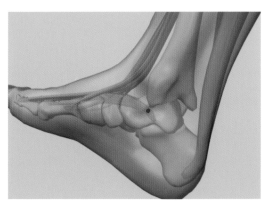

L: Location   T: Insertion Technique   P: Properties   A: Clinical Applications   Pec: Peculiarities

Ki

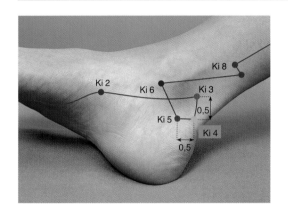
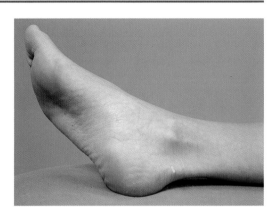

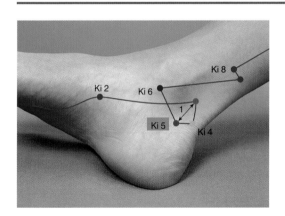
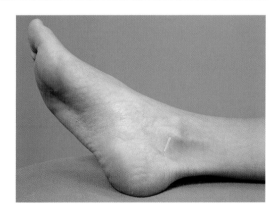

Ki

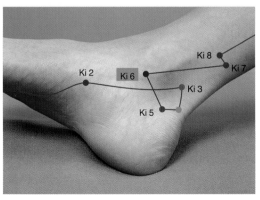
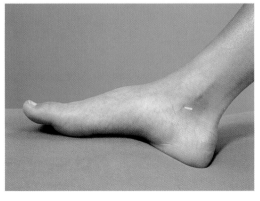

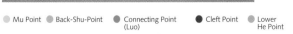

● Mu Point ● Back-Shu-Point ● Connecting Point (Luo) ● Cleft Point ● Lower He Point   ● Qi-Source-Point (Yuan) ● Confluent Point ● Converging Point

Ki 7 Fu Liu Returning Current

L: 2 cun proximal to Ki 3, ventral to the Achilles tendon

T: 0.5–1 cun perpendicular; moxibustion

P: replenishes the kidney, promotes urination, restores balance to sweat and body fluids

A: 1. insufficient or excessive sweating
2. edema

Pec: Jing (river) point (4th Shu-point)

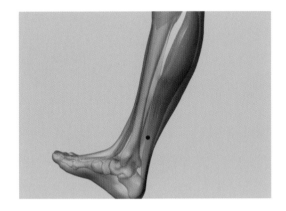

Ki 8 Jiao Xin Exchange Belief

L: 2 cun proximal to Ki 3, 0.5 cun ventral to Ki 7, at the posterior border of the tibia

T: 0.5–1.2 cun perpendicular; moxibustion

P: supports the kidney and regulates menstruation

A: 1. certain gynecological disorders, e.g. anovulatory dysfunctional uterine bleeding, uterine prolapse
2. acute and chronic inflammation of the urinary tract

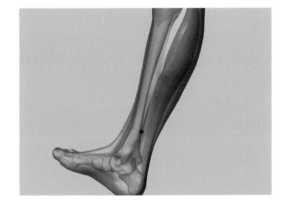

Ki 9 Zhu Bin Guest House

L: 5 cun proximal to Ki 3, on the connecting line between Ki 3 and Ki 10

T: 1–1.5 cun perpendicular; moxibustion

P: supports the kidney and pacifies the spirit, regulates Qi and alleviates pain

A: 1. psychic and psychosomatic disorders
2. external abdominal hernias

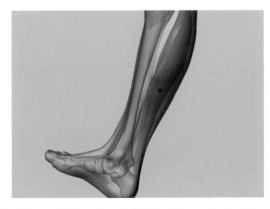

L: Location   T: Insertion Technique   P: Properties   A: Clinical Applications   Pec: Peculiarities

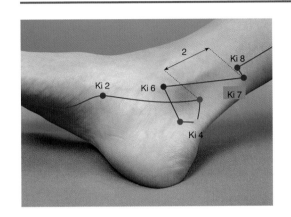

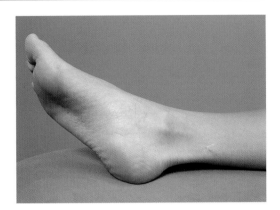

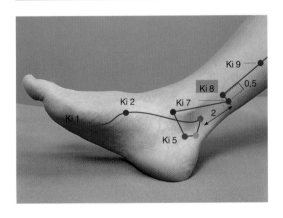

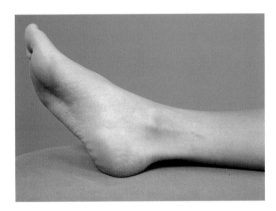

Ki

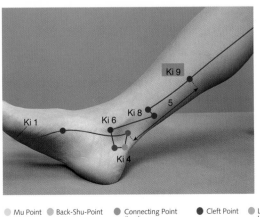

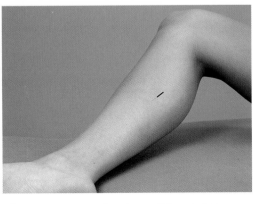

● Mu Point ● Back-Shu-Point ● Connecting Point (Luo) ● Cleft Point ● Lower He Point ● Qi-Source-Point (Yuan) ● Confluent Point ● Converging Point

Ki 10 Yin Gu   Yin Valley

L: with the patient's knee flexed, in the medial part of the popliteal fossa between the tendons of the semi-tendinosus and the semi-membranosus muscles

T: 1–1.5 cun perpendicular; moxibustion

P: supports the kidney and helps the Yang

A: 1. male sexual dysfunction e.g. impotence
2. anovulatory, dysfunctional uterine bleeding
3. pain in the knee joint

Pec: He (sea) point (5th Shu-point)

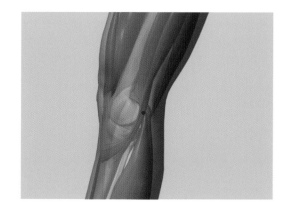

Ki 11 Heng Gu   Pubic Bone

L: 5 cun inferior to the umbilicus, 0.5 cun lateral to the ventral midline, on the superior border of the symphisis pubis

T: 1–1.5 cun perpendicular; moxibustion

P: supports the kidney and helps the Yang

A: 1. male sexual dysfunction e.g. impotence
2. prostatitis
3. urinary incontinence

Pec: CAUTION IN PREGNANCY!

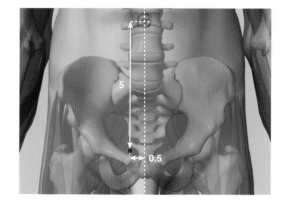

Ki

Ki 12 Dahe   Great Luminance

L: 4 cun inferior to the umbilicus, 0.5 cun lateral to the ventral midline

T: 1–1.5 cun perpendicular; moxibustion

P: replenishes the kidney and strengthens the essence, regulates menstruation and alleviates discharge

A: 1. male sexual dysfunction e.g. impotence
2. prostatitis
3. certain gynecological disorders, e.g. uterine myoma, inflammation of the small pelvis

Pec: CAUTION IN PREGNANCY!

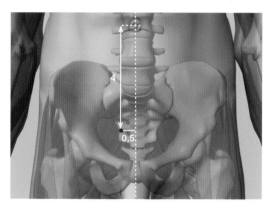

L: Location   **T:** Insertion Technique   **P:** Properties   **A:** Clinical Applications   **Pec:** Peculiarities

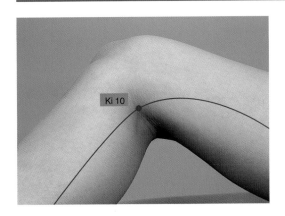

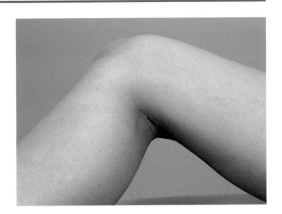

Ki

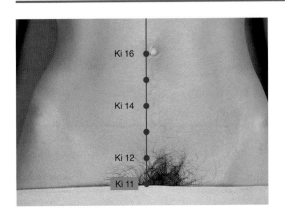

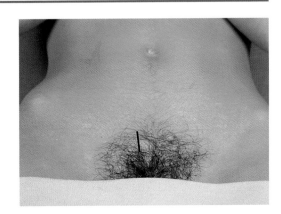

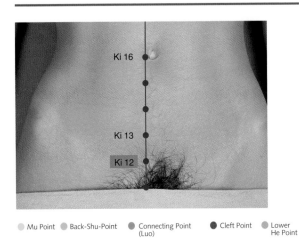

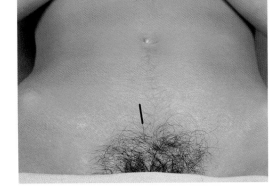

○ Mu Point ○ Back-Shu-Point ● Connecting Point (Luo) ● Cleft Point ○ Lower He Point ● Qi-Source-Point (Yuan) ● Confluent Point ● Converging Point

179

Ki 13 Qi Xue   Qi Cave

L: 3 cun inferior to the umbilicus, 0.5 cun lateral to the ventral midline

T: 1–1.5 cun perpendicular; moxibustion

P: regulates and replenishes the Chong Mai

A: 1. certain gynecological disorders, e.g. irregular menstruation, leucorrhoea
2. urinary retention

Pec: CAUTION IN PREGNANCY!

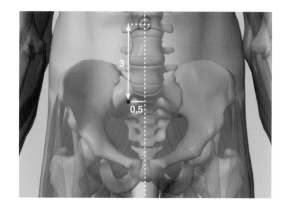

Ki 14 Si Man   Four Fullnesses

L: 2 cun inferior to the umbilicus, 0.5 cun lateral to the ventral midline

T: 1–1.5 cun perpendicular; moxibustion

P: regulates Qi and regulates menstruation

A: certain gynecological disorders, e.g. irregular menstruation, anovulatory, dysfunctional uterine bleeding, post-partum infections, fertility disorders

Pec: CAUTION IN PREGNANCY!

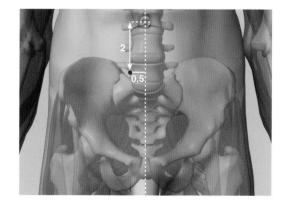

Ki 15 Zhong Zhu   Middle Flow

L: 1 cun inferior to the umbilicus, 0.5 cun lateral to the ventral midline

T: 1–1.5 cun perpendicular; moxibustion

P: regulates menstruation and activates defecation

A: 1. irregular menstruation
2. constipation

Pec: CAUTION IN PREGNANCY!

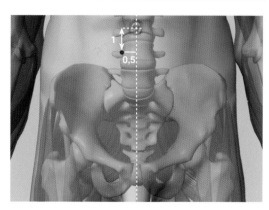

Ki

L: Location   **T:** Insertion Technique   **P:** Properties   **A:** Clinical Applications   **Pec:** Peculiarities

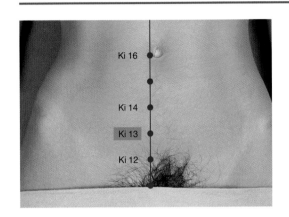
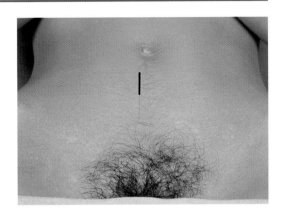

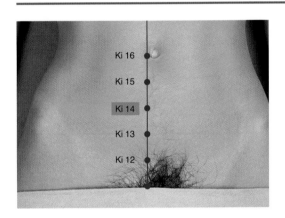
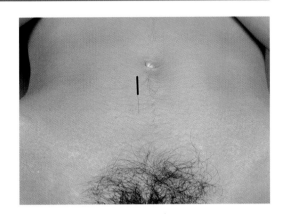

Ki

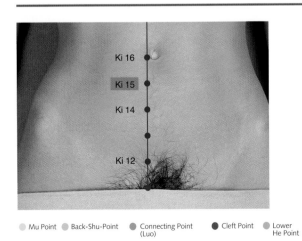
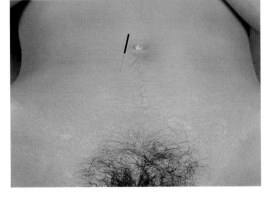

○ Mu Point ○ Back-Shu-Point ● Connecting Point (Luo) ● Cleft Point ○ Lower He Point   ● Qi-Source-Point (Yuan) ● Confluent Point ● Converging Point

181

Ki 16 Huang Shu   Vitals Shu

L: 0.5 cun lateral to the umbilicus

T: 1–1.5 cun perpendicular;
moxibustion

P: regulates Qi and promotes defecation

A: 1. sensation of abdominal swelling and tension,
abdominal pain
2. constipation

Pec: CAUTION IN PREGNANCY!

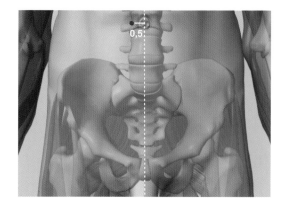

Ki 17 Shang Qu   Shang Bend

L: 2 cun superior to the umbilicus, 0.5 cun lateral to
the ventral midline

T: 1–1.5 cun perpendicular;
moxibustion

P: harmonizes the stomach and stimulates digestion

A: abdominal pain in digestive disorders

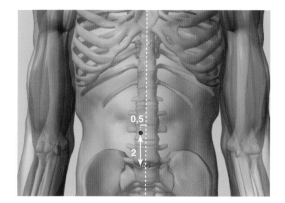

Ki 18 Shi Guan   Stone Pass

L: 3 cun superior to the umbilicus, 0.5 cun lateral to
the ventral midline

T: 1–1.5 cun perpendicular;
moxibustion

P: regulates Qi and strengthens the spleen

A: 1. pain in the upper abdomen
2. acute gastritis

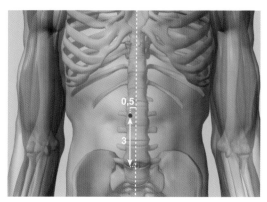

Ki

L: Location   T: Insertion Technique   P: Properties   A: Clinical Applications   Pec: Peculiarities

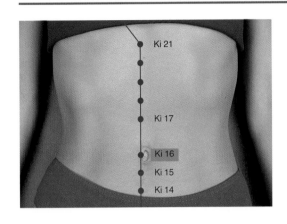

Ki 21
Ki 17
Ki 16
Ki 15
Ki 14

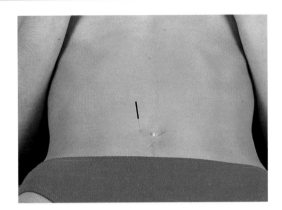

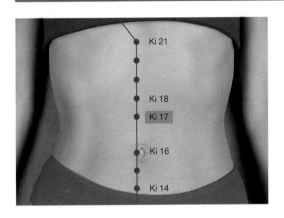

Ki 21
Ki 18
Ki 17
Ki 16
Ki 14

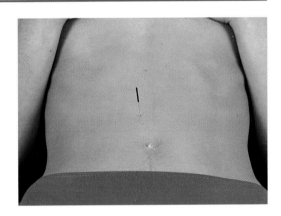

Ki

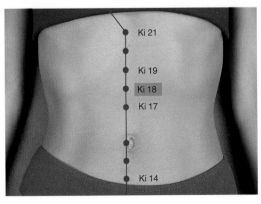

Ki 21
Ki 19
Ki 18
Ki 17
Ki 14

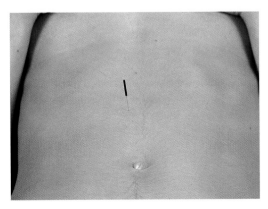

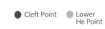

● Mu Point　● Back-Shu-Point　● Connecting Point (Luo)　● Cleft Point　● Lower He Point　　● Qi-Source-Point (Yuan)　● Confluent Point　● Converging Point

183

Ki 19 Yin Du   Yin Metropolis

L: 4 cun superior to the umbilicus, 0.5 cun lateral to the ventral midline

T: 1–1.5 cun perpendicular; moxibustion

P: regulates Qi and alleviates pain, strengthens the spleen and promotes digestion

A: 1. acute and chronic gastritis
2. pain in the upper abdomen

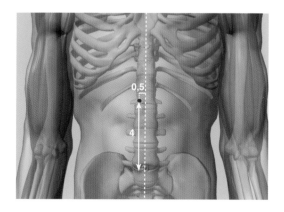

Ki 20 Fu Tong Gu   Abdomen Connecting Valley

L: 5 cun superior to the umbilicus, 0.5 cun lateral to the ventral midline

T: 0.5–1 cun perpendicular; moxibustion

P: harmonizes the stomach and alleviates pain

A: acute and chronic gastritis

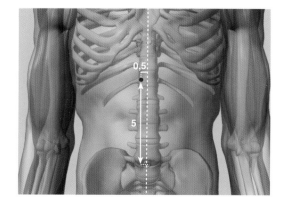

Ki 21 You Men   Hidden gate

L: 6 cun superior to the umbilicus, 0.5 cun lateral to the ventral midline

T: 0.5–1 cun perpendicular; moxibustion

P: strengthens the spleen and harmonizes the stomach, descends inverted Qi and alleviates nausea

A: 1. acute and chronic gastritis
2. esophagitis
3. hiccups

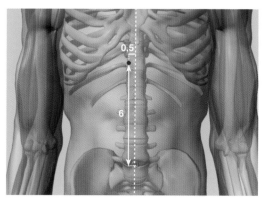

L: Location   T: Insertion Technique   P: Properties   A: Clinical Applications   Pec: Peculiarities

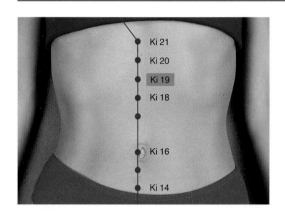
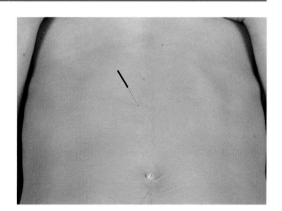

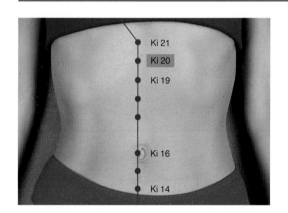
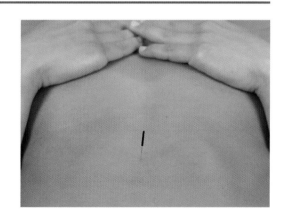

Ki

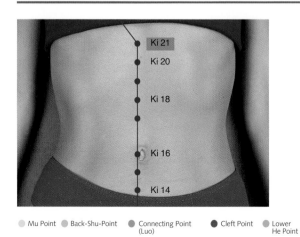
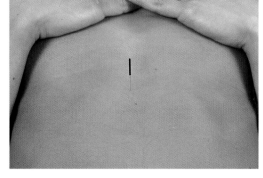

● Mu Point ● Back-Shu-Point ● Connecting Point (Luo) ● Cleft Point ● Lower He Point ● Qi-Source-Point (Yuan) ● Confluent Point ● Converging Point

Ki 22 Bu Lang   Walking on the Veranda

L: in the fifth ICR, 2 cun lateral to the ventral midline

T: 0.5–0.8 cun oblique or subcutaneously; moxibustion

P: unbinds the chest and regulates Qi, alleviates coughing and soothes breathing difficulty

A: 1. thoracic pain
2. acute and chronic inflammation of the respiratory tract

Pec: CAUTION, AVOID PNEUMOTHORAX!

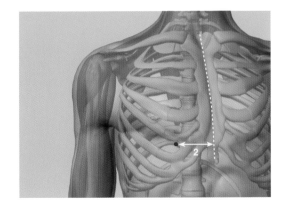

Ki 23 Shen Feng   Spirit Seal

L: in the fourth ICR, 2 cun lateral to the ventral midline

T: 0.5–0.8 cun oblique or subcutaneously; moxibustion

P: unbinds the chest and alleviates coughing

A: 1. thoracic pain
2. acute and chronic inflammation of the bronchia and lungs
3. acute mastitis

Pec: CAUTION, AVOID PNEUMOTHORAX!

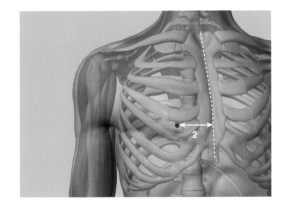

Ki 24 Ling Xu   Spirit Burial Ground

L: in the third ICR, 2 cun lateral to the ventral midline

T: 0.5–0.8 cun oblique or subcutaneously; moxibustion

P: alleviates coughing and soothes breathing difficulty

A: acute and chronic inflammation of the respiratory tract

Pec: CAUTION, AVOID PNEUMOTHORAX!

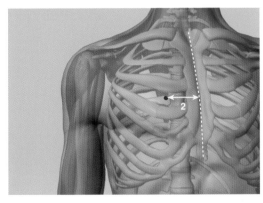

L: Location   **T:** Insertion Technique   **P:** Properties   **A:** Clinical Applications   **Pec:** Peculiarities

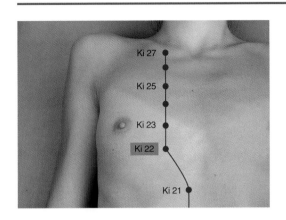

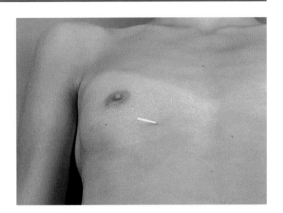

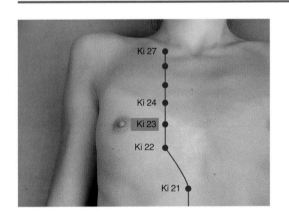

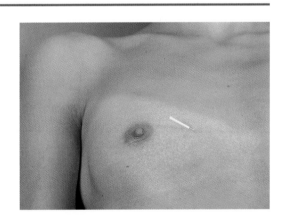

Ki

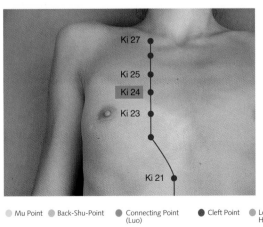

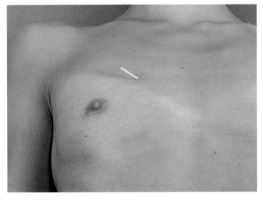

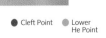

● Mu Point   ● Back-Shu-Point   ● Connecting Point (Luo)   ● Cleft Point   ● Lower He Point   ● Qi-Source-Point (Yuan)   ● Confluent Point   ● Converging Point

Ki 25 Shen Cang   Spirit Storehouse

L: in the second ICR, 2 cun lateral to the ventral midline

T: 0.5–0.8 cun oblique or subcutaneously; moxibustion

P: unbinds the chest and alleviates breathing difficulty

A: 1. acute and chronic inflammation of the respiratory tract
2. bronchial asthma
3. thoracic pain

Pec: CAUTION, AVOID PNEUMOTHORAX!

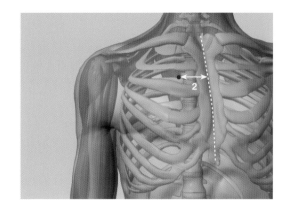

Ki 26 Yu Zhong   Comfortable Chest

L: in the first ICR, 2 cun lateral to the ventral midline

T: 0.5–0.8 cun oblique or subcutaneously; moxibustion

P: alleviates coughing and breathing difficulty

A: 1. acute and chronic inflammation of the respiratory tract
2. bronchial asthma

Pec: CAUTION, AVOID PNEUMOTHORAX!

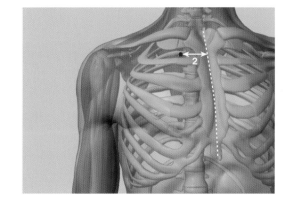

Ki 27 Shu Fu   Shu Mansion

L: on the inferior border of the clavicle, 2 cun lateral to the ventral midline

T: 0.5–0.8 cun oblique or subcutaneously; moxibustion

P: alleviates coughing and breathing difficulty, descends inverted Qi and alleviates pain

A: 1. acute and chronic inflammation of the respiratory tract
2. thoracic pain

Pec: CAUTION, AVOID PNEUMOTHORAX!

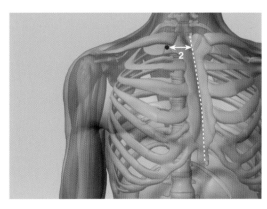

L: Location   T: Insertion Technique   P: Properties   A: Clinical Applications   Pec: Peculiarities

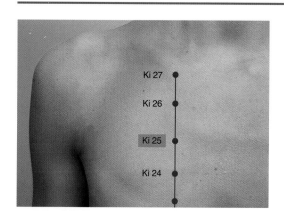

Ki 27
Ki 26
Ki 25
Ki 24

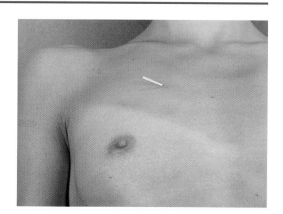

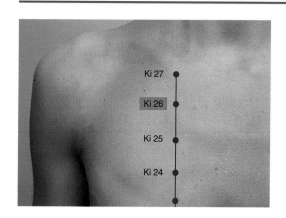

Ki 27
Ki 26
Ki 25
Ki 24

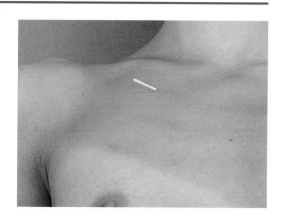

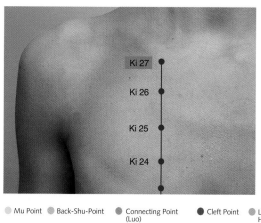

Ki 27
Ki 26
Ki 25
Ki 24

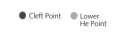

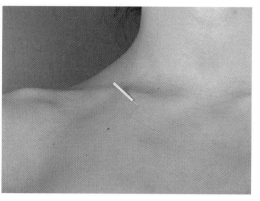

● Mu Point   ● Back-Shu-Point   ● Connecting Point (Luo)   ● Cleft Point   ● Lower He Point   ● Qi-Source-Point (Yuan)   ● Confluent Point   ● Converging Point

2.2.9   The pericardium channel (P)

Synonyms

- The pericardium-meridian (circulation-meridian; circulation-sexus-meridian)

- The Hand-Jueyin-Pericardium Channel (Hand-Jueyin-Heart cover-Channel)

Channel pathway

There are 9 acupuncture points on the surface pathway of the pericardium channel.

The inner pathway originates at the chest, where it serves its organ, the pericardium. The channel descends through the diaphragm to the abdomen and then connects with the upper, middle, and lower Jiao.

The surface pathway emerges from the chest near the nipple at point P 1. From here the channel ascends to the axilla and follows the antero-medial aspect of the upper arm, via the vessel-nerve street, to the cubital fossa. The channel then ascends further the middle of the antero-medal aspect of the lower arm, between the tendons of the palmaris longus and flexor carpi radialis, to the palm of the hand and the tip of the middle finger.

A branch leads from point P 8 to the tip of the ring finger and connects with the San Jiao channel.

P

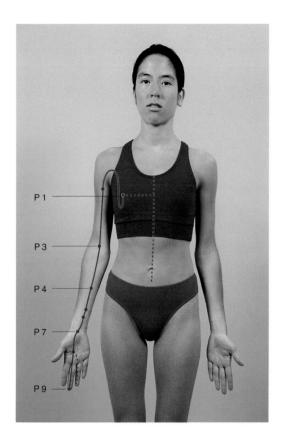

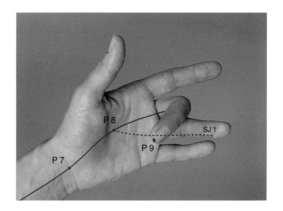

P 1 Tian Chi Heavenly Pool

L: in the fourth ICR, 1 cun lateral to the nipple, 5 cun lateral to the ventral midline

T: 0.3–0.5 cun oblique or subcutaneously; moxibustion

P: unbinds the chest and regulates Qi, alleviates coughing and breathing difficulty

A: 1. pectoral angina, sensation of bloated thorax, palpitations in coronary heart diseases
2. coughing and asthmatic complaints in lung and bronchial diseases

Pec: CAUTION, AVOID PNEUMOTHORAX!

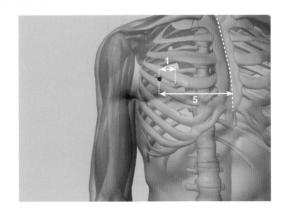

P 2 Tian Quan Heavenly Spring

L: on the inside of the arm, 2 cun lateral to the ventral end of the axillary fold, between the long and short heads of the biceps brachii muscle.

T: 1–1.5 cun perpendicular; moxibustion

P: unbinds the chest and regulates Qi; alleviates coughing

A: 1. pectoral angina
2. acute and chronic bronchitis

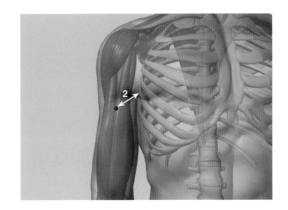

P 3 Qu Ze Marsh at the Crook

L: at the midpoint of the cubital crease, ulnar to the biceps brachii tendon

T: 1–1.5 cun perpendicular; prick to bleed; moxibustion

P: regulates Qi and alleviates pain, harmonizes the stomach, and descends inverted Qi

A: 1. pectoral angina, sensation of thoracic bloatedness and palpitations in coronary heart disease
2. stomach pain, nausea and vomiting in acute gastritis

Pec: He (sea) point (5th Shu-point)

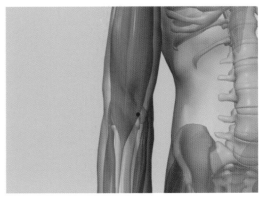

L: Location   T: Insertion Technique   P: Properties   A: Clinical Applications   Pec: Peculiarities

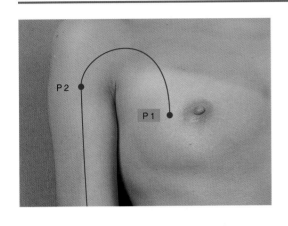

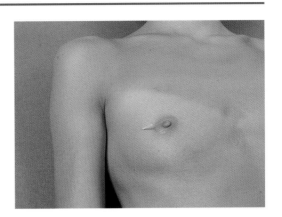

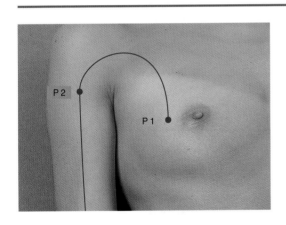

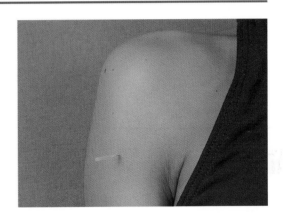

P

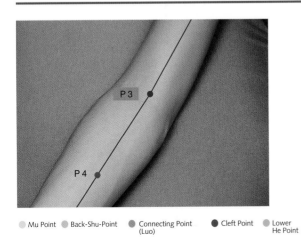

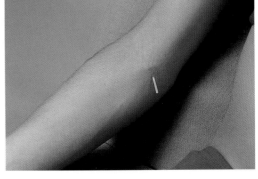

⬤ Mu Point   ⬤ Back-Shu-Point   ⬤ Connecting Point (Luo)   ⬤ Cleft Point   ⬤ Lower He Point   ⬤ Qi-Source-Point (Yuan)   ⬤ Confluent Point   ⬤ Converging Point

193

P 4 Xi Men Xi-Cleft Gate

L: on the inside of the arm, 5 cun proximal to the distal wrist crease, on the connecting line between P 3 and P 7 between the palmaris longus and flexor carpi radialis tendons

T: 0.8–1.2 cun perpendicular; moxibustion

P: clears the heart and suppresses pain, cools and soothes the blood

A: 1. pectoral angina, sensation of thoracic bloatedness and palpitations in coronary heart disease
2. stops nose-bleeds, coughing or spitting blood, hemotemesis

Pec: cleft (Xi) point

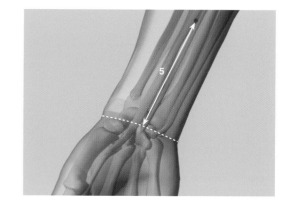

P 5 Jian Shi Intermediate Messenger

L: 3 cun proximal to the distal wrist crease, on the connecting line between P 3 and P 7, between the palmaris longus and flexor carpi radialis tendons

T: 0.5–1 cun perpendicular; moxibustion

P: unbinds the chest and alleviates pain, cools and soothes the blood

A: 1. pains in the heart region, palpitations, breathlessness, and sensation of thoracic bloatedness in heart disease
2. psychic and psychosomatic disorders; epileptic fits (sedative effect)

Pec: Jing (river) point (4th Shu-point)

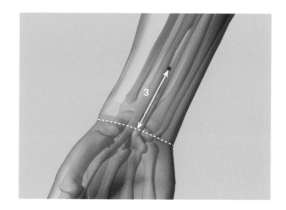

P 6 Nei Guan Inner Pass

L: 2 cun proximal to the distal wrist crease, on the connecting line between P 3 and P 7, between the palmaris longus and flexor carpi radialis tendons

T: 0.5–1 cun perpendicular; moxibustion

P: restores clarity to the brain and suppresses pain, strengthens the spleen and harmonizes the centre, decongests and activates the channel and its vessels

A: 1. pectoral angina, sensation of thoracic bloatedness
2. restricted movement and lateral paralysis in cerebro-vascular disease
3. stomach pain, nausea and vomiting
4. pain and restricted movement of the forearm

Pec: connecting point (Luo), confluent point (Ba Mai Jiao Hui) of the Yin Wei Mai

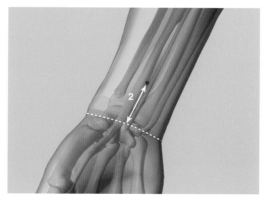

P

L: Location   T: Insertion Technique   P: Properties   A: Clinical Applications   Pec: Peculiarities

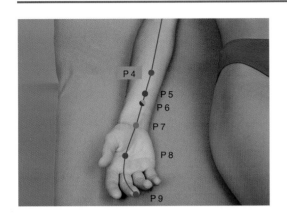

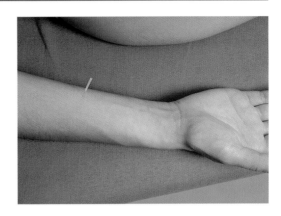

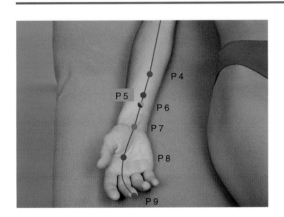

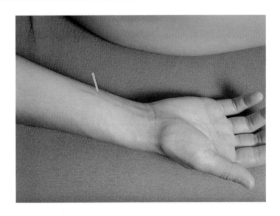

P

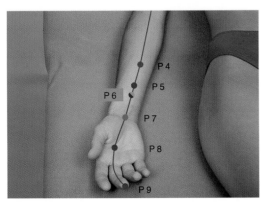

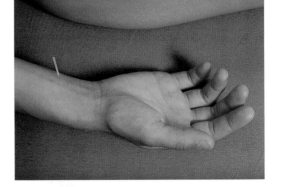

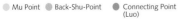

⬤ Mu Point ⬤ Back-Shu-Point ⬤ Connecting Point (Luo) ⬤ Cleft Point ⬤ Lower He Point ⬤ Qi-Source-Point (Yuan) ⬤ Confluent Point ⬤ Converging Point

P 7 Da Ling Great Mound

L: in the middle of the distal wrist crease, between the palmaris longus and flexor carpi radialis tendons

T: 0.5–0.8 cun perpendicular; moxibustion

P: calms the heart and alleviates pain, produces all-round calmness and releases cramps

A: 1. pectoral angina, sensation of thoracic bloatedness

2. psychic and psychosomatic disorders, epileptic fits (sedative and cramp-releasing effect)

Pec: Shu (stream) point (3rd Shu-point), Qi-source-point (Yuan)

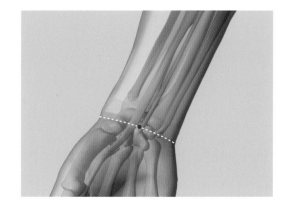

P 8 Lao Gong Palace of Toil

L: on the point of the palm of the hand, between the second and third metacarpal bones, where the middle finger rests when the patient's hand is closed into a fist

T: 0.3–0.5 cun perpendicular; moxibustion

P: clears the heart, pacifies the spirit, cools and soothes the blood, reduces edema and alleviates pain

A: 1. pectoral angina, sensation of thoracic bloatedness
2. psychic and psychosomatic disorders, epileptic fits (sedative and cramp-releasing effect)
3. stops bleeding in hemotemesis, epistaxis, anal bleeding
4. inflammations of the mouth

Pec: Xing (spring) point (2nd Shu-point)

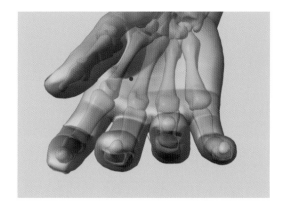

P 9 Zhong Chong Middle Rushing

L: in the middle of the tip of the middle finger

T: 0.1 cun perpendicular; moxibustion

P: restores clarity to the brain and opens the senses, drains and expels heat, clears the heart

A: loss of consciousness in cerebro-vascular diseases, heat-stroke, vagovasal syncope and high fever (also in children) as a complementary and emergency measure

Pec: Jing (well) point (1st Shu-point)

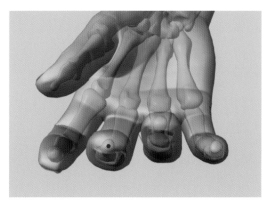

P

L: Location   T: Insertion Technique   P: Properties   A: Clinical Applications   Pec: Peculiarities

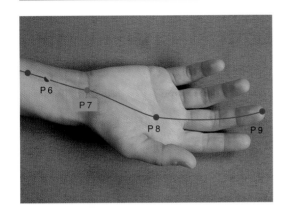

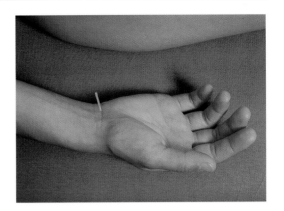

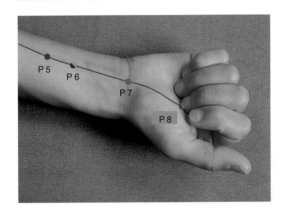

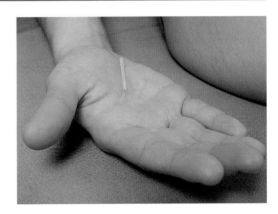

P

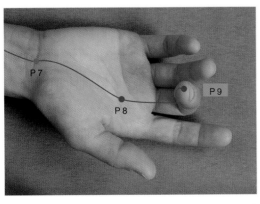

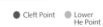

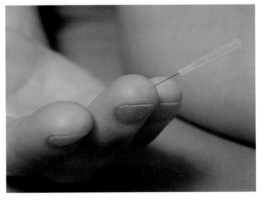

● Mu Point   ● Back-Shu-Point   ● Connecting Point (Luo)   ● Cleft Point   ● Lower He Point   ● Qi-Source-Point (Yuan)   ● Confluent Point   ● Converging Point

2.2.10 The San Jiao channel (SJ)

Synonyms

• San Jiao Meridian

• Hand-Shaoyang San Jiao Channel

Channel pathway

There are 23 acupuncture points in the surface pathway of the San Jiao channel.

The surface pathway of the San Jiao channel originates at the ulnar corner of the nail of the ring finger. From here the channel ascends via the dorsum of the hand between the fourth and fifth metacarpal bones and the central part of the outer aspect of the lower arm between the ulna and the radius, to the tip of the elbow. The channel further ascends via the posterior aspect of the upper arm and reaches the posterior aspect of the shoulder, traversing points of other channels such as SI 12 and GB 21. From point GB 21 the channel runs first to the superior fossa of the clavicle and from here returns to the seventh cervical vertebra (Du 14).

From the superior fossa of the clavicle the inner pathway of the channel descends to the centre of the chest, connects with the pericardium and traverses the diaphragm, thereby connecting all the parts of its organ, the upper, middle, and lower San Jiao.

From the seventh cervical vertebra (Du 14) the channel ascends to the region behind the ear. It branches at point SJ 17 directly into the ear and leaves the ear again in front of the ear at point SJ 21. From here it connects with point SJ 23 lateral to the eyebrow and the gall bladder channel lateral to the eye socket in the region of point GB 1.

SJ

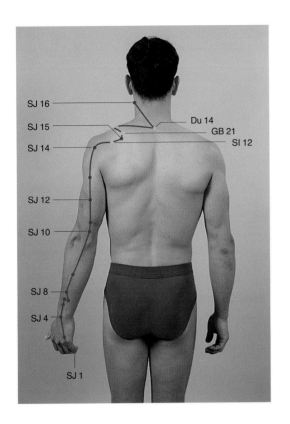

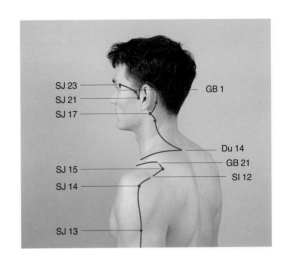

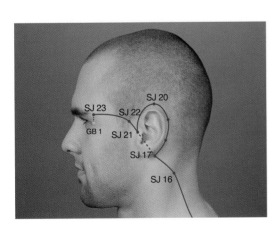

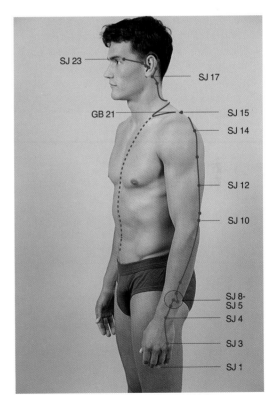

SJ

SJ 1 Guan Chong Rushing Pass

L: 0.1 cun proximal and lateral to the base and corner
of the nail of the ring finger

T: 0.1 cun perpendicular; prick to bleed;
moxibustion

P: clears heat and decongests the pharynx, sharpens
hearing and activates the orifices of the upper body

A: 1. acute inflammation of the pharynx and throat,
acute tonsillitis

2. diseases of the ear, e.g. deafness, tinnitus

Pec: Jing (well) point (1st Shu-point)

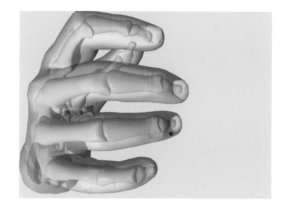

SJ 2 Ye Men Fluid Gate

L: distal to the fourth metacarpo-phalangeal joint, at
the border of the skin between the ring and little
finger, at the dividing line between red and white
flesh

T: 0.3–0.5 cun perpendicular;
moxibustion

P: clears heat and expels wind, sharpens hearing and
activates the orifices of the upper body

A: 1. one-sided headache

2. diseases of the ear, e.g. deafness, tinnitus

Pec: Xing (spring) point (2nd Shu-point)

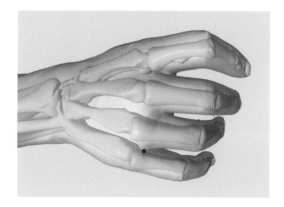

SJ

SJ 3 Zhong Zhu Central Islet

L: on the dorsum of the hand proximal to the fourth
metacarpo-phalangeal joint at the angle between the
heads of the fourth and fifth metacarpal bones

T: 0.3–0.5 cun perpendicular; moxibustion

P: clears heat and activates the channel, sharpens
eyesight and hearing

A: 1. one-sided headache

2. acute inflammation of the eye, e.g. conjunctivitis,
ceratitis

3. diseases of the ear, e.g. deafness, tinnitus

4. pain and restricted movement of the upper
extremity and the hand

Pec: Shu (stream) point (3rd Shu-point)

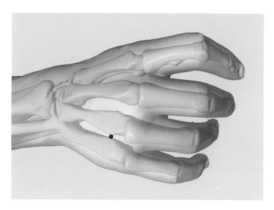

L: Location   T: Insertion Technique   P: Properties   A: Clinical Applications   Pec: Peculiarities

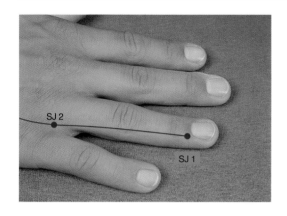

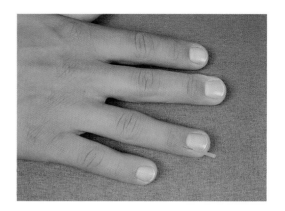

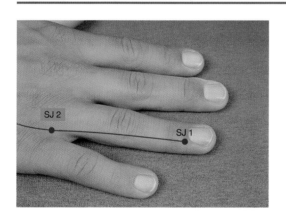

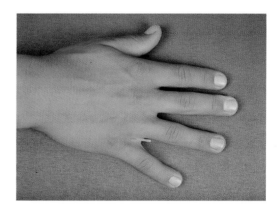

SJ

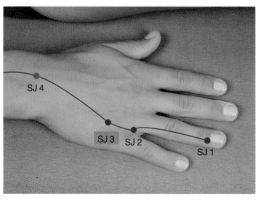

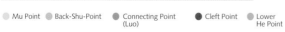

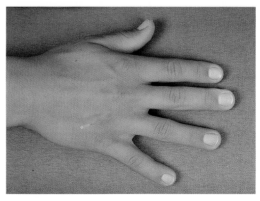

⬤ Mu Point ⬤ Back-Shu-Point ⬤ Connecting Point (Luo) ⬤ Cleft Point ⬤ Lower He Point ⬤ Qi-Source-Point (Yuan) ⬤ Confluent Point ⬤ Converging Point

SJ 4 Yang Chi   Yang Pool

L: in the centre of the dorsum, at the wrist joint, in the depression below the tendon of the extensor digitorum communis

T: 0.3–0.5 cun perpendicular; moxibustion

P: activates the channel and alleviates pain

A: shoulder, back, and wrist pain

Pec: Qi-source-point (Yuan)

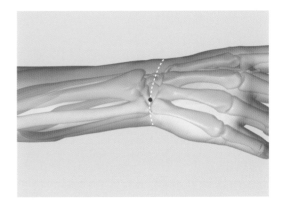

SJ 5 Wai Guan   Outer Pass

L: 2 cun proximal to the dorsal wrist crease between the ulna and radius

T: 0.5–1 cun perpendicular; moxibustion

P: clears heat and liberates the surface, sharpens eyesight and hearing, decongest, and activates the channel

A: 1. fever and headaches in infections of the upper respiratory tract
2. diseases of the ear, e.g. deafness, tinnitus
3. acute inflammation of the eye
4. pain and restricted movement in the shoulder, back, upper extremity, and hand

Pec: connecting point (Luo), confluent point (Ba Mai Jiao Hui) of the Yang Wei Mai

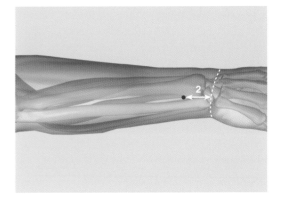

SJ 6 Zhi Gou   Branch Ditch

L: 3 cun proximal to the dorsal wrist crease, between the ulna and radius, on the connecting line between SJ 4 and the olecranon

T: 0.8–1.2 cun perpendicular; moxibustion

P: sharpens hearing and activates the upper body orifices, activates the channel and alleviates pain

A: 1. diseases of the ear, e.g. deafness, tinnitus
2. intercostal neuralgia

Pec: Jing (river) point (4th Shu-point)

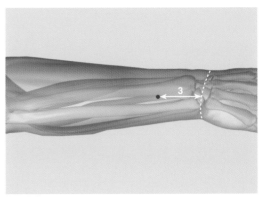

SJ

L: Location   T: Insertion Technique   P: Properties   A: Clinical Applications   Pec: Peculiarities

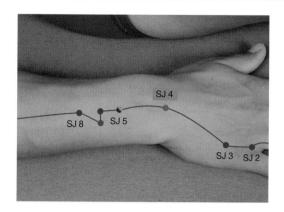

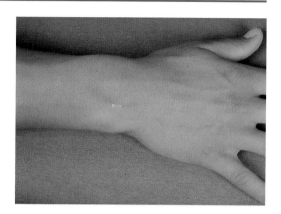

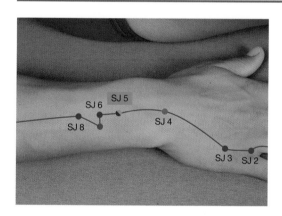

SJ

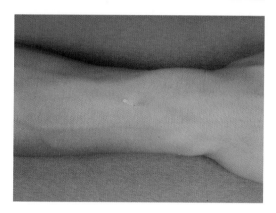

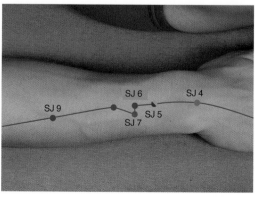

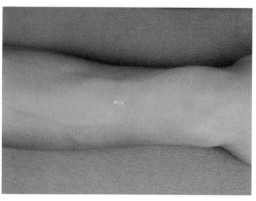

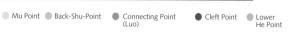

● Mu Point ● Back-Shu-Point ● Connecting Point (Luo) ● Cleft Point ● Lower He Point ● Qi-Source-Point (Yuan) ● Confluent Point ● Converging Point

SJ 7 Hui Zhong Ancestral Meeting

L: 3 cun proximal to the dorsal wrist crease, ulnar to point SJ 6, on the radial edge of the ulna

T: 0.5–1 cun perpendicular; moxibustion

P: sharpens hearing and releases cramp

A: 1. deafness
2. epilepsy

Pec: cleft (Xi) point

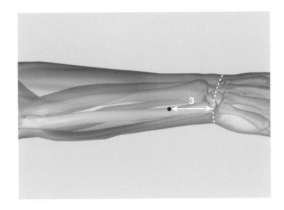

SJ 8 San Yang Luo Three Yang Luo

L: 4 cun proximal to the dorsal wrist crease, between the radius and ulna on the connecting line between SJ 4 and the olecranon

T: 0.8–1.2 cun perpendicular; moxibustion

P: activates the channel and sharpens hearing

A: 1. deafness
2. pain in the lower arm

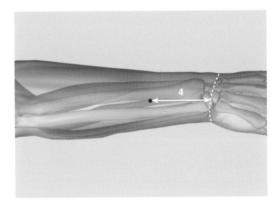

SJ

SJ 9 Si Du Four Rivers

L: 5 cun distal to the tip of the olecranon, between the radius and uilna, on the connecting line between SJ 4 and the olecranon

T: 0.5–1 cun perpendicular; moxibustion

P: sharpens hearing and eliminates deafness, activates the vessels and alleviates pain

A: 1. loss of hearing
2. acute chorditis vocalis
3. pain in the lower arm

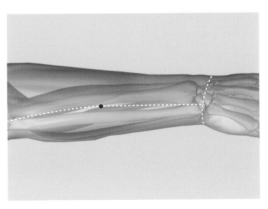

L: Location   T: Insertion Technique   P: Properties   A: Clinical Applications   Pec: Peculiarities

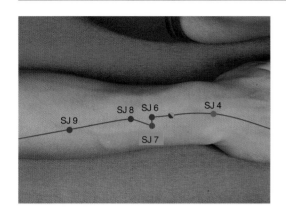
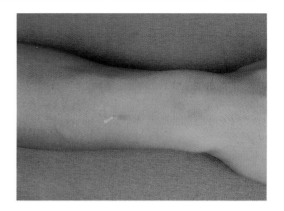

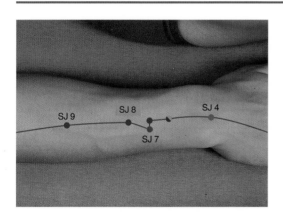
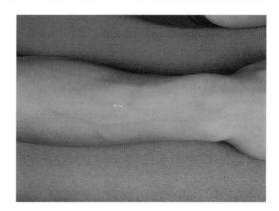

SJ

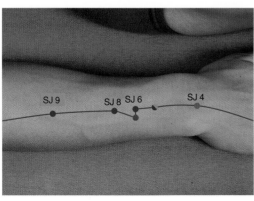
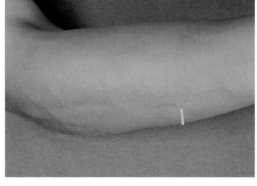

● Mu Point ● Back-Shu-Point ● Connecting Point (Luo) ● Cleft Point ● Lower He Point ● Qi-Source-Point (Yuan) ● Confluent Point ● Converging Point

SJ 10 Tiean Jing Heavenly Well

L: with the patient's elbow flexed, in the depression
1 cun proximal to the tip of the olecranon

T: 0.5–1 cun perpendicular;
moxibustion

P: regulates Qi and transforms phlegm, activates the
channel and alleviates pain

A: 1. pains in the shoulder, upper arm, and elbow joint
2. epilepsy
3. unspecific lymphadenitis and lymphadenitis
tuberculosa in the region of the neck and axilla

Pec: He (sea) point (5th Shu-point)

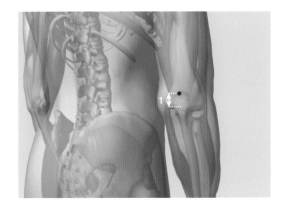

SJ 11 Qing Leng Yuan Clear Cold Abyss

L: with the patient's elbow flexed, 2 cun proximal to
the tip of the olecranon, 1 cun proximal to SJ 10

T: 0.8–1.2 cun perpendicular;
moxibustion

P: activates the channel and alleviates pain

A: pains in the shoulder and upper arm

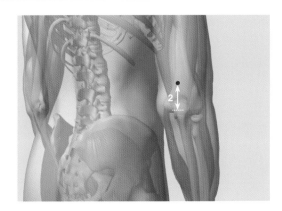

SJ 12 Xiao Luo Dispersing Luo River

L: at the midpoint between SJ 11 and SJ 13, on the
connecting line between the tip of the olecranon
and SJ 14

T: 1–1.5 cun perpendicular;
moxibustion

P: activates the channel and alleviates pain

A: pain in the upper arm

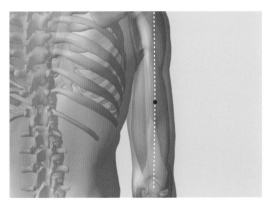

L: Location   **T:** Insertion Technique   **P:** Properties   **A:** Clinical Applications   **Pec:** Peculiarities

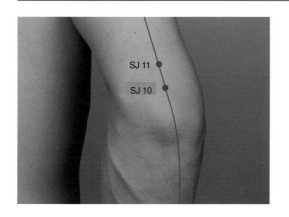

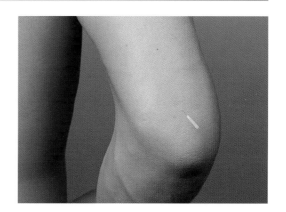

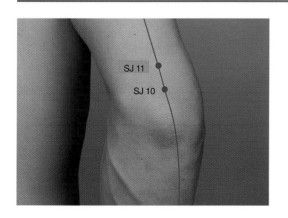

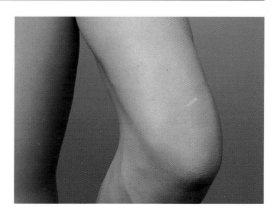

SJ

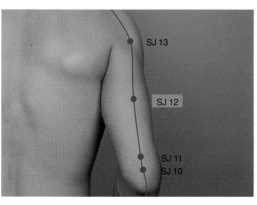

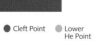

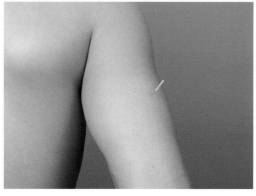

⬤ Mu Point   ⬤ Back-Shu-Point   ⬤ Connecting Point (Luo)   ⬤ Cleft Point   ⬤ Lower He Point   ⬤ Qi-Source-Point (Yuan)   ⬤ Confluent Point   ⬤ Converging Point

SJ 13 Nao Hui Upper Arm Meeting

L: 3 cun distal to SJ 14, on the connecting line between SJ 14 and the tip of the olecranon, on the posterior border of the deltoid muscle

T: 1–1.5 cun perpendicular; moxibustion

P: regulates Qi and transforms phlegm, activates the channel and alleviates pain

A: 1. pains in the shoulder, neck, and upper arm
2. diseases of the thyroid gland
3. unspecific lymphadenitis and lymphadenitis tuberculosa in the region of the neck and axilla

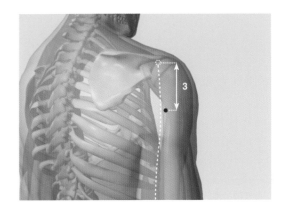

SJ 14 Jian Liao Shoulder Crevice

L: with the patient's arm abducted, in the depression dorsal and distal to the acromion dorsal to point LI 15

T: 1–1.5 cun perpendicular; moxibustion

P: improves joint mobility and activates the channel

A: periarthropia humeroscapularis

Pec: CAUTION, AVOID SPREADING GERMS TO THE SHOULDER JOINT!

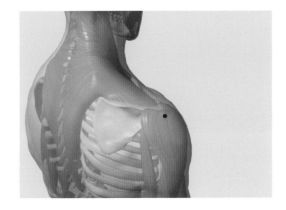

SJ 15 Tian Liao Heavenly Crevice

L: at the midpoint between GB 21 and SI 13, at the superior corner of the scapula

T: 0.5–0.8 cun perpendicular; moxibustion

P: activates the channel and alleviates pain

A: 1. pain in the shoulder and back
2. disorders of the cervical-spinal column

Pec: CAUTION, AVOID PNEUMOTHORAX!

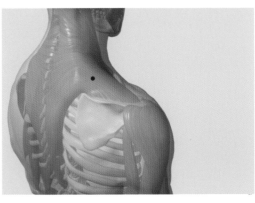

L: Location   **T:** Insertion Technique   **P:** Properties   **A:** Clinical Applications   **Pec:** Peculiarities

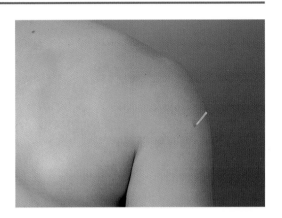

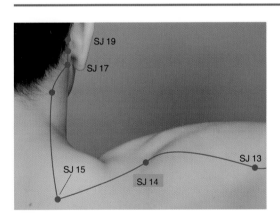

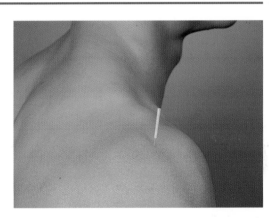

SJ

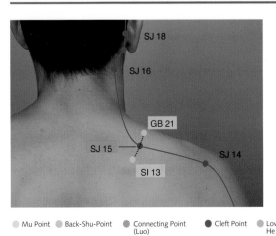

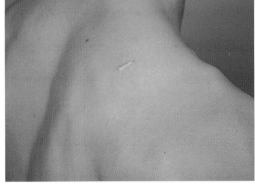

○ Mu Point ○ Back-Shu-Point ○ Connecting Point (Luo) ● Cleft Point ○ Lower He Point ● Qi-Source-Point (Yuan) ● Confluent Point ● Converging Point

SJ 16 Tian You   Window of Heaven

L: on the posterior border of the sternocleidomastoid muscle, caudal to the posterior border of the mastoid process, at the level of the corner of the jaw

T: 0.5–1 cun perpendicular; moxibustion

P: activates the channel and alleviates pain, sharpens hearing and activates the upper body orifices

A: 1. local pain of the cervical-spinal column
2. loss of hearing

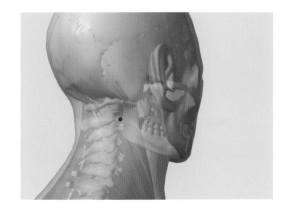

SJ 17 Yi Feng   Wind Screen

L: dorsal to the earlobe, in the depression between the mastoid process and the lower jaw

T: 0.8–1.2 cun perpendicular; moxibustion

P: sharpens hearing and corrects what is not straight

A: 1. diseases of the ear, e.g. deafness, tinnitus
2. facial paresis

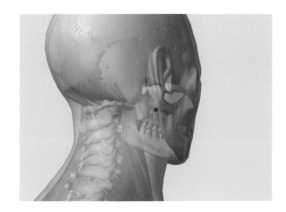

SJ

SJ 18 Chi Mai   Spasm Vessel

L: in the centre of the mastoid process, at the line between the lower and middle third of the connecting line, between SJ 17 and SJ 20, alongside the helix rim

T: 0.3–0.5 cun subcutaneously; prick to bleed; moxibustion

P: sharpens hearing and alleviates pain

A: 1. diseases of the ear, e.g. deafness, tinnitus
2. one-sided headache

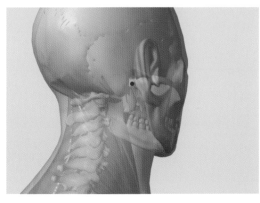

L: Location   **T:** Insertion Technique   **P:** Properties   **A:** Clinical Applications   **Pec:** Peculiarities

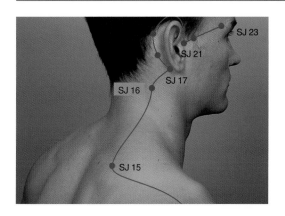

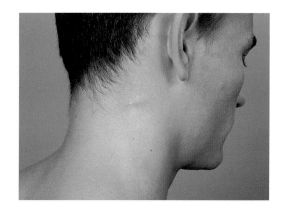

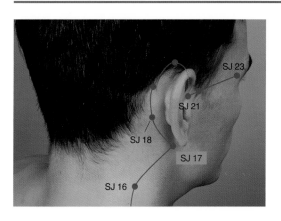

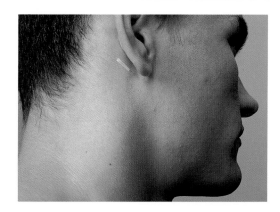

SJ

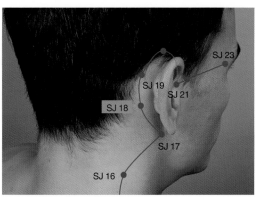

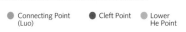

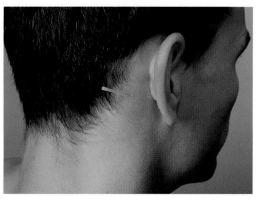

● Mu Point ● Back-Shu-Point ● Connecting Point (Luo) ● Cleft Point ● Lower He Point ● Qi-Source-Point (Yuan) ● Confluent Point ● Converging Point

SJ 19 Lu Xi   Skull's Rest

L: at the line between the middle and upper third of the connecting line, between SJ 17 and SJ 20, alongside the helix rim

T: moxibustion

P: expels wind and alleviates pain

A: 1. tinnitus

2. one-sided headache

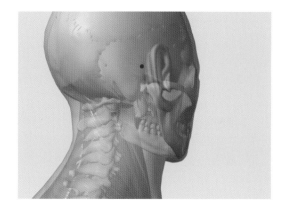

SJ 20 Jiao Sun   Minute Angle

L: directly above the auricular apex, on the hairline

T: 0.3–0.5 cun subcutaneously; moxibustion

P: alleviates pain and corrects dim vision

A: 1. one-sided headache
2. diseases of the cornea

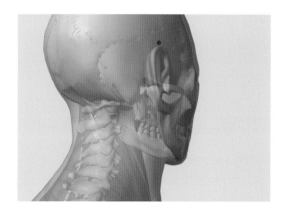

SJ

SJ 21 Er Men   Ear Gate

L: ventral to the supratragic notch, in the depression dorsal and cranial to the condyloid process of the mandible

T: 0.5–1 cun perpendicular; moxibustion

P: activates the channel and sharpens hearing

A: 1. diseases of the ear

2. trigeminal neuralgia

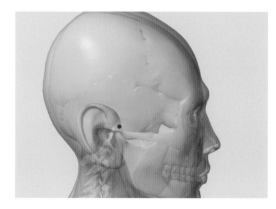

L: Location   T: Insertion Technique   P: Properties   A: Clinical Applications   **Pec:** Peculiarities

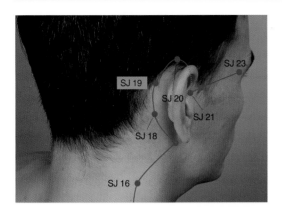

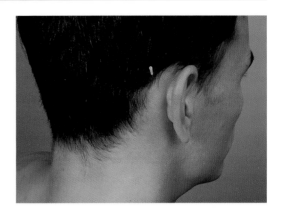

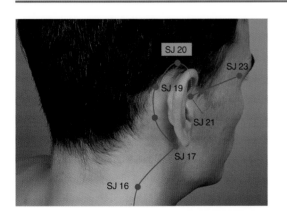

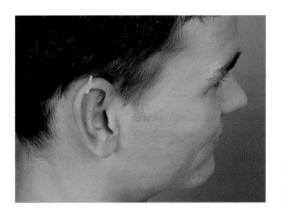

SJ

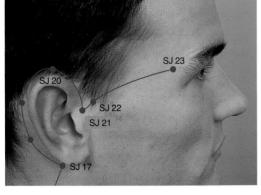

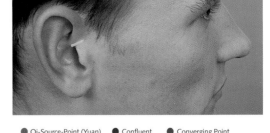

● Mu Point ● Back-Shu-Point ● Connecting Point (Luo) ● Cleft Point ● Lower He Point ● Qi-Source-Point (Yuan) ● Confluent Point ● Converging Point

213

SJ 22 Er He Liao   Ear Harmony Crevice

L: on the posterior border where the temple meets the hairline, ventral to the anterior border of the root of the ear muscle, dorsal to the A. temporalis superficialis

T: 0.3–0.5 cun subcutaneously; avoid the A. temporalis superficialis; moxibustion

P: activates the channel and sharpens hearing

A: 1. oromandibular dysfunction
2. tinnitus

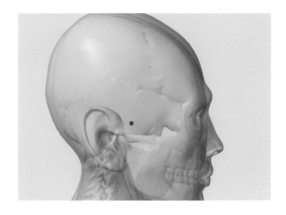

SJ 23 Si Zhu Kong   Silken Bamboo Hollow

L: in the depression at the lateral end of the eyebrow, near the bony limit of the orbit

T: 0.2–0.3 cun perpendicular or 0.5–1 cun subcutaneously; avoid the A. temporalis superficialis; moxibustion

P: expels wind and clears heat, sharpens eyesight and alleviates pain

A: 1. one-sided headache
2. diseases of the eye
3. tics of the eye

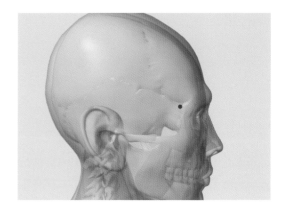

SJ

L: Location   T: Insertion Technique   P: Properties   A: Clinical Applications   Pec: Peculiarities

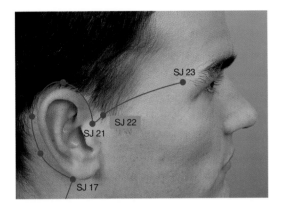

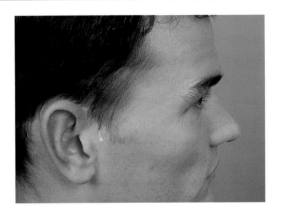

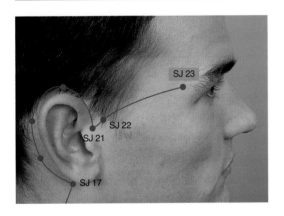

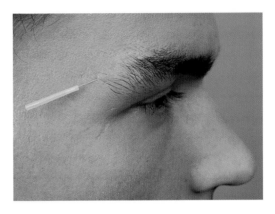

SJ

○ Mu Point   ○ Back-Shu-Point   ○ Connecting Point (Luo)   ● Cleft Point   ○ Lower He Point   ● Qi-Source-Point (Yuan)   ● Confluent Point   ● Converging Point

215

2.2.11　The gall bladder channel (GB)

Synonyms

• Gall Bladder Meridian

• Foot-Shaoyang Gall Bladder Channel

Channel pathway

There are 44 acupuncture points on the surface pathway of the gall bladder channel.

The surface pathway of the channel originates at the bony limit of the outer canthus and runs in front of the ear, before ascending to the region of the temple. From here the channel returns to the anterior part of the helix and passes the ear to the region of the mastoid process. From here the channel again arches over the temples to the forehead, before returning at a slightly more medial level over the skull and reaching the neck region at point GB 20.

A branch from the principal channel departs from below GB 20, just below point GB 12. It then runs through point SJ 17 through the ear and point SI 19 in front of the ear, to GB 1.

A further branch leads from point GB 1 to the lower jaw at point St 5, before ascending to the cheek at point SI 18 and descending back to point St 6 at the corner of the jaw. From here the branch runs to the superior clavicular fossa, where it reconnects with principal channel from point GB 20.

From the superior clavicular fossa the inner pathway of the channel winds its way into the chest, traverses the diaphragm, connecting with the liver and entering its organ, the gall bladder. The channel descends further down the flank, where it makes contact with the deep layers of point Lv 13 before entering the superficial layers in the region above the groin and descending past the hip to point GB 30.

The further surface pathway of the channel covers the channel from GB 20 in the region of the neck, via the seventh cervical vertebra (Du 14), to point GB 21 on the descending aspect of the trapezius muscle, and from here to the upper shoulder region and point SI 12 to the superior clavicular fossa. The channel zig-zags over the axillar region to the side of the chest and flank to point GB 29 in the region of the hip. From here, a branch runs to the sacral bone, via points BL 31–BL 34, before reconnecting with the inner branch and the surface pathway of the principal channel at point GB 30. From point GB 30 the channel descends alongside the middle region of the antero-lateral aspect of the thigh, passing the outside of the knee to the middle part of the antero-lateral aspect of the lower leg and in front of the outside ankle bone, via the dorsum, to the outside corner of the nail of the fourth toe.

From point GB 41 on the dorsum of the foot a branch runs between the first and second metatarsal bones to the big toe, where it connects with the liver channel.

GB

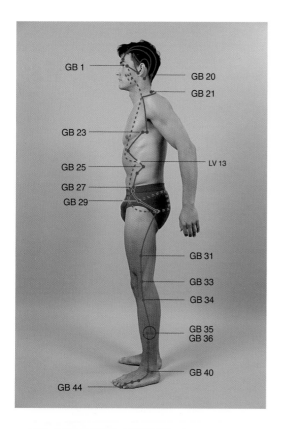

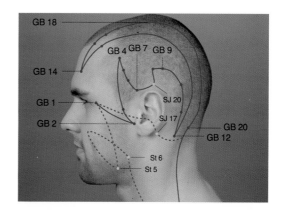

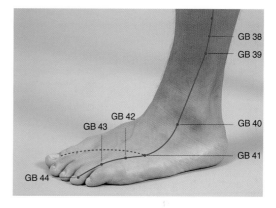

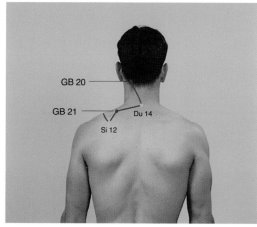

GB

GB 1 Tong Zi Liao Pupil Crevice

L: 0.5 cun lateral to the outer canthus of the eye, in the depression at the lateral end of the orbit

T: 0.3–0.5 cun subcutaneously; moxibustion

P: sharpens eyesight and improves dim eyesight

A: diseases of the eye

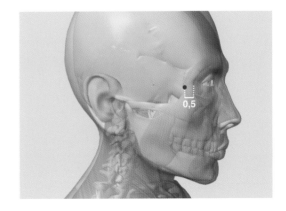

GB 2 Ting Hui Meeting of Hearing

L: with the patient's mouth open, in front of the intertragic notch, in the depression below the condyloid process of the mandible

T: 0.5–1 cun perpendicular; moxibustion

P: opens the senses and sharpens hearing, activates the channel and alleviates pain

A: 1. diseases of the ear, e.g. deafness, tinnitus, infections of the auditory canal
2. trigeminal neuralgia

Pec: CAUTION, AVOID SPREADING GERMS TO THE JAW JOINT!

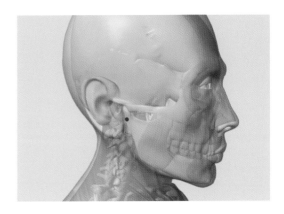

GB 3 Shang Guan Above the Joint

L: directly above St 7, in the depression at the superior border of the zygomatic arch

T: 0.5–1 cun perpendicular; moxibustion

P: sharpens hearing and alleviates pain

A: 1. tinnitus, deafness
2. toothache in the upper jaw

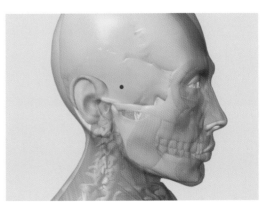

L: Location   **T:** Insertion Technique   **P:** Properties   **A:** Clinical Applications   **Pec:** Peculiarities

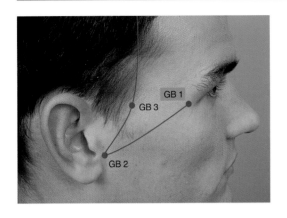

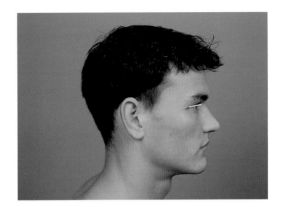

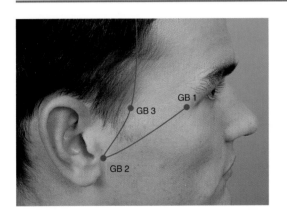

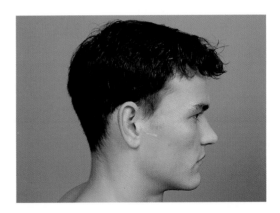

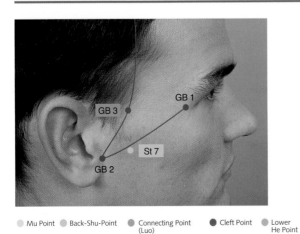

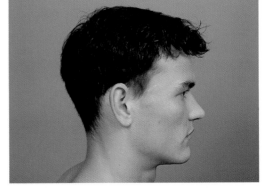

GB

○ Mu Point   ○ Back-Shu-Point   ● Connecting Point (Luo)   ● Cleft Point   ○ Lower He Point   ● Qi-Source-Point (Yuan)   ● Confluent Point   ● Converging Point

GB 4 Han Yan Jaw Serenity

L: in the temporal region within the hairline, at the dividing line between the upper and second quarter of the shortened connecting line between St 8 and GB 7

T: 0.5–0.8 cun subcutaneously; moxibustion

P: soothes the liver and expels wind, activates the vessels and alleviates pain

A: 1. hypertension
2. one-sided headache

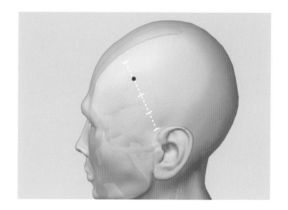

GB 5 Xuan Lu Suspended Skull

L: in the temporal region within the hairline, in the middle of the shortened connecting line between St 8 and GB 7

T: 0.5–0.8 cun subcutaneously; moxibustion

P: expels wind and alleviates pain

A: one-sided headache

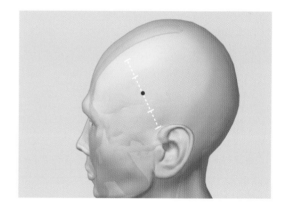

GB 6 Xuan Li Suspended Hair

L: in the temporal region within the hairline, at the dividing line between the lower and next quarter of the shortened connecting line between St 8 and GB 7

T: 0.5–0.8 cun subcutaneously; moxibustion

P: expels wind and alleviates pain

A: one-sided headache

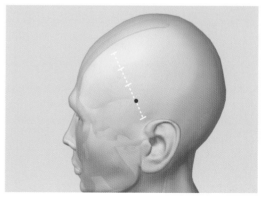

GB

L: Location   T: Insertion Technique   P: Properties   A: Clinical Applications   **Pec:** Peculiarities

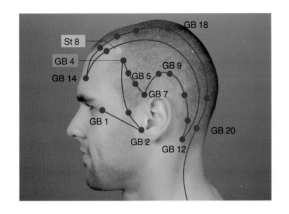

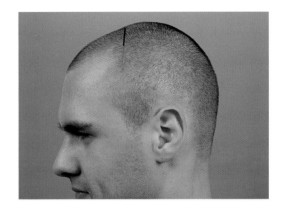

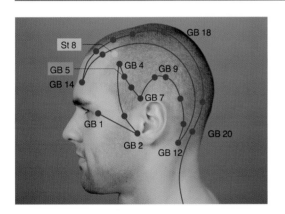

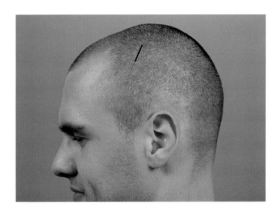

GB

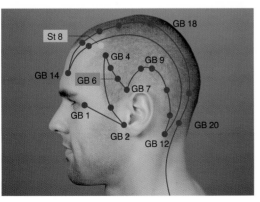

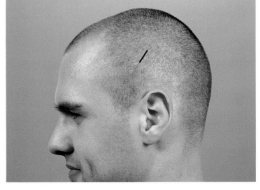

● Mu Point   ● Back-Shu-Point   ● Connecting Point (Luo)   ● Cleft Point   ● Lower He Point   ● Qi-Source-Point (Yuan)   ● Confluent Point   ● Converging Point

GB 7 Qu Bin   Crook of the Temple

L: at the point of intersection of one horizontal through the auricular apex with a vertical alongside the dorsal hairline in front of the ear

T: 0.5–0.8 cun subcutaneously; moxibustion

P: expels wind and alleviates pain, clears heat, and reduces edema

A: 1. one-sided headache
2. parotitis and inflammation of other salival glands

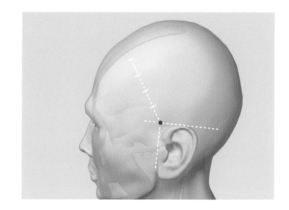

GB 8 Shuai Gu   Leading Valley

L: directly above the auricular apex, above point SJ 20, 1.5 cun within the ideal hairline

T: 0.5–0.8 cun subcutaneously; moxibustion

P: soothes the liver and expels wind, descends inverted Qi

A: 1. hypertension
2. one-sided headache
3. morbus meniére

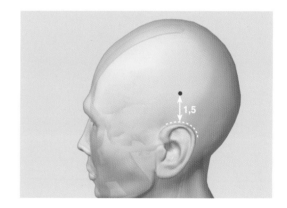

GB 9 Tian Chong   Heavenly Rushing

GB

L: directly above the posterior border of the root of the ear muscle, 2 cun within the hairline, 0.5 cun dorsal to GB 8

T: 0.5–0.8 cun subcutaneously; moxibustion

P: pacifies the spirit and releases cramp, reduces edema and alleviates pain

A: 1. one-sided headache
2. epilepsy
3. acute parodonitis

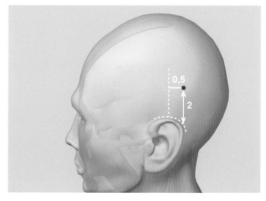

L: Location   T: Insertion Technique   P: Properties   A: Clinical Applications   **Pec:** Peculiarities

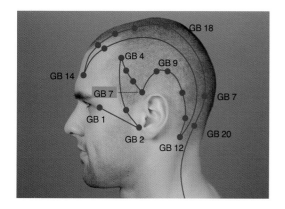

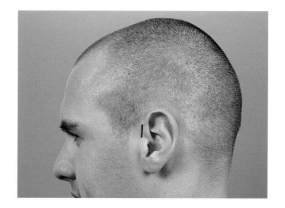

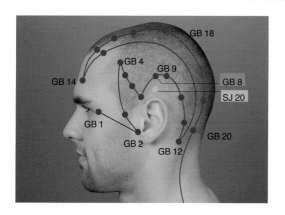

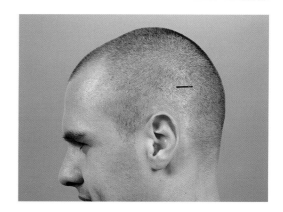

GB

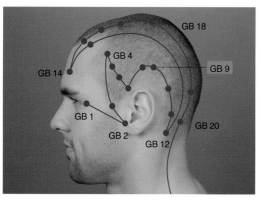

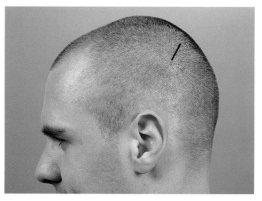

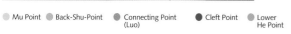

● Mu Point ● Back-Shu-Point ● Connecting Point (Luo) ● Cleft Point ● Lower He Point ● Qi-Source-Point (Yuan) ● Confluent Point ● Converging Point

223

GB 10 Fu Bai   Floating White

L: dorso-cranial to the mastoid process, at the dividing line between the middle to the upper third of the shortened connecting line between GB 9 and GB 12

T: 0.5–0.8 cun subcutaneously; moxibustion

P: expels wind and alleviates pain

A: 1. hypertension
2. tinnitus, deafness

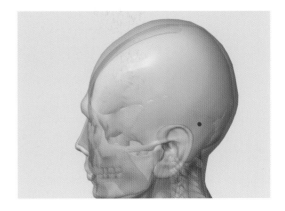

GB 11 Tou Qiao Yin   Yin Portals of the Head

L: dorso-cranial to the mastoid process, at the dividing line between the middle to the lower third of the shortened connecting line between GB 9 and GB 12

T: 0.5–0.8 cun subcutaneously; moxibustion

P: soothes the liver and expels wind, activates the vessels and alleviates pain

A: 1. one-sided headache
2. disorders of the cervical-spinal column
3. tinnitus, deafness

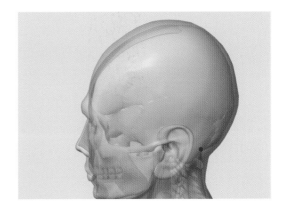

GB 12 Wan Gu   Mastoid Process

L: in the depression dorso-cranial to the mastoid process

T: 0.5–0.8 cun perpendicular; moxibustion

P: expels wind and alleviates pain, activates the vessels and strengthens the brain

A: 1. one-sided headache
2. headache, dizziness, and numbness in vertebro-basiliar insufficiency
3. disorders of the cervical-spinal column

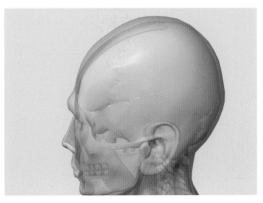

L: Location   T: Insertion Technique   P: Properties   A: Clinical Applications   Pec: Peculiarities

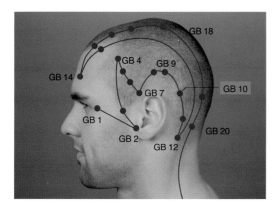

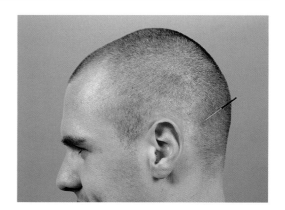

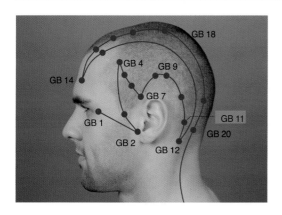

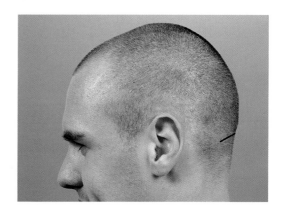

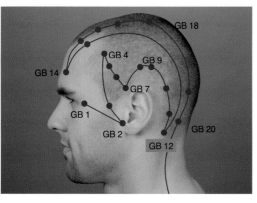

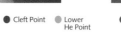

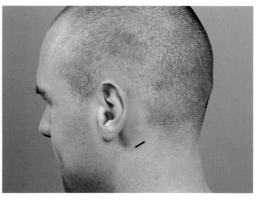

GB

● Mu Point ● Back-Shu-Point ● Connecting Point (Luo) ● Cleft Point ● Lower He Point ● Qi-Source-Point (Yuan) ● Confluent Point ● Converging Point

GB 13 Ben Shen   Root of the Spirit

L: 0.5 cun within the ideal anterior hairline, 3 cun
lateral to the midline (Du 24), at the dividing line
between the middle and lateral third of the
connecting line between Du 24 and St 8

T: 0.5–0.8 cun subcutaneously;
moxibustion

P: pacifies the spirit and suppresses cramp, expels wind
and alleviates pain

A: 1. headache, dizziness, and numbness in vertebro-
basiliar insufficiency
2. epilepsy
3. fever cramps in children

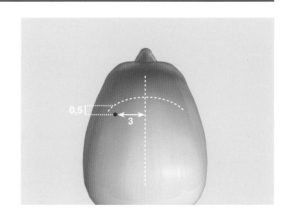

GB 14 Yang Bai   Yang White

L: directly above the pupil, 1 cun above the eyebrow

T: 0.3–0.5 cun subcutaneously;
moxibustion

P: expels wind and alleviates pain, clears heat and
sharpens eyesight

A: 1. headache
2. diseases of the eye
3. peripheral facial paresis

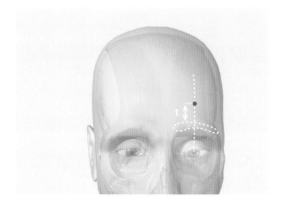

GB

GB 15 Tou Lin Qi   Head Governor of Tears

L: directly above the pupil, 0.5 cun within the ideal
anterior hairline, in the middle between Du 24 and
St 8

T: 0.3–0.5 cun subcutaneously;
moxibustion

P: expels wind and clears heat, sharpens eyesight and
activates the upper body orifices

A: 1. headache
2. diseases of the eye, e.g. conjunctivitis, ceratitis,
dacryocystitis
3. rhinitis

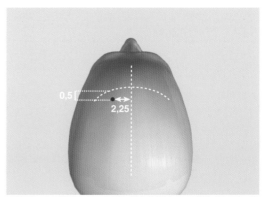

L: Location   T: Insertion Technique   P: Properties   A: Clinical Applications   Pec: Peculiarities

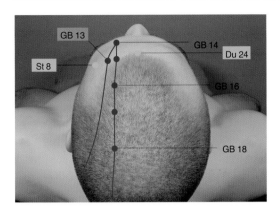

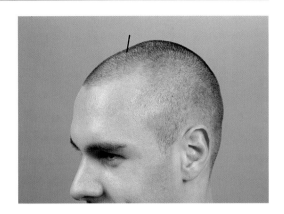

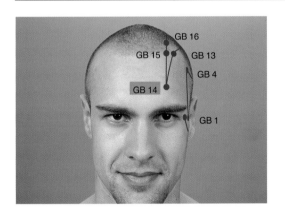

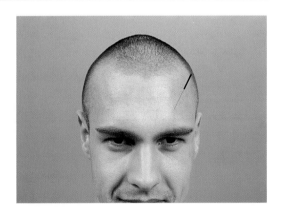

GB

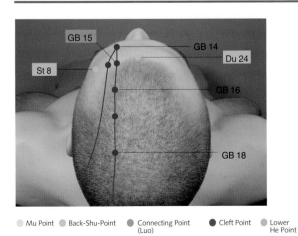

○ Mu Point ○ Back-Shu-Point ○ Connecting Point (Luo) ● Cleft Point ○ Lower He Point   ● Qi-Source-Point (Yuan) ● Confluent Point ● Converging Point

GB 16 Mu Chuang Window of the Eye

L: 1.5 cun within the ideal anterior hairline, 2.25 cun lateral to the midline, on the connecting line between GB 15 and GB 20

T: 0.3–0.5 cun subcutaneously; moxibustion

P: expels wind and sharpens eyesight

A: 1. headache
2. diseases of the eye, e.g. refraction disorders, conjunctivitis

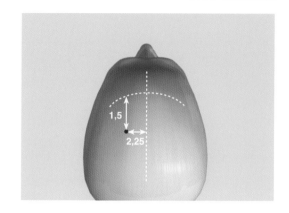

GB 17 Zheng Ying Upright Nutrition

L: 2.5 cun within the ideal anterior hairline, 2.25 cun lateral to the midline, on the connecting line between GB 15 and GB 20

T: 0.3–0.5 cun subcutaneously; moxibustion

P: soothes the liver and expels wind, clears heat and alleviates pain

A: 1. hypertension
2. toothache in the upper jaw

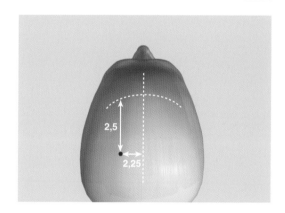

GB 18 Cheng Ling Support Spirit

L: 4 cun within the ideal anterior hairline, 2.25 cun lateral to the midline, on the connecting line between GB 15 and GB 20

T: 0.3–0.5 cun subcutaneously; moxibustion

P: clears heat and alleviates pain

A: headache, dizziness, and numbness

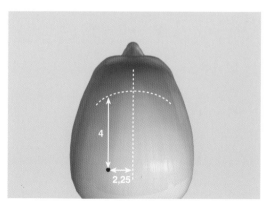

L: Location　　T: Insertion Technique　　P: Properties　　A: Clinical Applications　　**Pec:** Peculiarities

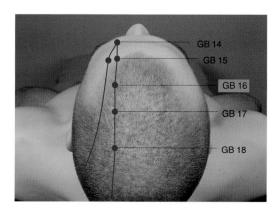

GB 14
GB 15
GB 16
GB 17
GB 18

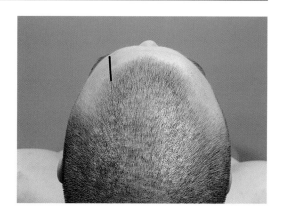

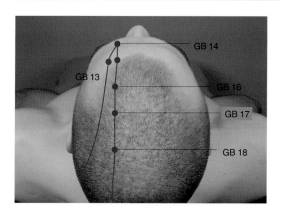

GB 14
GB 13
GB 16
GB 17
GB 18

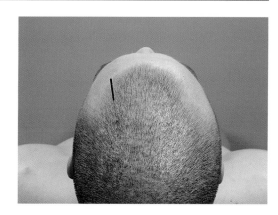

GB

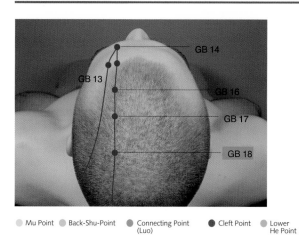

GB 14
GB 13
GB 16
GB 17
GB 18

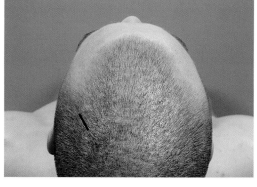

● Mu Point   ● Back-Shu-Point   ● Connecting Point (Luo)   ● Cleft Point   ● Lower He Point   ● Qi-Source-Point (Yuan)   ● Confluent Point   ● Converging Point

GB 19 Nao Kong Brain Hollow

L: at the level of the superior border of the external occipital protuberance (Du 17), 2.25 cun lateral to the midline

T: 0.3–0.5 cun subcutaneously; moxibustion

P: clears heat and alleviates pain

A: 1. headache in the neck
2. conjunctivitis

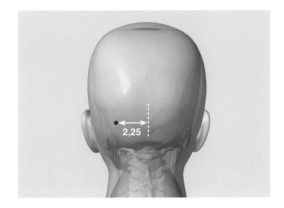

GB 20 Feng Chi Wind Pool

L: below the occipital bone at the level of Du 16, in the depression between the start of the sternocleido-mastoid process and the trapezius muscle

T: 0.8–1.2 cun oblique towards the tip of the nose or towards Du 16; moxibustion

P: disseminates wind and alleviates pain, clears heat and liberates the surface, soothes the liver and expels wind

A: 1. all forms of headache
2. infections of the superior respiratory tract
3. hypertension
4. cerebro-vascular diseases, vertebro-basiliar insufficiency
5. disorders of the cervical-spinal column

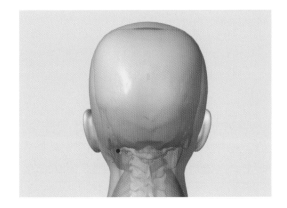

GB 21 Jian Jing Shoulder Well

L: at the midpoint between the depression below the spinous process C7 (Du 14) and the acromion

T: 0.5–0.8 cun perpendicular; moxibustion

P: clears heat and expels wind, reduces edema and alleviates pain

A: 1. mastitis
2. protracted labour
3. pain in the shoulder and back

Pec: CAUTION, AVOID PNEUMOTHORAX!
CAUTION IN PREGNANCY!

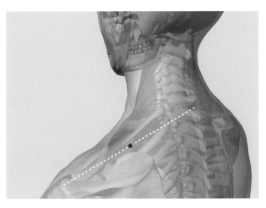

L: Location   T: Insertion Technique   P: Properties   A: Clinical Applications   Pec: Peculiarities

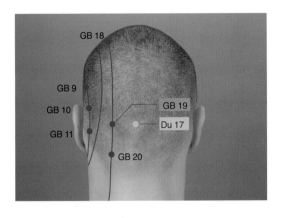

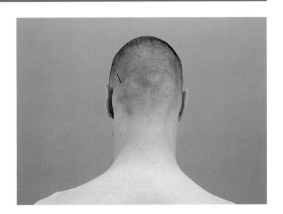

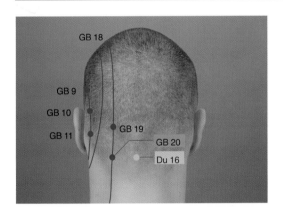

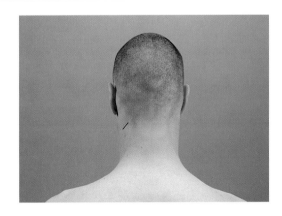

GB

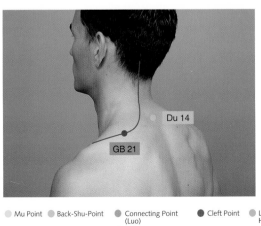

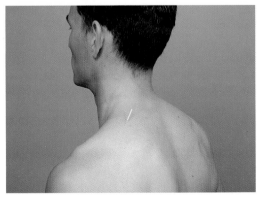

● Mu Point ● Back-Shu-Point ● Connecting Point (Luo) ● Cleft Point ● Lower He Point   ● Qi-Source-Point (Yuan) ● Confluent Point ● Converging Point

231

GB 22 Yuan Ye Armpit Abyss

L: with the patient's arm lifted, in the mid-axillary line, 3 cun below the axilla in the fourth ICR

T: 0.5–0.8 cun oblique or subcutaneously; moxibustion

P: alleviates pain and reduces edema

A: 1. intercostal neuralgia

2. herpes zoster

3. lymphadenitis in the axilla

Pec: CAUTION, AVOID PNEUMOTHORAX!

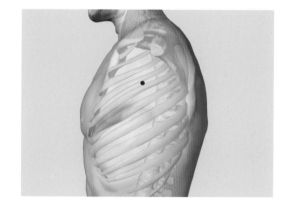

GB 23 Zhe Jin Flank Sinews

L: 1 cun ventral to GB 22, in the fourth ICR, at the level of the nipple

T: 0.5–0.8 cun oblique or subcutaneously; moxibustion

P: regulates Qi and alleviates pain, descends inverted Qi and alleviates breathing difficulty

A: 1. intercostal neuralgia

2. herpes zoster

3. asthmatic complaints

Pec: CAUTION, AVOID PNEUMOTHORAX!

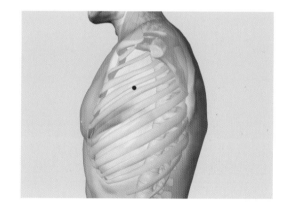

GB

GB 24 Ri Yue Sun and Moon

L: directly below the nipple, in the seventh ICR, 4 cun lateral to the ventral midline

T: 0.5–0.8 cun oblique or subcutaneously; moxibustion

P: promotes the gall bladder and descends inverted Qi

A: diseases of the gall bladder

Pec: Mu point of the gall bladder
CAUTION, AVOID PNEUMOTHORAX!

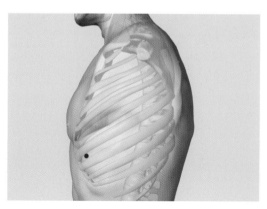

L: Location   T: Insertion Technique   P: Properties   A: Clinical Applications   Pec: Peculiarities

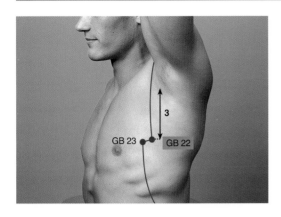

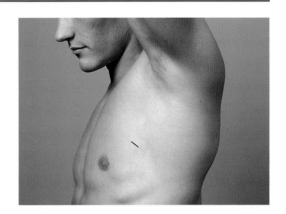

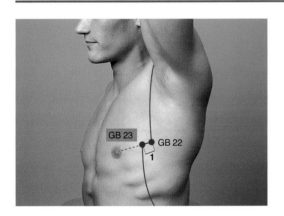

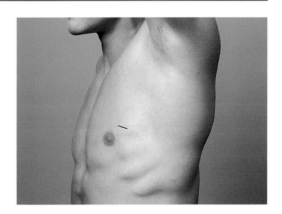

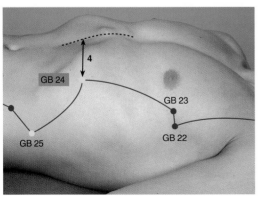

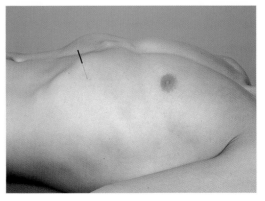

GB

● Mu Point ● Back-Shu-Point ● Connecting Point (Luo) ● Cleft Point ● Lower He Point ● Qi-Source-Point (Yuan) ● Confluent Point ● Converging Point

GB 25 Jing Men   Capital Gate

L: on the inferior border of the free end of the twelfth rib, 1.8 cun dorso-caudal to Lv 13

T: 0.5–1 cun perpendicular; moxibustion

P: supports the kidney and strengthens the lumbar region

A: 1. chronic enteritis
2. pain in the lumbar and rib regions

Pec: Mu point of the kidney

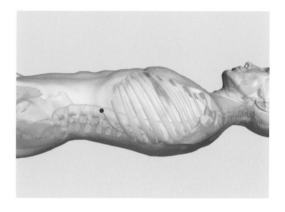

GB 26 Dai Mai   Girdling Vessel

L: at the point of intersection of one vertical through the free end of the eleventh rib, and one horizontal through the umbilicus, 1.8 cun ventro-caudal to Lv 13

T: 1–1.5 cun perpendicular; moxibustion

P: regulates menstruation and soothes discharge

A: certain gynecological disorders, e.g. irregular menstruation, leucorrhoea, chronic inflammation of the internal female genitalia

Pec: CAUTION IN PREGNANCY!

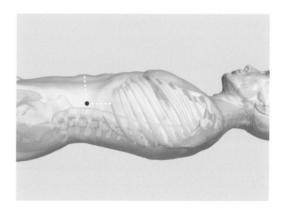

GB 27 Wu Shu   Five Pivots

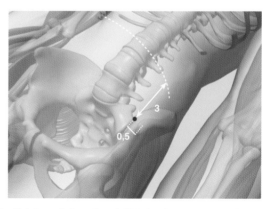

L: at the level 3 cun caudal to the umbilicus, 0.5 cun ventral to the anterior superior iliac spine

T: 1–1.5 cun perpendicular or oblique; moxibustion

P: regulates menstruation and soothes discharge, regulates Qi and alleviates pain

A: 1. gynecological disorders, e.g. uterine prolapse, irregular menstruation, leucorrhoea
2. external abdominal hernias

Pec: CAUTION IN PREGNANCY!

GB

L: Location   T: Insertion Technique   P: Properties   A: Clinical Applications   Pec: Peculiarities

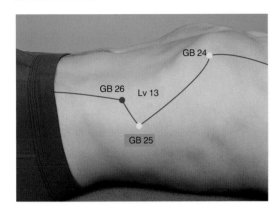

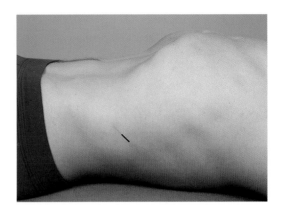

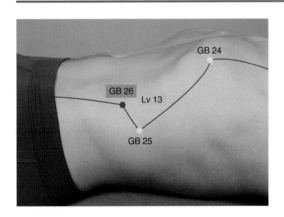

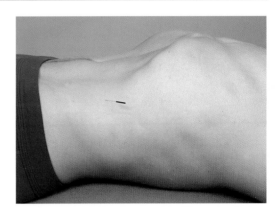

GB

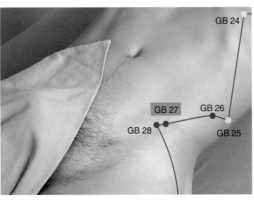

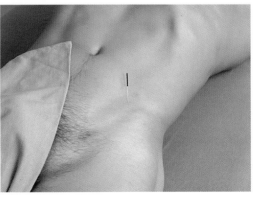

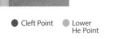

○ Mu Point ○ Back-Shu-Point ○ Connecting Point (Luo) ● Cleft Point ○ Lower He Point ● Qi-Source-Point (Yuan) ● Confluent Point ● Converging Point

235

GB 28 Wei Dao   Linking Path

L: ventro-caudal to the anterior superior iliac spine, 0.5 cun ventro-caudal to GB 27

T: 1–1.5 cun perpendicular; moxibustion

P: regulates menstruation and soothes discharge, regulates Qi and alleviates pain

A: 1. gynecological disorders, e.g. uterine prolapse, irregular menstruation, leucorrhoea

2. external abdominal hernias

Pec: CAUTION IN PREGNANCY!

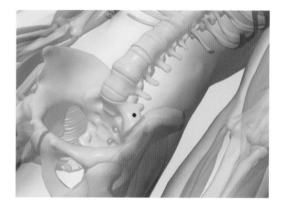

GB 29 Ju Liao   Stationary Crevice

L: at the midpoint between the anterior superior iliac spine and the highest point of the major femoral trochanter

T: 1–1.5 cun perpendicular; moxibustion

P: decongests and activates the channel and its vessels

A: 1. pain in the lumbar region and the legs
2. pareses of the lower extremity

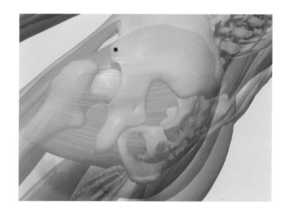

GB 30 Huan Tiao   Jumping Circle

L: with the patient lying down with hip lifted, in the hip joint, at the dividing line between the middle and lateral third of the connecting line between the major femoral trochanter and the sacral hiatus

T: 2–3 cun perpendicular; moxibustion

P: activates the channel and its vessels and alleviates pain

A: 1. pain in the lumbo-sacral region
2. ischialgia
3. restricted movement of the lower extremity

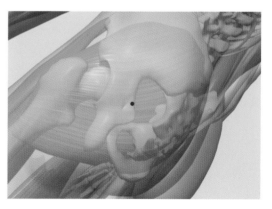

GB

L: Location   T: Insertion Technique   P: Properties   A: Clinical Applications   Pec: Peculiarities

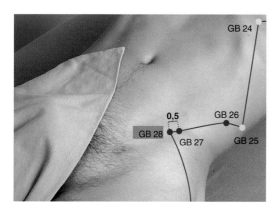

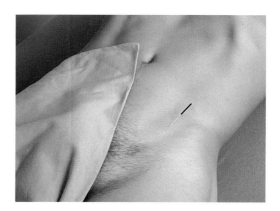

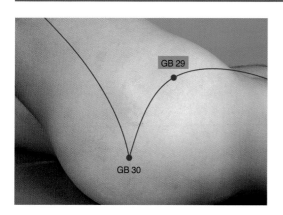

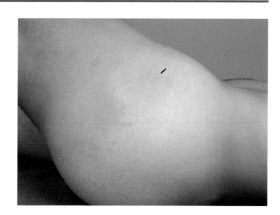

GB

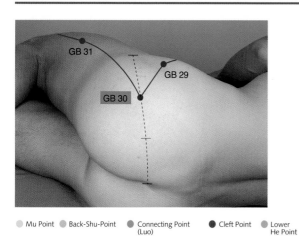

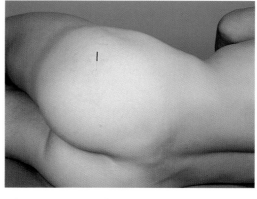

● Mu Point ● Back-Shu-Point ● Connecting Point (Luo) ● Cleft Point ● Lower He Point ● Qi-Source-Point (Yuan) ● Confluent Point ● Converging Point

GB 31 Feng Shi   Wind Market

L: 7 cun proximal to the popliteal crease, on the lateral aspect of the upper leg; with the patient standing, the tip of the middle finger of a relaxed arm indicates the point

T: 1–2 cun perpendicular; moxibustion

P: decongests and activates the channel and its vessels, expels wind and alleviates pain

A: 1. one-sided paralysis in cerebro-vascular diseases
2. pain and parestheses of the lower extremity

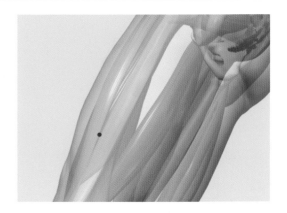

GB 32 Zhong Du   Middle Ditch

L: 5 cun proximal to the popliteal crease, between the vastus lateralis and the biceps femoris muscles, 2 cun below GB 31

T: 1–2 cun perpendicular; moxibustion

P: decongests and activates the channel and its vessels

A: 1. one-sided paralysis in cerebro-vascular diseases
2. paraestheses of the lower extremity

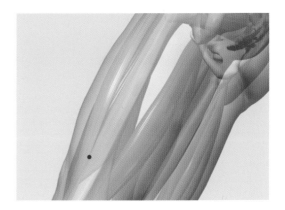

GB 33 Xi Yang Guan   Knee Yang Gate

L: 3 cun proximal to GB 34, in the depression proximal to the lateral epicondyle of the femur

T: 1–1.5 cun perpendicular; moxibustion

P: activates the channel and alleviates pain

A: 1. pain in the region of the knee joint
2. paraestheses of the lower leg

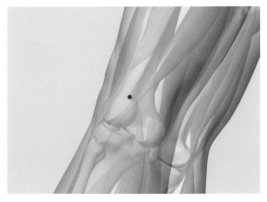

L: Location   T: Insertion Technique   P: Properties   A: Clinical Applications   Pec: Peculiarities

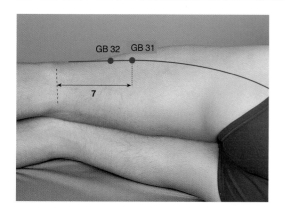

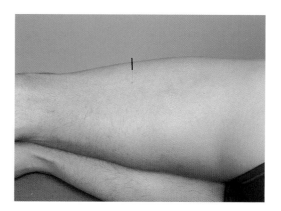

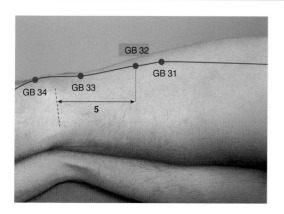

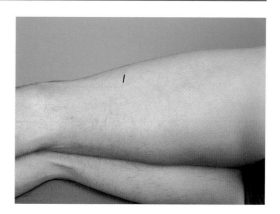

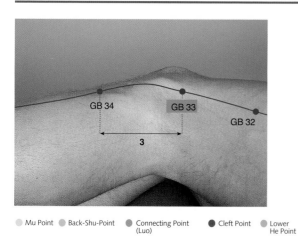

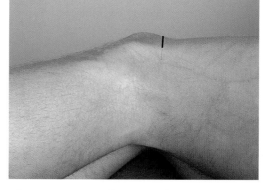

GB

○ Mu Point ○ Back-Shu-Point ○ Connecting Point (Luo) ● Cleft Point ○ Lower He Point   ● Qi-Source-Point (Yuan) ● Confluent Point ● Converging Point

239

GB 34 Yang Ling Quan   Yang Mound Spring

L: in the depression ventral and distal to the head of the fibula

T: 1–1.5 cun perpendicular; moxibustion

P: decongests the liver and promotes the gall bladder, makes the tendons supple, and alleviates pain

A: 1. diseases of the gall bladder, e.g. cholecystitis, cholelithiasis
2. pains in the region of the knee joint
3. one-sided paralysis, paraestheses, and pain in cerebro-vascular diseases

Pec: He (sea) point (5th Shu-point), meeting (master) point (Hui) of the tendons

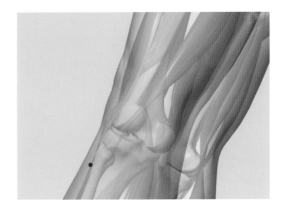

GB 35 Yang Jiao   Yang Intersection

L: 7 cun proximal to the prominence of the lateral malleolus on the posterior border of the fibula at the level of GB 36

T: 1–1.5 cun perpendicular; moxibustion

P: pacifies the spirit and promotes all-round calmness, activates the channel and alleviates pain

A: 1. psychic and pyschosomatic disorders (sedative effect)
2. diseases of the gall bladder
3. pain on the outside of the lower leg

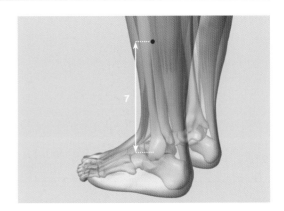

GB 36 Wai Qiu   Outer Hill

L: 7 cun proximal to the prominence of the lateral malleolus on the anterior border of the fibula at the level of GB 35

T: 1–1.5 cun perpendicular; moxibustion

P: pacifies the spirit and activates the channel

A: 1. depressive disorders
2. intercostal neuralgia

Pec: cleft (Xi) point

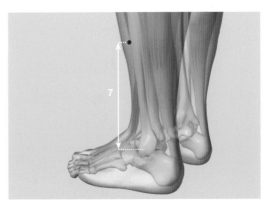

L: Location   T: Insertion Technique   P: Properties   A: Clinical Applications   Pec: Peculiarities

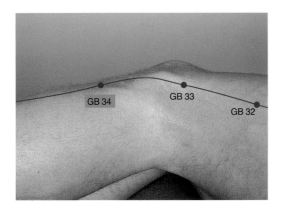

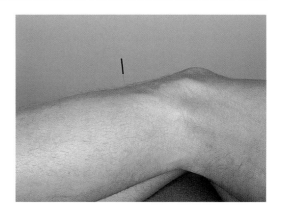

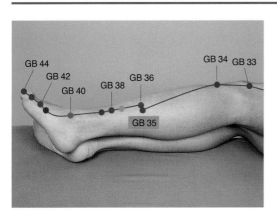

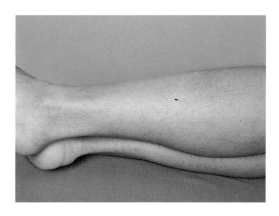

GB

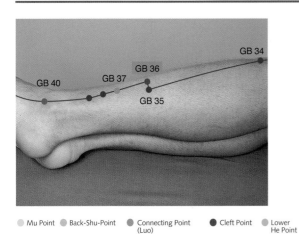

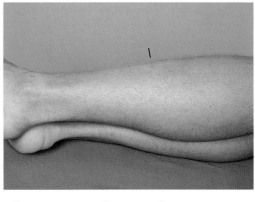

● Mu Point ● Back-Shu-Point ● Connecting Point (Luo) ● Cleft Point ● Lower He Point ● Qi-Source-Point (Yuan) ● Confluent Point ● Converging Point

GB 37 Guang Ming Bright Light

L: 5 cun proximal to the maximum prominence of the lateral malleolus, on the anterior border of the fibula

T: 1–1.5 cun perpendicular; moxibustion

P: clears the liver and sharpens eyesight, eliminates sensation of tension and alleviates pain

A: 1. certain diseases of the eye, e.g. ceratitis, glaucoma, night blindness
2. sense of tension and pain in the breast in the early stage of mastitis

Pec: connecting point (Luo)

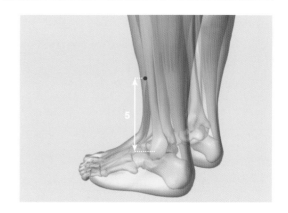

GB 38 Yang Fu Yang Assistance

L: 4 cun proximal to the maximum prominence of the lateral malleolus, on the anterior border of the fibula

T: 1–1.5 cun perpendicular; moxibustion

P: expels wind and clears heat, decongests and activates the channel and its vessels

A: 1. one-sided headache
2. pains in the lateral thorax, flank, and the lower extremity
3. one-sided paralysis in cerebro-vascular disease

Pec: Jing (river) point (4th Shu-point)

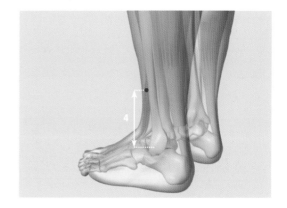

GB

GB 39 Xuan Zhong Suspended Bell

L: 3 cun proximal to the maximum prominence of the lateral malleolus on the anterior border of the fibula

T: 1–1.5 cun perpendicular; moxibustion

P: decongests and activates the channel and its vessels

A: 1. one-sided paralysis in cerebro-vascular diseases
2. disorders of the cervical-spinal column
3. pains and loss of strength in the lower leg

Pec: meeting (master) point (Hui) of the marrow

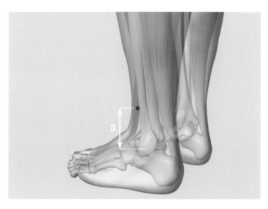

L: Location   **T:** Insertion Technique   **P:** Properties   **A:** Clinical Applications   **Pec:** Peculiarities

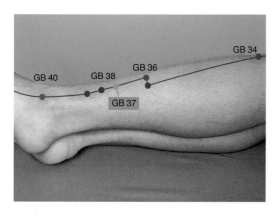

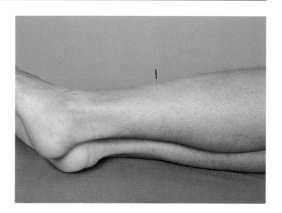

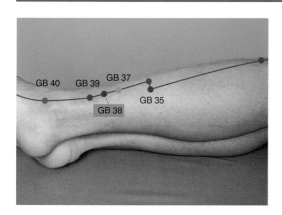

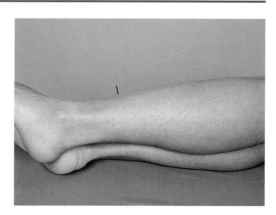

GB

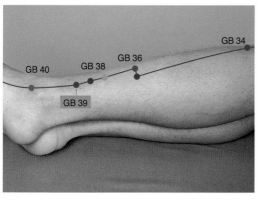

● Mu Point　　● Back-Shu-Point　　● Connecting Point (Luo)　　● Cleft Point　　● Lower He Point　　　　● Qi-Source-Point (Yuan)　　● Confluent Point　　● Converging Point

GB 40 Qiu Xu Mound of Ruins

L: ventral and distal to the lateral malleolus, in the depression lateral to the tendon of the extensor digitorum longus

T: 0.5–0.8 cun perpendicular; moxibustion

P: clears heat and sharpens eyesight, benefits the gall bladder and activates the channel

A: 1. certain acute inflammations of the eye
2. diseases of the gall bladder
3. pain in the lateral malleolus, supination position of the foot in one-sided paralysis

Pec: Qi-source-point (Yuan)
CAUTION, AVOID SPREADING GERMS TO THE ANKLE!

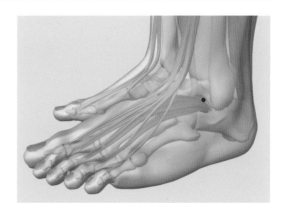

GB 41 Zu Lin Qi Foot Governor of Tears

L: on the dorsum of the foot, in the proximal angle between the fourth and fifth metatarsal bones, in the depression lateral to the tendon of the extensor digiti minimi longus

T: 0.5–0.8 cun perpendicular; moxibustion

P: clears heat and expels wind, activates the channel and alleviates pain

A: 1. one-sided headache
2. one-sided paralysis and loss of sensation after apoplexy
3. foot pain
4. pain in the lumbar and abdominal regions

Pec: Shu (stream) point (3rd Shu-point), confluent point (Ba Mai Jiao Hui) of the Dai Mai

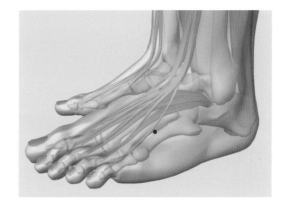

GB 42 Di Wu Hui Earth Five Meetings

L: on the dorsum of the foot, between the fourth and fifth metatarsal bones, proximal to the fourth metatarso-phalangeal joint, in the depression medial to the tendon of the extensor digiti minimi longus

T: 0.3–0.5 cun perpendicular; moxibustion

P: clears heat and expels wind, sharpens eyesight and hearing

A: 1. diseases of the ear, e.g. deafness, tinnitus
2. acute conjunctivitis

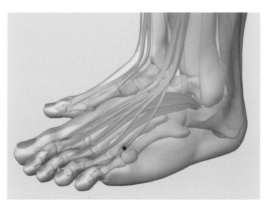

L: Location   T: Insertion Technique   P: Properties   A: Clinical Applications   Pec: Peculiarities

GB

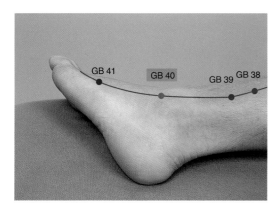

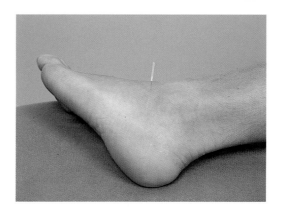

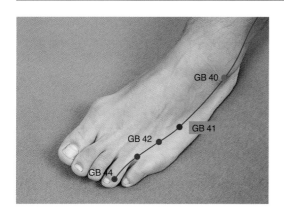

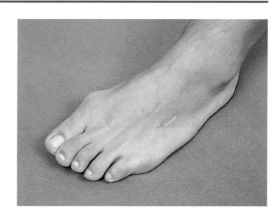

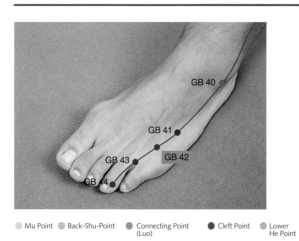

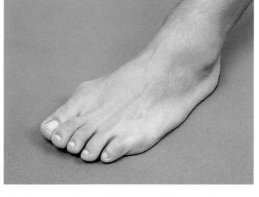

● Mu Point　● Back-Shu-Point　● Connecting Point (Luo)　● Cleft Point　● Lower He Point　● Qi-Source-Point (Yuan)　● Confluent Point　● Converging Point

GB

245

GB 43 Xia Xi   Clamped Stream

L: between the fourth and fifth metatarso-phalangeal joints, on the border of the interdigital skin between the fourth and fifth toes, on the dividing line between white and red flesh

T: 0.3–0.6 cun perpendicular; moxibustion

P: clears and drains liver and gall bladder

A: 1. hypertension
2. diseases of the ear, e.g. deafness, tinnitus
3. diseases of the gall bladder

Pec: Xing (spring) point (2nd Shu-point)

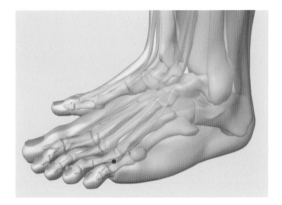

GB 44 Zu Qiao Yin   Yin Portals of the Foot

L: 1 cun proximal and lateral to the base and border of the nail of the fourth toe

T: 0.1 cun perpendicular; moxibustion

P: clears heat and alleviates pain, sharpens hearing and eyesight

A: 1. one-sided headache
2. certain acute inflammations of the eye
3. tinnitus

Pec: Jing (well) point (1st Shu-point)

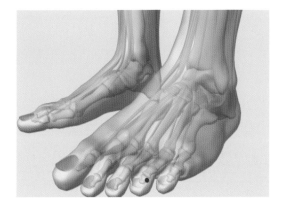

GB

L: Location   T: Insertion Technique   P: Properties   A: Clinical Applications   Pec: Peculiarities

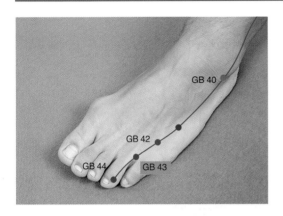

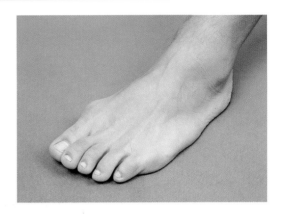

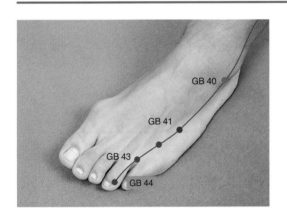

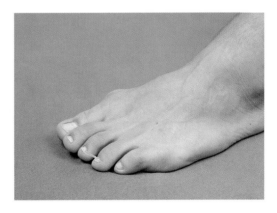

● Mu Point ● Back-Shu-Point ● Connecting Point (Luo) ● Cleft Point ● Lower He Point ● Qi-Source-Point (Yuan) ● Confluent Point ● Converging Point

GB

2.2.12   The liver channel (Lv)

Synonyms

• Liver Meridian

• Foot-Jueyin-Liver Channel

Channel pathway

There are 14 acupuncture points on the surface pathway of the liver channel.

The surface pathway of the channel originates at the outside corner and base of the nail of the big toe and ascends via the dorsum of the foot, between the first and second metatarsal bones, to the region in front of the inside ankle bone. From here the channel connects with Sp 6 and ascends via the centre of the inside of the shin bone. Below the knee the channel crosses behind the spleen channel and runs inside, past the knee over the central aspect of the inside of the upper leg, to the groin, where it passes over the points Sp 12 and Sp 13 before rounding the external genitalia and the pubic region over the abdomen in the region of the points Ren 3 and Ren 4. From here the surface pathway of the channel ascends to the ribcage at point Lv 13 and ends at point Lv 14 below the nipple.

The internal pathway of the channel originates at point Lv 14, where it connects with the liver and gall bladder. A branch traverses the diaphragm and ascends to the lung before descending through the diaphragm again to the epigastrium. Another branch runs cranially alongside the side of the ribcage, touching the larynx and pharynx, and ascends via the cheeks to the "eye system," that is the eyeball with all related structures. From here a branch ascends to the apex, and another descends to the corner of the mouth and circles the lips from within.

Lv

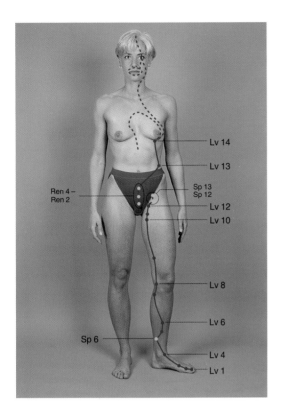

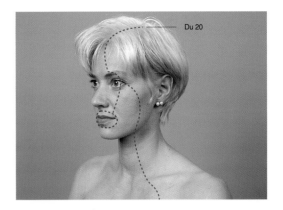

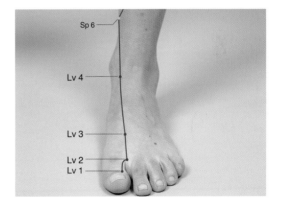

Lv

Lv 1 Da Dun Big Mound

L: 0.1 cun proximal to and lateral to the base and corner of the nail of the big toe

T: 0.1–0.2 cun oblique; prick to bleed; moxibustion

P: decongests the liver and regulates Qi, regulates menstruation and promotes urination

A: 1. external abdominal hernias
2. anovulatory dysfunctional uterine bleeding
3. diseases of the bladder, e.g. urinary retention, urinary incontinence, infections of the urinary tract (restores balance)

Pec: Jing (well) point (1st Shu-point)

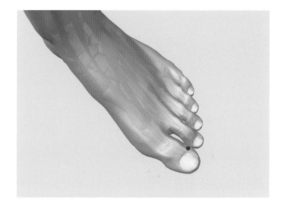

Lv 2 Xing Jian Moving Between

L: between the first and second metatarso-phalangeal joints, at the border of the interdigital skin between the first and second toe, at the dividing line between red and white flesh

T: 0.5–0.8 cun oblique; moxibustion

P: soothes the liver and expels wind, regulates menstruation and promotes urination

A: 1. hypertension
2. certain gynecological disorders, e.g. anovulatory dysfunctional uterine bleeding, dysmenorrhoea, amenorrhoea
3. diseases of the bladder, urinary incontinence
4. cerebro-vascular diseases, apoplexy

Pec: Xing (spring) point (2nd Shu-point)

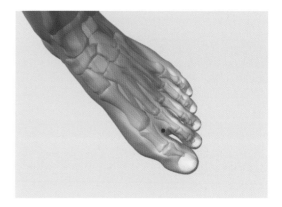

Lv 3 Tai Chong Great Rushing

L: on the dorsum of the foot, in the depression distal to the proximal corner between the first and second metatarsal bones

T: 0.5–0.8 cun perpendicular; moxibustion

P: soothes the liver and expels wind, decongests the liver and regulates Qi, strengthens the spleen, and transforms dampness

A: 1. hypertension
2. irregular menstruation
3. urinary incontinence, urinary retention
4. psychic and psychosomatic disorders, epileptic fits
5. pain and restricted movement in the lower extremity and the foot

Pec: Shu (stream) point (3rd Shu-point), Qi-source-point (Yuan)

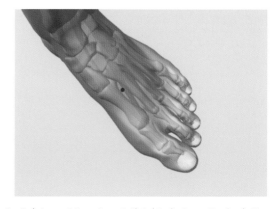

L: Location **T:** Insertion Technique **P:** Properties **A:** Clinical Applications **Pec:** Peculiarities

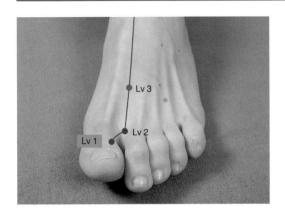

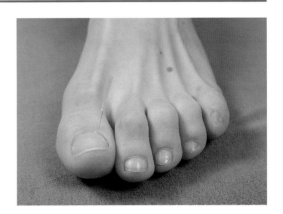

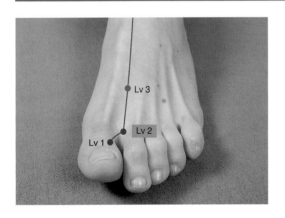

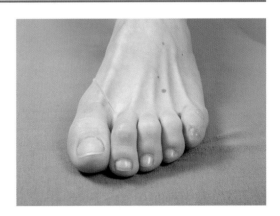

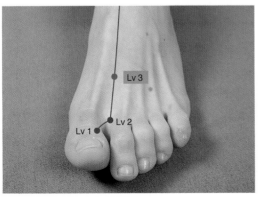

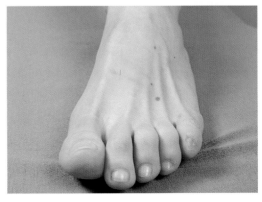

Lv

○ Mu Point ○ Back-Shu-Point ○ Connecting Point (Luo) ● Cleft Point ○ Lower He Point ● Qi-Source-Point (Yuan) ● Confluent Point ● Converging Point

Lv 4 Zhong Feng Middle Seal

L: ventral to the medial malleolus, on the connecting line between Sp 5 and St 41, in the depression medial to the anterior tibialis tendon

T: 0.5–0.8 cun perpendicular; moxibustion

P: decongests the liver and regulates Qi, activates the channel and alleviates pain

A: 1. external abdominal hernias
2. urinary retention, acute urinary infection
3. restricted movement and pain on the medial malleolus

Pec: Jing (river) point (4th Shu-point)

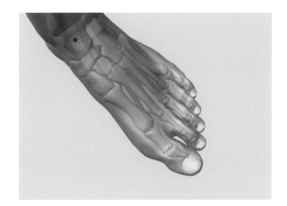

Lv 5 Li Gou Woodworm Canal

L: 5 cun proximal to the greatest prominence of the medial malleolus in the centre of the medial surface of the tibia

T: 0.5–0.8 cun subcutaneously; moxibustion

P: nourishes the blood and regulates menstruation, reduces edema and alleviates pain

A: 1. gynecological disorders, e.g. irregular menstruation, inflammation of the pelvis, uterine prolapse
2. acute inflammation of external male genitalia, scrotal hernias
3. pain in the lower leg

Pec: connecting point (Luo)

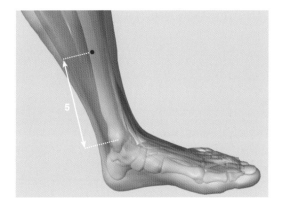

Lv 6 Zhong Du Central Capital

L: 7 cun proximal to the greatest prominence of the medial malleolus, in the centre of the medial surface of the tibia

T: 0.5–0.8 cun subcutaneously; moxibustion

P: nourishes and soothes the blood, mobilises Qi and alleviates pain

A: 1. anovulatory dysfunctional uterine bleeding
2. external abdominal hernias

Pec: cleft (Xi) point

Lv

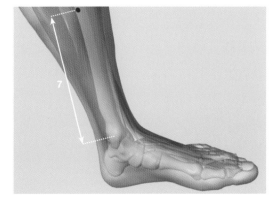

L: Location   T: Insertion Technique   P: Properties   A: Clinical Applications   Pec: Peculiarities

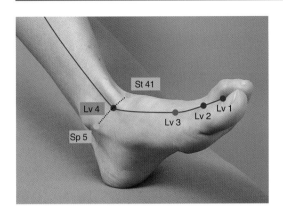

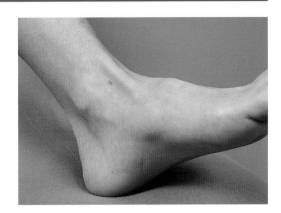

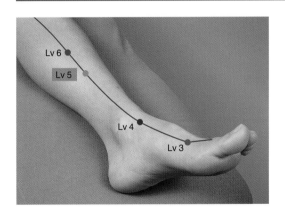

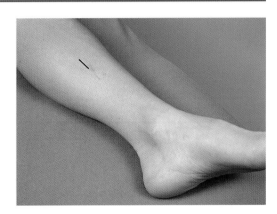

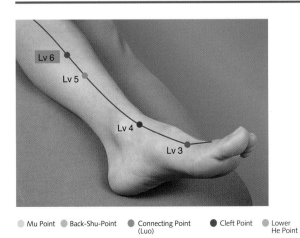

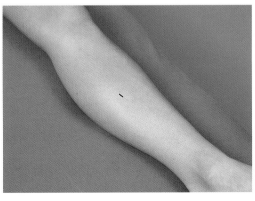

Lv

⬤ Mu Point　⬤ Back-Shu-Point　⬤ Connecting Point (Luo)　⬤ Cleft Point　⬤ Lower He Point　⬤ Qi-Source-Point (Yuan)　⬤ Confluent Point　⬤ Converging Point

Lv 7 Xi Guan   Knee Joint

L: dorsal and distal to the medial condyle of the tibia, 1 cun dorsal to Sp 9

T: 1–1.5 cun perpendicular; moxibustion

P: dispels wind and eliminates dampness, reduces edema and alleviates pain

A: 1. redness, swelling, and pain in the knee joint
2. restricted movement of the lower extremity

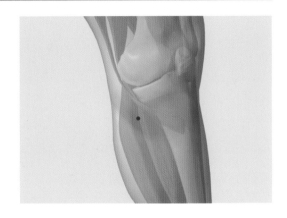

Lv 8 Qu Quan   Spring at the Crook

L: with the patient's knee flexed, at the medial end of the popliteal crease, dorsal to the medial condyle of the tibia, in the depression at the anterior border of the onset of the semi-membranosus and semi-tendinosus muscles

T: 1–1.5 cun perpendicular; moxibustion

P: regulates the liver and nourishes the blood, supports the kidney and expands the essence

A: 1. certain gynecological disorders, especially pruritus vulvae
2. male sexual dysfunction
3. pain and restricted movement of the knee joint and lower extremity

Pec: He (sea) point (5th Shu-point)

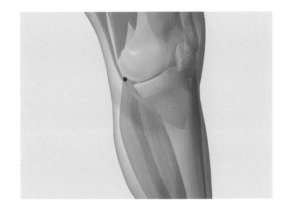

Lv 9 Yin Bao   Yin Wrapping

L: 4 cun proximal to the medial condyle of the tibia, between the vastus medialis and sartorius muscles

T: 1–1.5 cun perpendicular; moxibustion

P: regulates Qi, promotes urination

A: 1. urinary retention
2. irregular menstruation

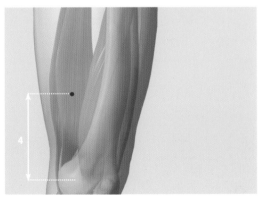
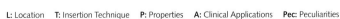

L: Location   T: Insertion Technique   P: Properties   A: Clinical Applications   Pec: Peculiarities

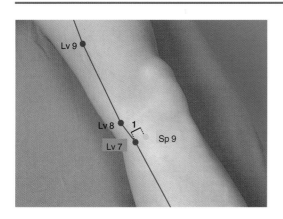

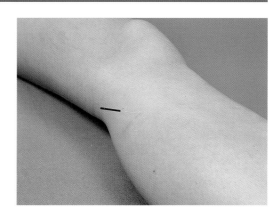

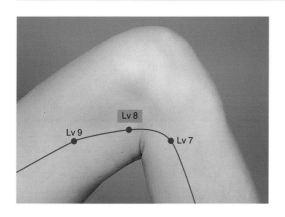

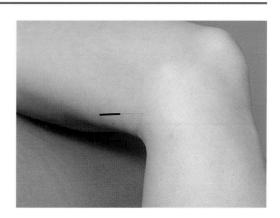

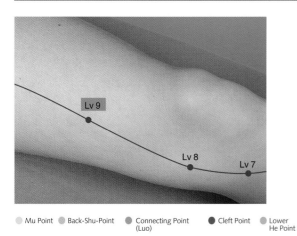

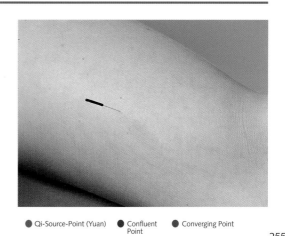

Lv

● Mu Point ● Back-Shu-Point ● Connecting Point (Luo) ● Cleft Point ● Lower He Point   ● Qi-Source-Point (Yuan) ● Confluent Point ● Converging Point

Lv 10 Zu Wu Li Leg Five Miles

L: 4 cun distal to the upper border of the pubic symphisis (St 30), at the edge of the M. adductor longus

T: 1–2 cun perpendicular; moxibustion

P: regulates Qi, promotes urination

A: 1. urinary retention
2. prostatitis, prostate adenoma

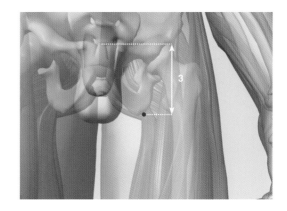

Lv 11 Yin Lian Yin Corner

L: 2 cun distal to the upper border of the pubic symphisis (St 30), at the edge of M. adductor longus

T: 1–2 cun perpendicular; moxibustion

P: regulates menstruation and promotes fertility

A: irregular menstruation, female fertility disorders

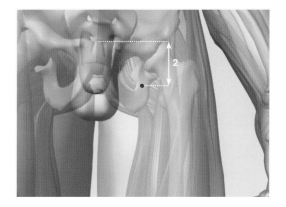

Lv 12 Ji Mai Urgent Pulse

L: lateral to the symphisis, 2.5 cun lateral to the ventral midline, lateral and distal to St 30, in the groin above the palpable femoral artery

T: 0.5–0.8 cun perpendicular above the palpable femoral artery; moxibustion

P: regulates Qi and alleviates pain

A: 1. srcotal hernias
2. orchitis

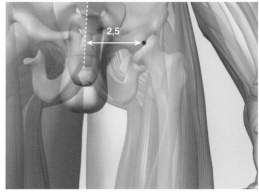

L: Location   T: Insertion Technique   P: Properties   A: Clinical Applications   Pec: Peculiarities

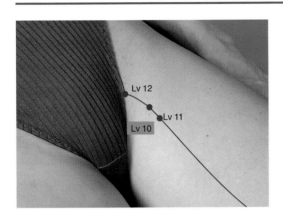

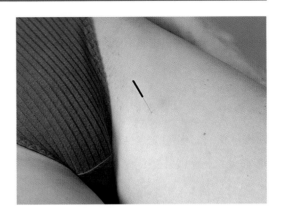

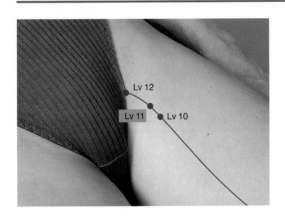

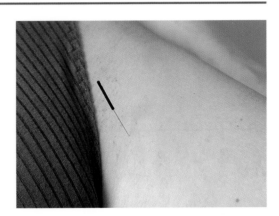

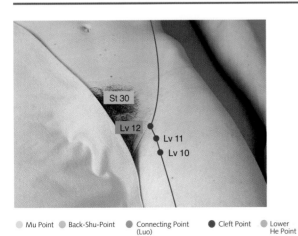

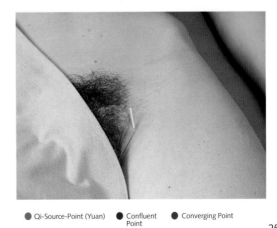

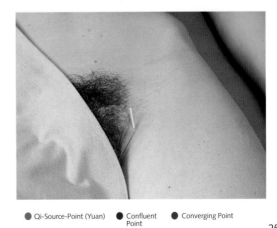

Lv

● Mu Point ● Back-Shu-Point ● Connecting Point (Luo) ● Cleft Point ● Lower He Point ● Qi-Source-Point (Yuan) ● Confluent Point ● Converging Point

Lv 13 Zhang Men   Completion Gate

L: the inferior border of the free end of the eleventh rib

T: 0.8–1 cun perpendicular;
moxibustion

P: strengthens the spleen and harmonizes the stomach,
eliminates tension and promotes the gall bladder

A: 1. acute and chronic gastroenteritis, chronic diarrhoea
2. acute and chronic cholecystitis
3. welling of the liver or spleen

Pec: Mu point of the spleen, meeting (master) point
(Hui) of the zhang (storage) organs

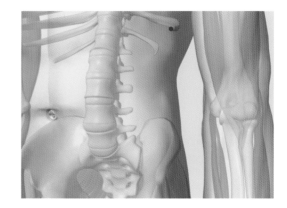

Lv 14 Qi Men   Cycle Gate

L: below the nipple in the sixth ICR, 4 cun lateral to the
ventral midline

T: 0.5–0.8 cun oblique or subcutaneously;
moxibustion

P: decongests the liver and strengthens the spleen,
harmonizes the stomach and descends inverted Qi

A: 1. liver disease, e.g. hepatitis, swelling of the liver
2. swelling of the spleen

Pec: Mu point of the liver
CAUTION, AVOID PNEUMOTHORAX!

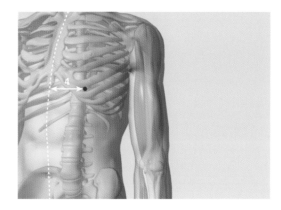

Lv

L: Location   T: Insertion Technique   P: Properties   A: Clinical Applications   Pec: Peculiarities

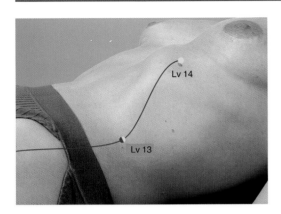

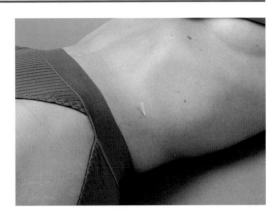

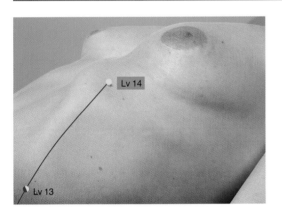

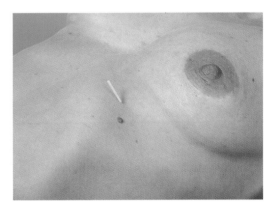

Lv

○ Mu Point ○ Back-Shu-Point ● Connecting Point (Luo) ● Cleft Point ○ Lower He Point ● Qi-Source-Point (Yuan) ● Confluent Point ● Converging Point

2.3 The Points of the Extraordinary Vessels Du Mai and Ren Ma

2.3.1 The Du Mai (Du)

Synonyms

• Governing Vessel
• Steering Channel

Channel Pathway

There are 28 acupuncture points on the surface pathway of the Du Mai.

The surface pathway of the Du Mai originates in the region of the uterus and lower abdomen, where the Ren Mai and Chong Mai also originate. In the region of the perineum, a mixture with the Qi of the kidney and bladder channels takes place. On the inside of the spine a branch leads to the kidney and from here ascends further alongside the inside of the spine to the apex, where it enters the brain.

A second branch ascends from the abdomen to the umbilicus and heart. It ascends further, via the region of the throat and pharynx, where contact is made with the Chong Mai and Ren Mai, to the lower jaw and inferior border of the eye socket. A further branch ascends from the inner canthus to the apex.

The surface pathway of the channel leads from the perineum region via point Du 1 at the coccyx and sacrum and the entire spine to the region of the neck. Under the posterior nape of the neck at point Du 16 a branch runs to the brain. At the skull, the channel further descends via the midline and nose and philtrum to the frenum of the upper lip.

Du

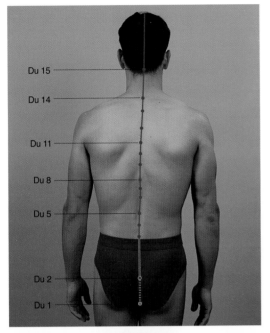

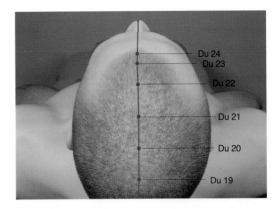

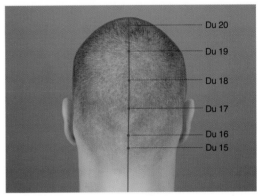

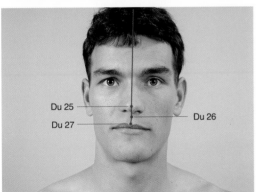

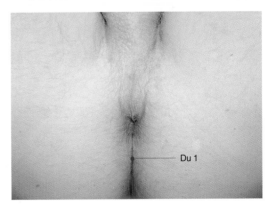

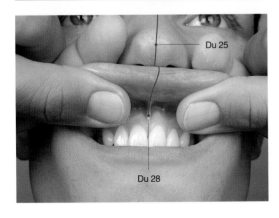

Du

Du 1 Chang Qiang Long Strong

L: on the midline, in the centre between the tip of the coccyx and the anus

T: 0.5–0.8 cun ventrally from the coccyx; moxibustion

P: pacifies the spirit and suppresses cramp, promotes defecation and eliminates hemorrhoids

A: 1. psychic and psychosomatic disorders, epileptic fits (sedative effect)
   2. constipation
   3. hemorrhoids

Pec: connecting point (Luo)

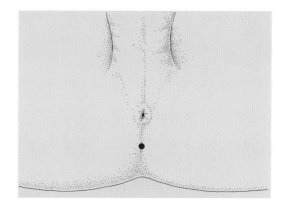

Du 2 Yao Shu Lumbar Shu

L: on the dorsal midline directly in the sacral hiatus

T: 0.5–1 cun oblique cranially; moxibustion

P: activates the channel and alleviates pain

A: pain in the lumbo-sacral region

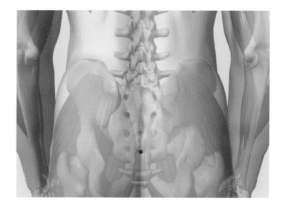

Du 3 Yao Yyang Guan Lumbar Yang Gate

L: on the dorsal midline, in the depression below spinous process L4

T: 0.5–1 cun oblique cranially; moxibustion

P: decongests and activates the channel and its vessels

A: 1. pain in the lumbo-sacral region
   2. pain and loss of strength in the lower extremities

Pec: CAUTION IN PREGNANCY!

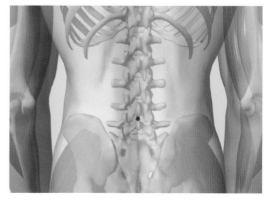

Du

L: Location   T: Insertion Technique   P: Properties   A: Clinical Applications   Pec: Peculiarities

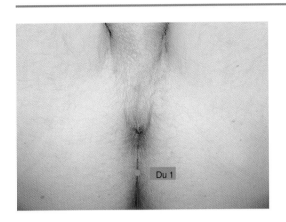

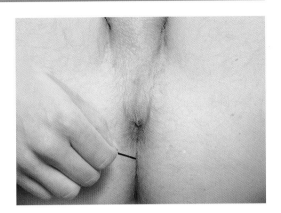

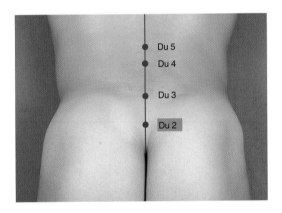

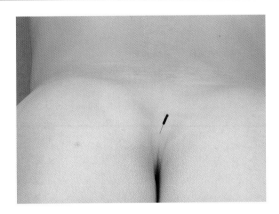

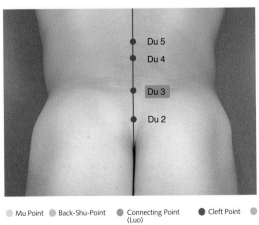

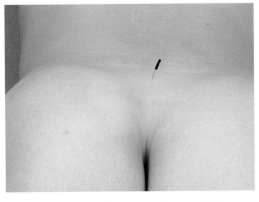

Du

● Mu Point   ● Back-Shu-Point   ● Connecting Point (Luo)   ● Cleft Point   ● Lower He Point   ● Qi-Source-Point (Yuan)   ● Confluent Point   ● Converging Point

263

Du 4 Ming Men Gate of Life

L: on the dorsal midline, in the depression below
spinous process L2

T: 0.5–1 cun oblique cranially;
moxibustion

P: warms and replenishes the kidney yang, relaxes the
tendons and suppresses cramp

A: 1. male sexual dysfunction, e.g. impotence
2. certain gynecological and obstetric disorders
3. epileptic fits
4. lumbalgia

Pec: CAUTION IN PREGNANCY!

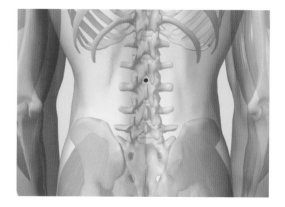

Du 5 Xuan Shu Suspended Pivot

L: on the dorsal midline, in the depression below
spinous process L1

T: 0.5–1 cun oblique cranially;
moxibustion

P: promotes the yang and strengthens the spleen

A: chronic enteritis, diarrhoea in digestive disorders

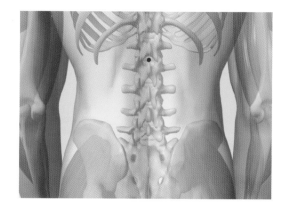

Du 6 Ji Zhong Centre of the Spine

L: on the dorsal midline in the depression below
spinous process Th11

T: 0.5–1 cun oblique cranially;
moxibustion

P: strengthens the spleen, promotes urination, pacifies
the spirit, and suppresses cramp

A: 1. chronic enteritis
2. hemorrhoids
3. epileptic fits (cramp-releasing function)

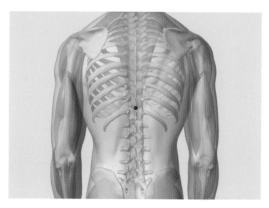

Du

L: Location   T: Insertion Technique   P: Properties   A: Clinical Applications   Pec: Peculiarities

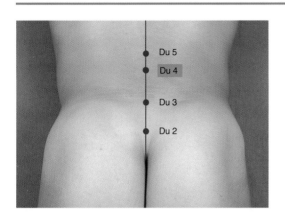

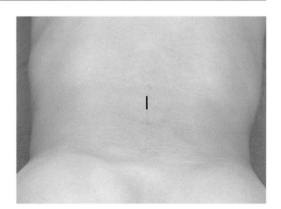

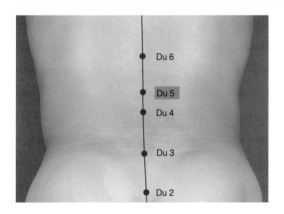

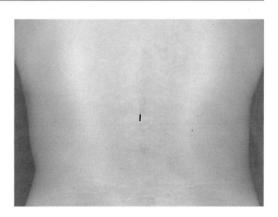

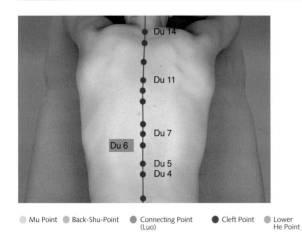

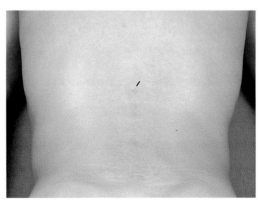

Du

⬤ Mu Point ⬤ Back-Shu-Point ⬤ Connecting Point (Luo) ⬤ Cleft Point ⬤ Lower He Point ⬤ Qi-Source-Point (Yuan) ⬤ Confluent Point ⬤ Converging Point

Du 7 Zhong Shu Central Pivot

L: on the dorsal midline, in the depression below
spinous process Th10

T: 0.5–1 cun oblique cranially;
moxibustion

P: strengthens the spleen, promotes urination

A: 1. loss of appetite
2. back pain

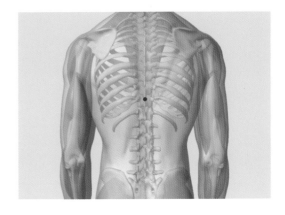

Du 8 Jin Suo Sinew Contraction

L: on the dorsal midline, in the depression below
spinous process Th9

T: 0.5–1 cun oblique cranially;
moxibustion

P: pacifies the spirit and suppresses cramp

A: psychic and psychosomatic disorders, epileptic fits,
fever cramps (sedative and cramp-releasing effect)

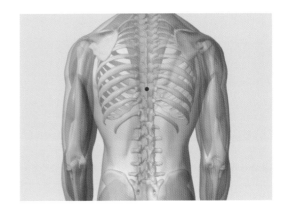

Du 9 Zhi Yang Reaching Yang

L: on the dorsal midline, in the depression below
spinous process Th7

T: 0.5–1 cun oblique cranially;
moxibustion

P: benefits the gall bladder and treats jaundice,
regulates Qi and unbinds the chest

A: 1. jaundice in diseases of the liver and gall bladder
2. feeling of tension, fullness or swelling of the
thorax and abdomen
3. acute mastitis

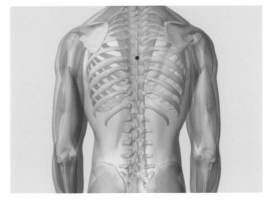

Du

L: Location   T: Insertion Technique   P: Properties   A: Clinical Applications   Pec: Peculiarities

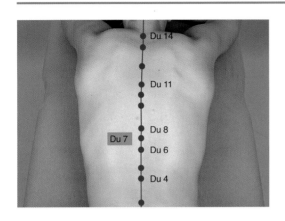

Du 14
Du 11
Du 8
Du 7
Du 6
Du 4

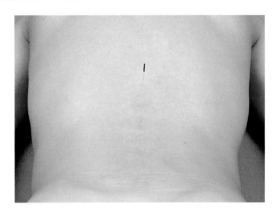

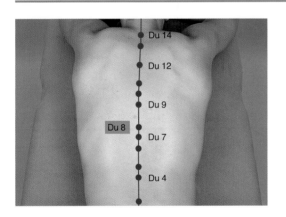

Du 14
Du 12
Du 9
Du 8
Du 7
Du 4

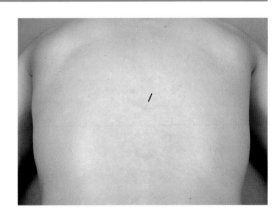

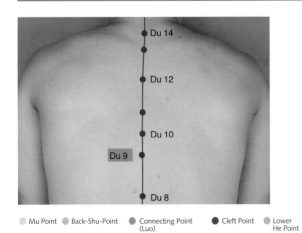

Du 14
Du 12
Du 10
Du 9
Du 8

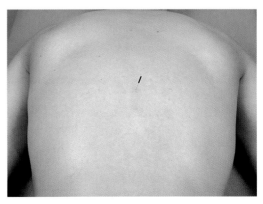

Du

● Mu Point ● Back-Shu-Point ● Connecting Point (Luo) ● Cleft Point ● Lower He Point ● Qi-Source-Point (Yuan) ● Confluent Point ● Converging Point

Du 10 Ling Tai Spirit Tower

L: on the dorsal midline, in the depression below spinous process Th6

T: 0.5–1 cun oblique cranially; moxibustion

P: alleviates coughing and breathing difficulty

A: 1. acute and chronic bronchitis
2. pain in the spine

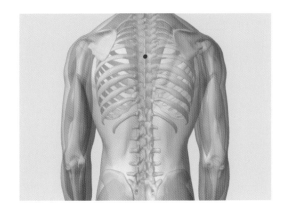

Du 11 Shen Dao Spirit Pathway

L: on the dorsal midline, in the depression below spinous process Th5

T: 0.5–1 cun oblique cranially; moxibustion

P: dispels wind and clears heat, pacifies the spirit and alleviates breathing difficulty

A: 1. neurasthenia
2. bronchial asthma

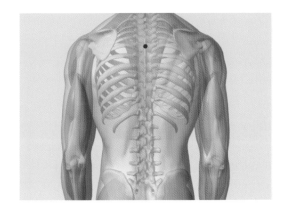

Du 12 Shen Zhu Body Pillar

L: on the dorsal midline, in the depression below spinous process Th3

T: 0.5–1 cun oblique cranially; moxibustion

P: pacifies the spirit and releases cramp, clears heat and extends lung Qi

A: 1. psychic and psychosomatic disorders, epileptic fits, fever cramps (sedative and cramp-releasing effect)
2. "colds," bronchitis

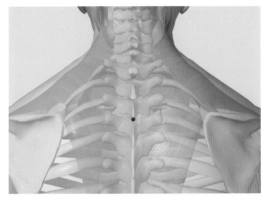

Du

L: Location   T: Insertion Technique   P: Properties   A: Clinical Applications   Pec: Peculiarities

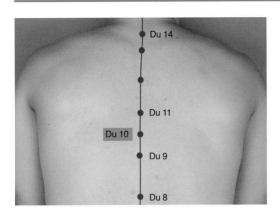

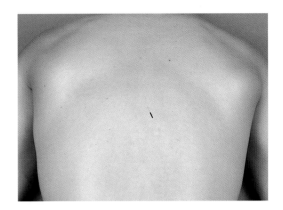

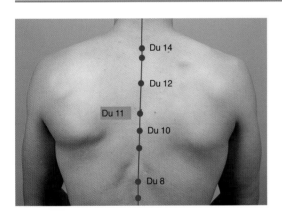

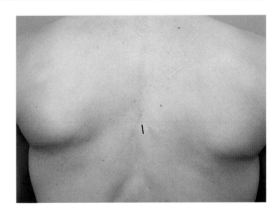

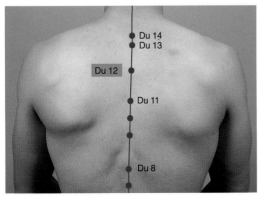

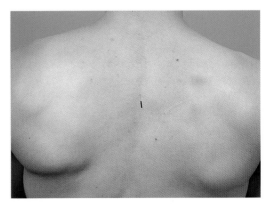

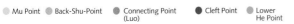

○ Mu Point   ○ Back-Shu-Point   ○ Connecting Point (Luo)   ● Cleft Point   ○ Lower He Point   ● Qi-Source-Point (Yuan)   ● Confluent Point   ● Converging Point

Du

Du 13 Tao Dao   Way of Happiness

L: on the dorsal midline, in the depression below spinous process Th1

T: 0.5–1 cun oblique cranially; moxibustion

P: clears heat and liberates the surface

A: "colds," influenza

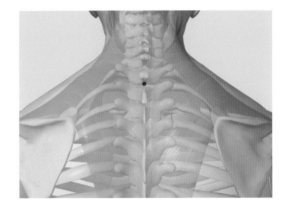

Du 14 Da Zhui   Great Vertebra

L: on the dorsal midline, in the depression below spinous process C7

T: 0.5–1 cun oblique cranially; moxibustion

P: clears heat and liberates the surface, generates all-round calmness and stops falling fever

A: 1. high, constant fever
2. "colds," influenza
3. disorders of the cervical-spinal column
4. epilepsy

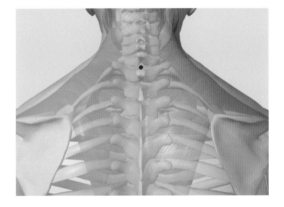

Du 15 Ya Men   Gate of Dumbness

L: on the dorsal midline, 0.5 cun cranial to the midpoint of the posterior hairline below C1

T: 0.2–0.5 cun perpendicular or oblique caudally; deep and cranial needle insertion prohibited; moxibustion

P: restores clarity to the brain and opens the senses, disseminates and expels wind

A: 1. sudden loss of voice, deaf-and-dumbness
2. apoplexy
3. epilepsy

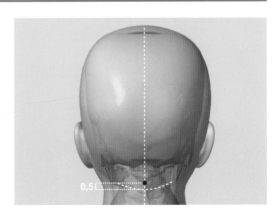

Du

L: Location   T: Insertion Technique   P: Properties   A: Clinical Applications   Pec: Peculiarities

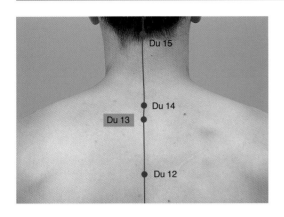

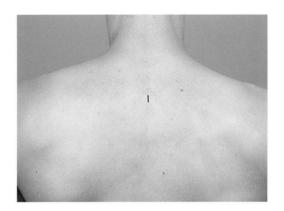

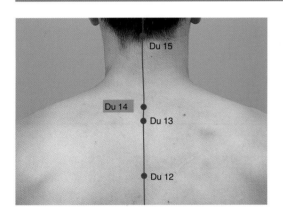

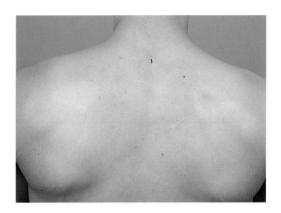

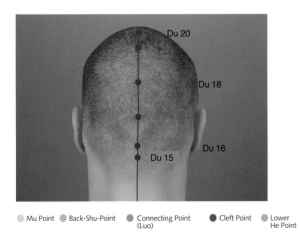

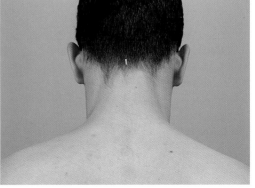

Du

● Mu Point   ● Back-Shu-Point   ● Connecting Point (Luo)   ● Cleft Point   ● Lower He Point   ● Qi-Source-Point (Yuan)   ● Confluent Point   ● Converging Point

271

Du 16 Feng Fu   Palace of Wind

L: on the dorsal midline, 1 cun within the midpoint of the posterior hairline, below the external occipital protuberance, in the gap between the right and left trapezius muscles

T: 0.5–1 cun perpendicular or oblique caudally; deep and cranial needle insertion prohibited; moxibustion

P: restores clarity to the brain and opens the senses, expels wind and releases cramp

A: 1. apoplexy
2. severe neck headache
3. agitation disorders

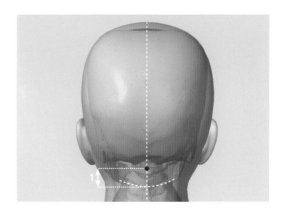

Du 17 Nao Hu   Brain's Door

L: on the dorsal midline, 2.5 cun within the midpoint of the posterior hairline, 1.5 cun cranial to Du 16, in the depression at the superior border of the external occipital protuberance

T: 0.5–0.8 cun subcutaneously; moxibustion

P: restores clarity to the brain and opens the senses, soothes the liver and expels wind

A: 1. psychic and psychosomatic disorders
2. hypertension

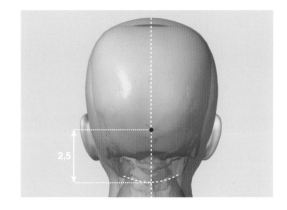

Du 18 Qiang Jian   Unyielding Space

L: on the dorsal midline, 4 cun within the midpoint of the posterior hairline, 1.5 cun cranial to Du 17

T: 0.5–0.8 cun subcutaneously; moxibustion

P: restores clarity to the brain and opens the senses, soothes the liver and expels wind

A: 1. psychic and psychosomatic disorders
2. hypertension
3. Parkinson's disease

Du

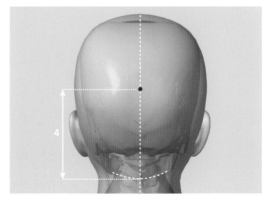

L: Location   T: Insertion Technique   P: Properties   A: Clinical Applications   Pec: Peculiarities

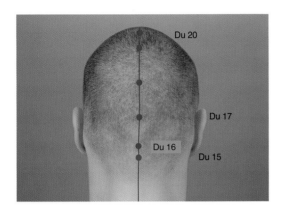
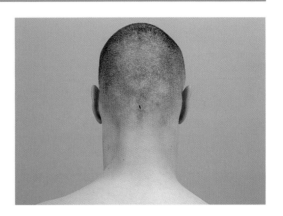

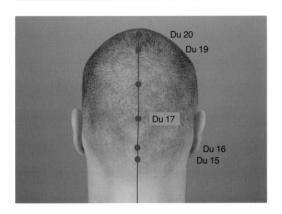
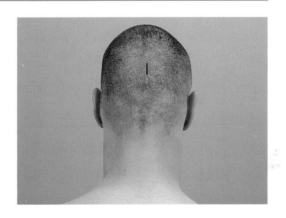

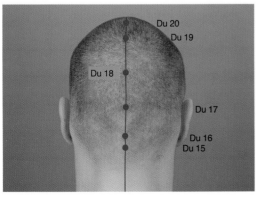
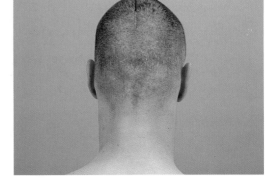

Du

⬤ Mu Point ⬤ Back-Shu-Point ⬤ Connecting Point (Luo) ⬤ Cleft Point ⬤ Lower He Point ⬤ Qi-Source-Point (Yuan) ⬤ Confluent Point ⬤ Converging Point

Du 19 Hou Ding Behind the Crown

L: on the dorsal midline, 5.5 cun within the midpoint of the posterior hairline, 3 cun cranial to Du 17

T: 0.5–0.8 cun subcutaneously; moxibustion

P: soothes the liver and expels wind, pacifies the spirit and releases cramps

A: 1. hypertension
2. psychic and psychosomatic disorders, epileptic fits (sedative and cramp-releasing effect)

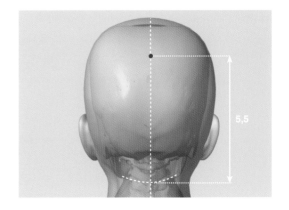

Du 20 Bai Hui Hundred Meetings

L: on the dorsal midline, 5.0 cun within the midpoint of the ideal anterior hairline, at the midpoint between the two auricular apices

T: 0.5–0.8 cun subcutaneously; moxibustion; prick to bleed

P: soothes the liver and expels wind, pacifies the spirit and releases cramps

A: 1. apoplexy
2. headache, dizziness, and numbness
3. anal and rectal prolapse
4. uterine prolapse

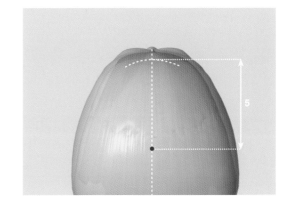

Du 21 Qian Ding In Front of the Crown

L: on the dorsal midline, 3.5 cun within the midpoint of the ideal anterior hairline, 1.5 cun frontal to Du 20

T: 0.5–0.8 cun subcutaneously; moxibustion

P: pacifies the spirit and releases cramps, soothes the liver and expels wind,

A: 1. depressive disorders, epileptic fits
2. hypertension

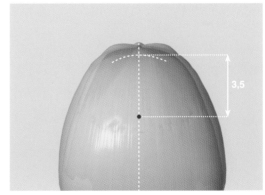

Du

L: Location T: Insertion Technique P: Properties A: Clinical Applications Pec: Peculiarities

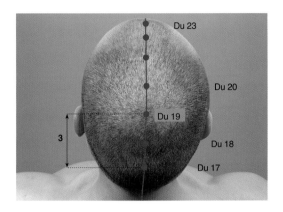

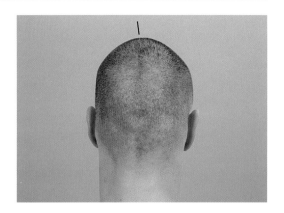

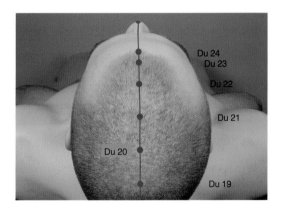

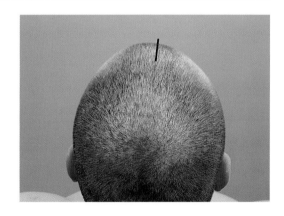

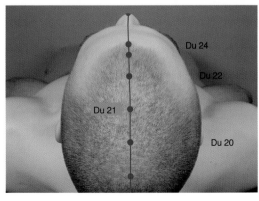

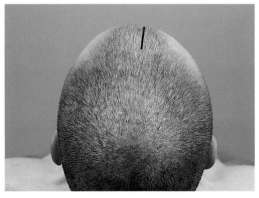

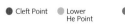

Mu Point   Back-Shu-Point   Connecting Point (Luo)   ● Cleft Point   Lower He Point   ● Qi-Source-Point (Yuan)   ● Confluent Point   ● Converging Point

Du

Du 22 Xin Hui Fontanelle meeting

L: on the midline, 2 cun within the midpoint of the ideal anterior hairline, 3 cun frontal to Du 20

T: 0.5–0.8 cun subcutaneously; moxibustion

P: pacifies the spirit and releases cramps, expels wind and alleviates pain

A: 1. epileptic fits
2. headache

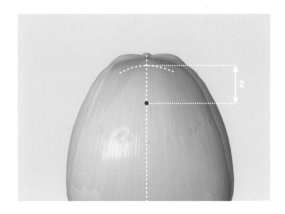

Du 23 Shang Xing Upper Star

L: on the midline, 1 cun within the midpoint of the ideal anterior hairline

T: 0.5–0.8 cun subcutaneously; moxibustion

P: strengthens the brain and regulates the spirit, alleviates pain and activates the upper body orifices

A: 1. apoplexy
2. headache
3. psychic and psychosomatic disorders
4. diseases of the nose, e.g. epistaxis, sinusitis

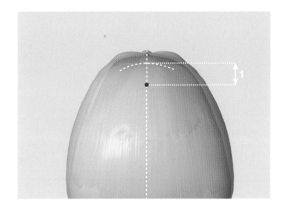

Du 24 Shen Ting Courtyard of the Spirit

L: on the midline, 0.5 cun within the midpoint of the ideal anterior hairline

T: 0.5–0.8 cun subcutaneously; moxibustion

P: promotes general calmness and pacifies the spirit, alleviates pain and opens the senses

A: 1. psychic and psychosomatic disorders, neurasthenia, insomnia (sedative effect)
2. apoplexy
3. headache

Du

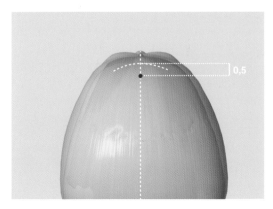

L: Location   T: Insertion Technique   P: Properties   A: Clinical Applications   Pec: Peculiarities

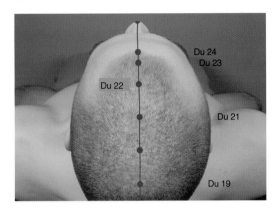

Du 24
Du 23
Du 22
Du 21
Du 19

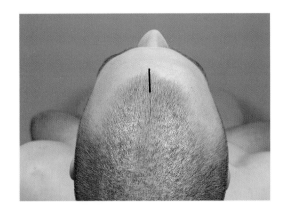

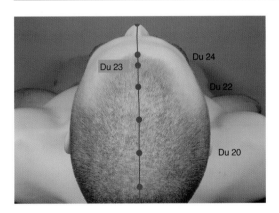

Du 24
Du 23
Du 22
Du 20

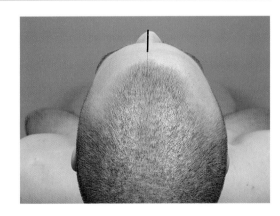

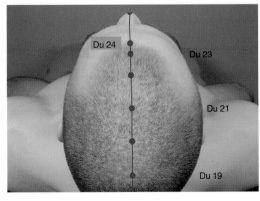

Du 24
Du 23
Du 21
Du 19

○ Mu Point   ○ Back-Shu-Point   ○ Connecting Point (Luo)   ● Cleft Point   ○ Lower He Point   ● Qi-Source-Point (Yuan)   ● Confluent Point   ● Converging Point

Du

Du 25 Su Liao   White Crevice

L: in the midpoint of the tip of the nose

T: 0.3–0.5 cun oblique cranially;
no moxibustion

P: restores the Yang and arrests inverted Qi, activates
the nose

A: 1. diseases of the nose, e.g. rhinitis, epistaxis, nasal
polyps
2. hypotonia also in states of shock

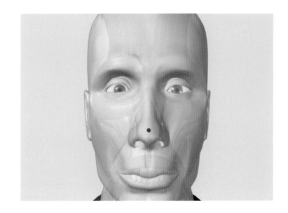

Du 26 Shui Gou   Water Ditch

L: on the ventral midline, at the dividing line between
the upper and middle thirds of the philtrum

T: 0.3–0.5 cun oblique cranially;
moxibustion

P: restores clarity to the brain and opens the senses,
expels wind and releases cramp

A: 1. apoplexy
2. loss of consciousness, syncopic states
(complementary or emergency measure)
3. psychic and psychosomatic disorders, epileptic fits,
fever cramps (sedative and cramp-releasing effect)
4. acute lumbalgia

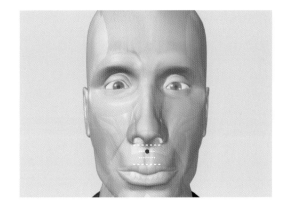

Du 27 Dui Duan   Extremity of the Mouth

L: on the ventral midline, on the tuberculum of the
upper lip, at the junction between the philtrum and
the red of the lip

T: 0.2–0.3 cun oblique cranially;
no moxibustion

P: pacifies the spirit and releases cramp

A: 1. epilepsy
2. tic disorders of the mouth

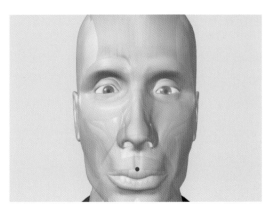

Du

L: Location   T: Insertion Technique   P: Properties   A: Clinical Applications   Pec: Peculiarities

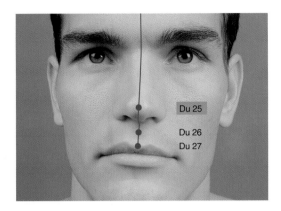

Du 25

Du 26
Du 27

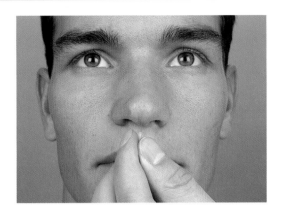

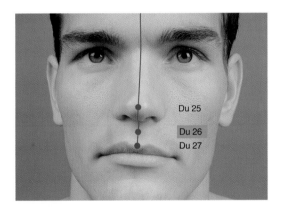

Du 25

Du 26
Du 27

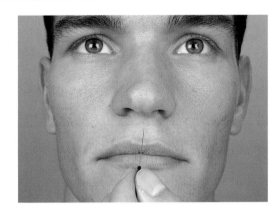

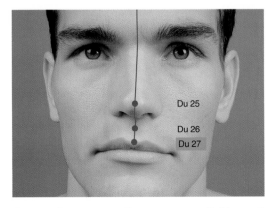

Du 25

Du 26

Du 27

Du

Mu Point ○ Back-Shu-Point ○ Connecting Point (Luo) ○ ● Cleft Point ○ Lower He Point ● Qi-Source-Point (Yuan) ● Confluent Point ● Converging Point

Du 28 Yin Jiao   Gum Intersection

L: on the ventral midline, on the inside of the upper lip, at the junction between the frenum of the upper lip and the gum

T: 0.2–0.3 cun oblique cranially; prick to bleed; no moxibustion

P: clears heat and reduces edema

A: 1. acute inflammations of the mouth cavity, e.g. acute pulpitis, acute parodonitis, stomatitis aphthosa

2. diseases of the nose, e.g. nasal polyps, rhinitis

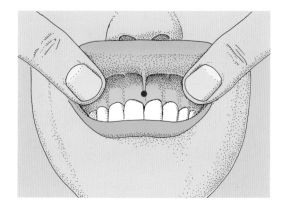

Du

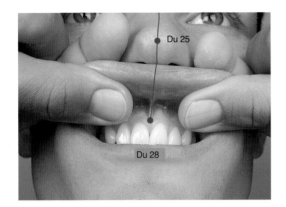

Du 25

Du 28

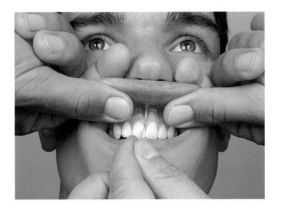

Mu Point   Back-Shu-Point   Connecting Point (Luo)   Cleft Point   Lower He Point   Qi-Source-Point (Yuan)   Confluent Point   Converging Point

2.3.2   Ren Mai (Ren)

Synonyms

• Conception Vessel

• Intake Channel

Channel pathway

There are 24 acupuncture points on the surface pathway of the Ren Mai.

The inner pathway of the Ren Mai originates at the uterus and the lower abdomen, where the Du Mai and Chong Mai also have their origins. The inner pathway intersects with the kidney channel and the Du Mai, and ascends with the other two channels internally alongside the spine. From the source region the Ren Mai runs to the perineum region.

The surface pathway of the Ren Mai begins at the region of the perineum at point Ren 1. The vessel ascends alongside the anterior midline via the lower abdomen, umbilicus, upper abdomen, ensiform process, and sternum to the jugular fossa. The Ren Mai traverses the midline in the region of the trachea and the larynx, where there is contact with the Chong Mai, to the chin dimple. Together with the Chong Mai, branches from the region of the chin encircle the lips and ascend to the area below the eye socket.

Ren

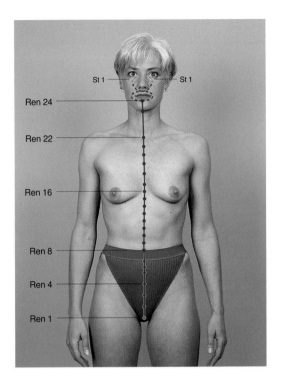

St 1 — St 1
Ren 24 —
Ren 22 —
Ren 16 —
Ren 8 —
Ren 4 —
Ren 1 —

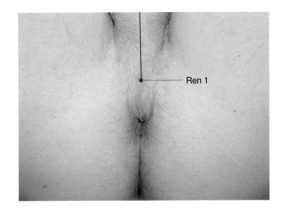

— Ren 1

Ren

Ren 1 Hui Yin   Meeting of Yin

L: on the midline, at the midpoint between the anus and the dorsal commisure of the major labia, or the posterior border of the scrotum

T: 0.5–1 cun perpendicular; moxibustion

P: restores clarity to the spirit and opens the senses

A: 1. movement disorders
2. psychic and psychosomatic disorders

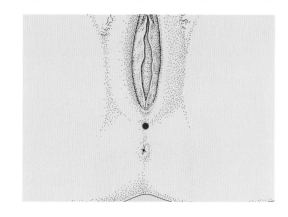

Ren 2 Qu Gu   Curved Bone

L: on the ventral midline, at the midpoint of the superior border of the pubic symphysis

T: 0.5–1 cun perpendicular; moxibustion

P: promotes urination and activates the urinary tract, regulates menstruation and alleviates pain

A: 1. diseases of the urinary tract, e.g. urinary retention, acute and chronic infections of the urinary tract, urinary incontinence
2. gynecological disorders, e.g. irregular menstruation, leucorrhoea, dysmenorrhoea
3. male sexual dysfunction

Pec: CAUTION IN PREGNANCY!

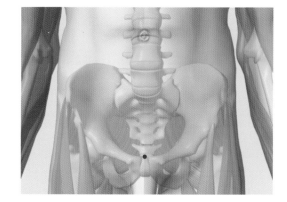

Ren 3 Zhong Ji   Middle Pole

L: on the ventral midline, 4 cun below the umbilicus, 1 cun above Ren 2

T: 0.5–1 cun perpendicular; moxibustion

P: helps the Yang and orders water, regulates menstruation and alleviates discharge

A: 1. male sexual dysfunction
2. diseases of the bladder, e.g. urinary retention, urinary incontinence
3. gynecological and obstetric disorders

Pec: Mu point of the bladder
CAUTION IN PREGNANCY!

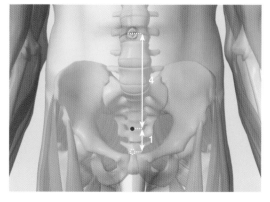

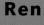
Ren

L: Location   T: Insertion Technique   P: Properties   A: Clinical Applications   Pec: Peculiarities

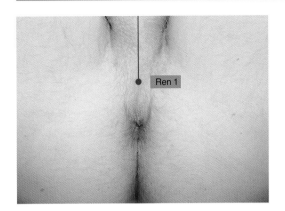

Ren 1

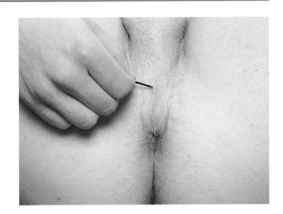

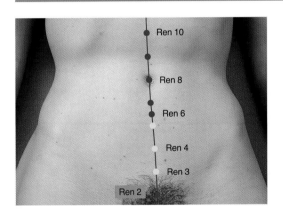

Ren 10

Ren 8

Ren 6

Ren 4

Ren 3

Ren 2

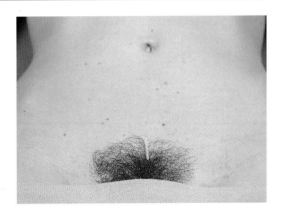

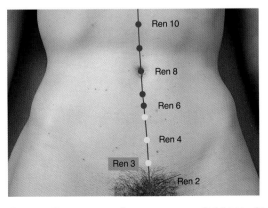

Ren 10

Ren 8

Ren 6

Ren 4

Ren 3

Ren 2

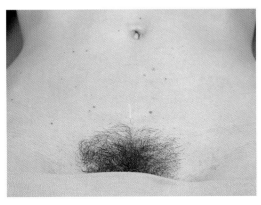

Ren

● Mu Point   ● Back-Shu-Point   ● Connecting Point (Luo)   ● Cleft Point   ● Lower He Point   ● Qi-Source-Point (Yuan)   ● Confluent Point   ● Converging Point

285

Ren 4 Guan Yuan Gate of Origin

L: on the ventral midline, 3 cun below the umbilicus, 2 cun above Ren 2

T: 1–2 cun perpendicular; moxibustion

P: expands and replenishes source Qi, regulates menstruation and promotes urination

A: 1. all states of weakness (strengthens the body and health)
2. diseases of the urinary tract, e.g. infections of the urinary tract, urinary retention, urinary incontinence
3. male sexual dysfunction, e.g. prostatitis
4. gynecological and obstetric disorders

Pec: Mu point of the small intestine
CAUTION IN PREGNANCY!

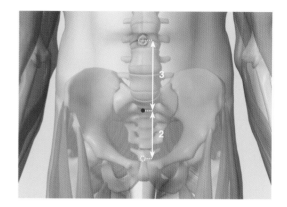

Ren 5 Shi Men Stone Gate

L: on the ventral midline, 2 cun below the umbilicus, 3 cun above Ren 2

T: 1–2 cun perpendicular; moxibustion

P: regulates Qi and alleviates pain, activates urination

A: 1. chronic enteritis, chronic dysentery
2. urinary retention
3. certain gynecological disorders, e.g. anovulatory dysfunctional uterine bleeding, amenorrhoea, post-partum bleeding

Pec: Mu point of the Sanjiao
CAUTION IN PREGNANCY!

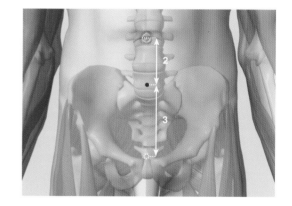

Ren 6 Qi Hai Sea of Qi

L: on the ventral midline, 1.5 cun below the umbilicus

T: 1–2 cun perpendicular; moxibustion

P: increases and regulates Qi, regulates menstruation, and strengthens essence

A: 1. all states of weakness (strengthens the organism and the immune function)
2. many gynecological disorders
3. male sexual disorder

Pec: CAUTION IN PREGNANCY!

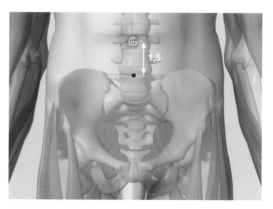

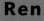
Ren

L: Location   T: Insertion Technique   P: Properties   A: Clinical Applications   Pec: Peculiarities

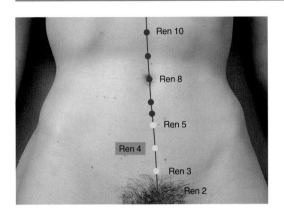
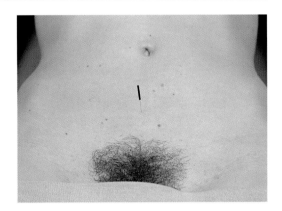

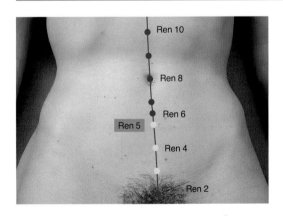
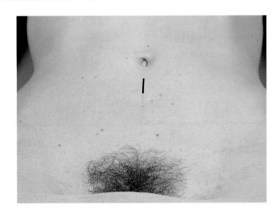

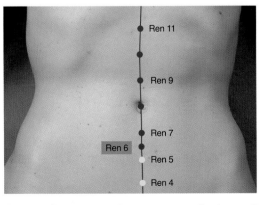
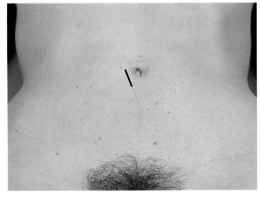

Ren

⬤ Mu Point ⬤ Back-Shu-Point ⬤ Connecting Point (Luo) ⬤ Cleft Point ⬤ Lower He Point ⬤ Qi-Source-Point (Yuan) ⬤ Confluent Point ⬤ Converging Point

Ren 7 Yin Jiao   Yin Intersection

L: on the ventral midline, 1 cun below the umbilicus

T: 1–2 cun perpendicular;
moxibustion

P: regulates menstruation and alleviates discharge,
mobilises Qi and alleviates essence

A: 1. certain gynecological disorders, e.g. irregular
menstruation
2. abdominal pains, feeling of abdominal tension,
swelling, and fullness

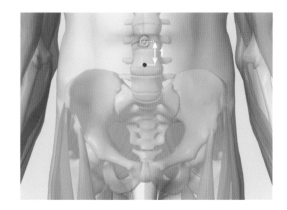

Ren 8 Shen Que   Spirit Gateway

L: in the umbilicus

T: no acupuncture;
moxibustion only

P: warms the yang, promotes urination, alleviates
diarrhoea, and firms prolapse conditions

A: 1. acute and chronic enteritis, periumbilical pains
2. ascites
3. anal and rectal prolapse

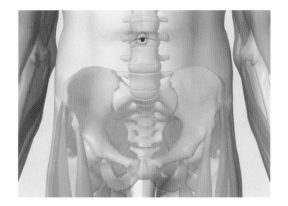

Ren 9 Shui Fen   Water Separation

L: on the ventral midline, 1 cun above the umbilicus

T: 1–2 cun perpendicular;
moxibustion

P: harmonizes the urinary system, regulates Qi, and
alleviates pain

A: 1. ascites, edemas
2. abdominal pain and diarrhoea in chronic
gastroenteritis

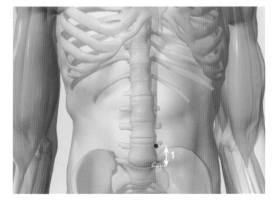

Ren

L: Location   **T:** Insertion Technique   **P:** Properties   **A:** Clinical Applications   **Pec:** Peculiarities

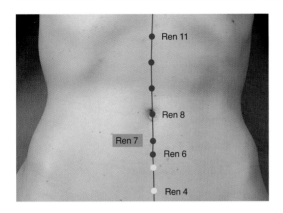

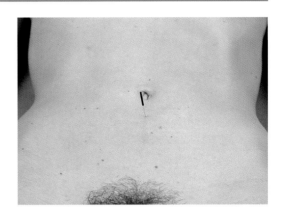

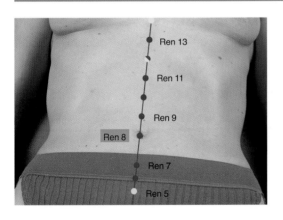

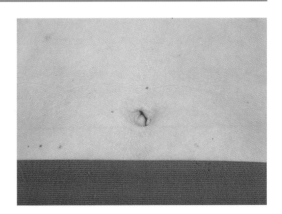

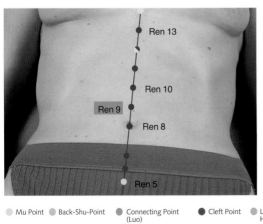

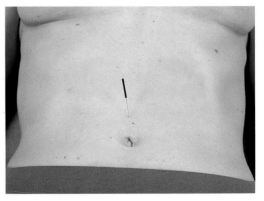

Ren

● Mu Point ● Back-Shu-Point ● Connecting Point (Luo) ● Cleft Point ● Lower He Point   ● Qi-Source-Point (Yuan) ● Confluent Point ● Converging Point

Ren 10 Xia Wan Lower Cavity

L: on the ventral midline, 2 cun above the umbilicus

T: 1–2 cun perpendicular;
moxibustion

P: strengthens the spleen and harmonizes the stomach,
alleviates nausea and diarrhoea

A: 1. acute and chronic gastroenteritis, diarrhoea in
digestive disorders
2. hiccups

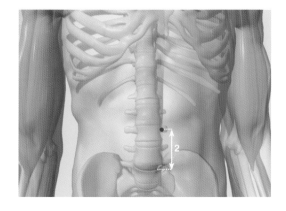

Ren 11 Jian Li Strenghten the Interior

L: on the ventral midline, 3 cun above the umbilicus

T: 1–2 cun perpendicular;
moxibustion

P: strengthens the spleen and harmonizes the centre,
restores balance to stomach and intestine

A: 1. stomach pains and chronic gastritis
2. gastric ulcers

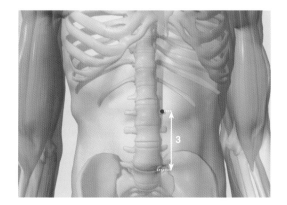

Ren 12 Zhong Wan Middle Cavity

L: on the ventral midline, 4 cun above the umbilicus

T: 1–1.5 cun perpendicular;
moxibustion

P: harmonizes the stomach and strengthens the spleen,
activates and descends Fu (palace) organ Qi

A: 1. acute and chronic gastroenteritis
2. gastric ulcers, stomach pains
3. acute and chronic cholecystitis, acute and chronic
cholelithiasis
4. hiccups

Pec: Mu point of the stomach, meeting (master) point
(Hui) of the Fu (palace) organs

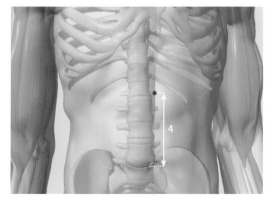

Ren

L: Location   T: Insertion Technique   P: Properties   A: Clinical Applications   Pec: Peculiarities

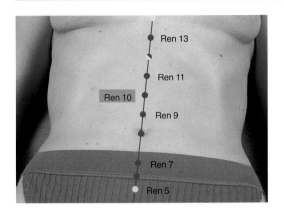

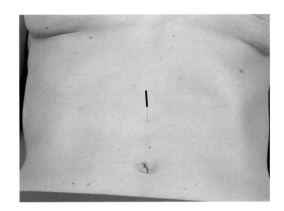

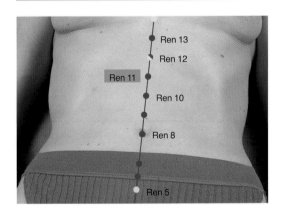

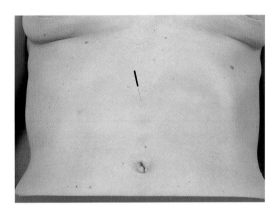

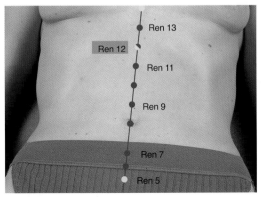

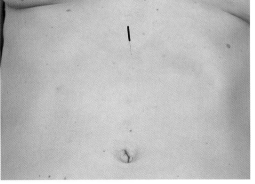

Ren

Mu Point   Back-Shu-Point   Connecting Point (Luo)   Cleft Point   Lower He Point   Qi-Source-Point (Yuan)   Confluent Point   Converging Point

Ren 13 Shang Wan   Upper Cavity

L: on the ventral midline, 5 cun above the umbilicus

T: 1–1.5 cun perpendicular;
moxibustion

P: harmonizes the stomach and descends inverted Qi

A: 1. acute and chronic gastritis
2. stomach pains
3. hiccups

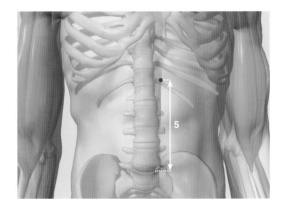

Ren 14 Ju Que   Great Gateway

L: on the ventral midline, 6 cun above the umbilicus

T: 0.5–1 cun oblique caudally;
moxibustion

P: pacifies the spirit and soothes the heart, unbinds the chest and alleviates pain

A: 1. coronary heart disease, pectoral angina, heartbeat disorders
2. psychic and psychosomatic disorders, epilepsy (sedative and cramp-releasing effect)

Pec: Mu point of the heart

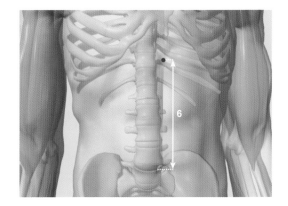

Ren 15 Jiu Wei   Turtledove Tail

L: on the ventral midline, 7 cun above the umbilicus, 1 cun below the xiphoid process

T: 0.4–0.6 cun oblique caudally;
moxibustion

P: soothes the heart and pacifies the spirit

A: 1. psychic and psychosomatic disorders, epilepsy
2. pains, itching of the abdominal skin

Pec: connecting point (Luo)

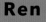

Ren

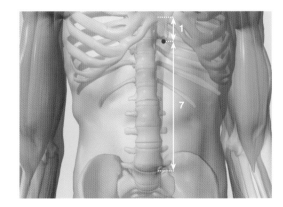

L: Location   T: Insertion Technique   P: Properties   A: Clinical Applications   Pec: Peculiarities

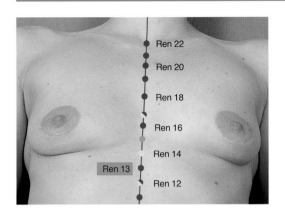

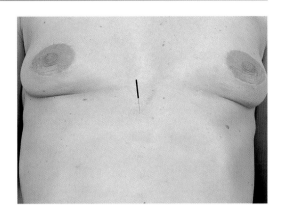

Ren 22
Ren 20
Ren 18
Ren 16
Ren 14
Ren 13
Ren 12

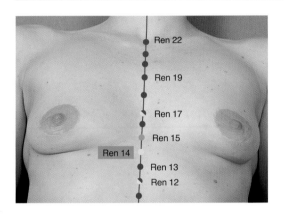

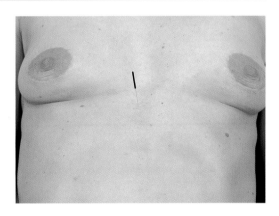

Ren 22
Ren 19
Ren 17
Ren 15
Ren 14
Ren 13
Ren 12

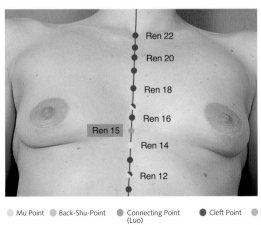

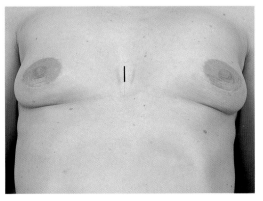

Ren 22
Ren 20
Ren 18
Ren 16
Ren 15
Ren 14
Ren 12

Ren

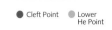

● Mu Point ● Back-Shu-Point ● Connecting Point (Luo) ● Cleft Point ● Lower He Point   ● Qi-Source-Point (Yuan) ● Confluent Point ● Converging Point

293

Ren 16 Zhong Ting   Central Courtyard

L: on the ventral midline, at the midpoint of the
xiphsternal joint

T: 0.3–0.5 cun subcutaneously;
moxibustion

P: unbinds the chest and descends inverted Qi

A: 1. precordial pain
2. nausea and vomiting in diseases of the stomach
and the gullet

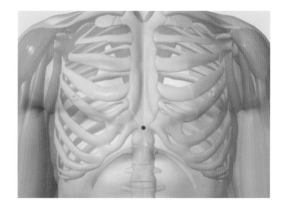

Ren 17 Dan Zhong   Chest Centre

L: on the ventral midline, at the level of the fourth ICR,
at the midpoint between the nipples

T: 0.3–0.5 cun subcutaneously caudally;
moxibustion

P: unbinds the chest and regulates Qi, alleviates pain,
and soothes breathing difficulty

A: 1. coronary heart disease
2. bronchial asthma, spastic bronchitis
3. insufficient lactation

Pec: Mu point of the pericardium, meeting (master)
point (Hui) of the Qi

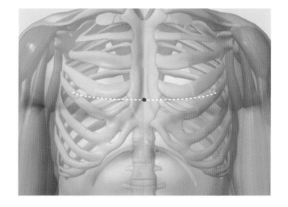

Ren 18 Yu Tang   Jade Hall

L: on the ventral midline, at the level of the third ICR

T: 0.3–0.5 cun subcutaneously;
moxibustion

P: unbinds the chest and alleviates pain, alleviates
coughing and soothes breathing difficulty

A: 1. pectoral angina in coronary heart disease
2. bronchial asthma, spastic bronchitis

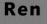
Ren

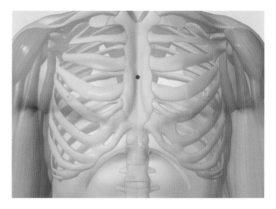

L: Location   T: Insertion Technique   P: Properties   A: Clinical Applications   Pec: Peculiarities

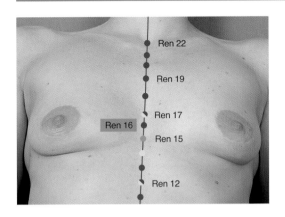

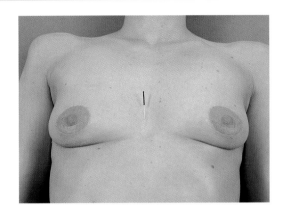

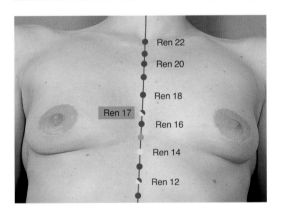

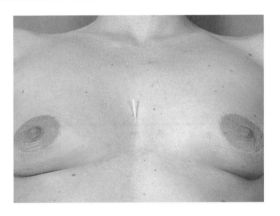

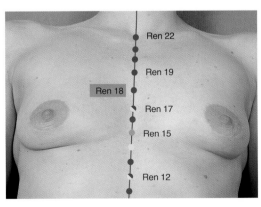

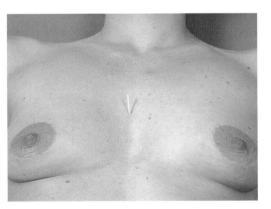

Ren

● Mu Point ● Back-Shu-Point ● Connecting Point (Luo) ● Cleft Point ● Lower He Point   ● Qi-Source-Point (Yuan) ● Confluent Point ● Converging Point

Ren 19 Zi Gong Purple Palace

L: on the ventral midline, at the level of the second ICR

T: 0.3–0.5 cun subcutaneously;
moxibustion

P: unbinds the chest and regulates Qi, alleviates coughing and soothes breathing difficulty

A: 1. bronchial asthma, spastic bronchitis
2. acute tonsillitis
3. diseases of the gullet

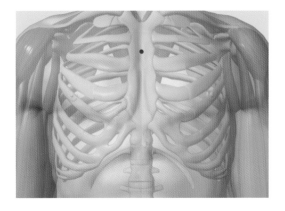

Ren 20 Hua Gai Magnificent Canopy

L: on the ventral midline, at the level of the first ICR, at the midpoint of the manubriosternal synchondrosis (angulus sterni)

T: 0.3–0.5 cun subcutaneously;
moxibustion

P: unbinds the chest and regulates Qi, alleviates coughing and soothes breathing difficulty

A: 1. bronchial asthma, spastic bronchitis
2. pectoral angina in coronary heart disease

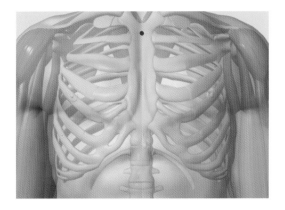

Ren 21 Xuan Ji Jade Pivot

L: on the ventral midline, 1 cun below Ren 22, at the midpoint of the sternal manubrium

T: 0.3–0.5 cun subcutaneously;
moxibustion

P: unbinds the chest and regulates Qi, alleviates coughing and soothes breathing difficulty

A: 1. dull, retrosternal pain in coronary heart disease
2. bronchial asthma
3. acute laryngitis, pharyngitis, tonsillitis

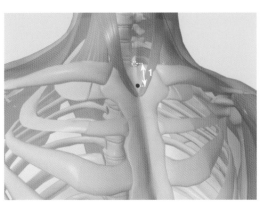

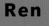
Ren

L: Location   T: Insertion Technique   P: Properties   A: Clinical Applications   Pec: Peculiarities

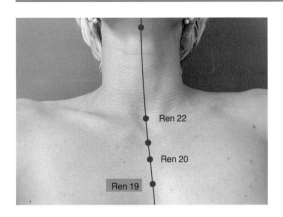

Ren 22
Ren 20
Ren 19

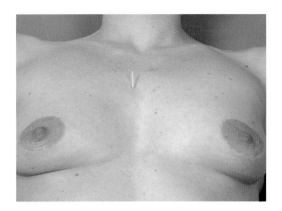

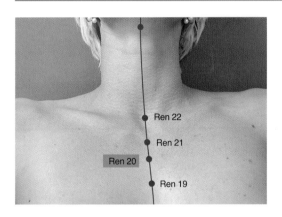

Ren 22
Ren 21
Ren 20
Ren 19

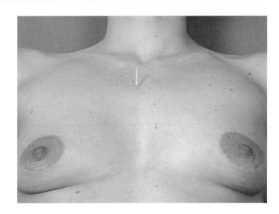

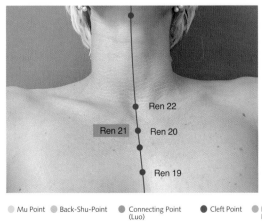

Ren 22
Ren 21
Ren 20
Ren 19

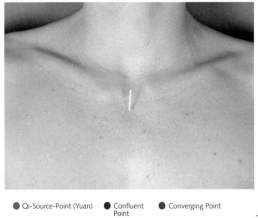

Ren

○ Mu Point ○ Back-Shu-Point ○ Connecting Point (Luo) ● Cleft Point ○ Lower He Point ● Qi-Source-Point (Yuan) ● Confluent Point ● Converging Point

297

Ren 22 Tian Tu   Heavenly Prominence

L: in the middle of the suprasternal fossa

T: 0.2 cun perpendicular, then 1–1.5 cun dorsal to the sternal manubrium caudally; moxibustion

P: activates lung and stomach Qi, descends inverted Qi and alleviates nausea

A: 1. diseases of the respiratory tract, e.g. bronchial asthma
2. anchone
3. sudden loss of voice

Pec: CAUTION, AVOID SPREADING GERMS TO THE MEDIASTINUM!

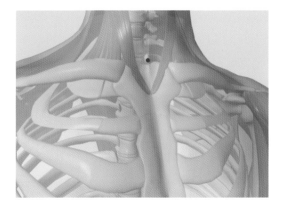

Ren 23 Lian Quan   Corner Spring

L: on the ventral midline, in the depression superior to the hyoid bone

T: 0.5–0.8 cun oblique, towards the base of the tongue; moxibustion

P: relieves the throat and regulates the tongue

A: 1. acute inflammations of the tissue at the base of the tongue
2. speech disorders after apoplexy
3. pseudobulbar paralysis

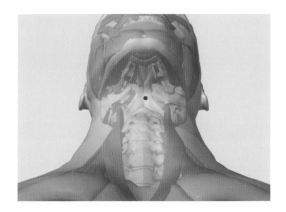

Ren 24 Cheng Jiang   Container of Fluids

L: on the ventral midline, in the middle of the mentolabial groove

T: 0.3–0.5 cun oblique or perpendicular; moxibustion

P: decongests and activates the channel and its vessels, reduces edema and alleviates pain

A: 1. facial pareses
2. acute toothache, pulpitis, parodontitis
3. facial edemas

Pec: symptomatic point for the suppression of the gagging reflex

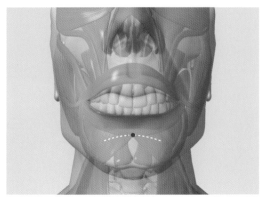

Ren

L: Location   T: Insertion Technique   P: Properties   A: Clinical Applications   Pec: Peculiarities

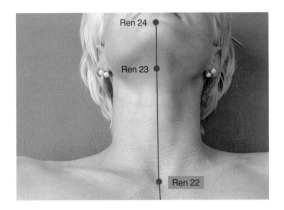

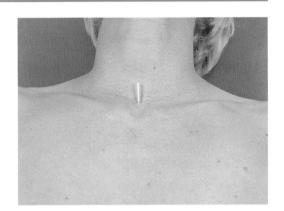

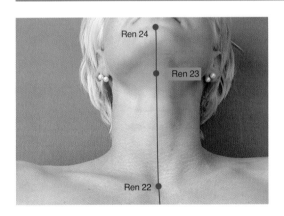

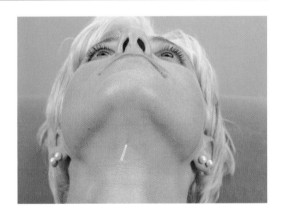

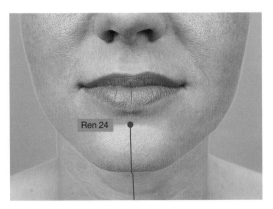

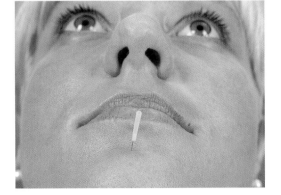

Ren

● Mu Point   ● Back-Shu-Point   ● Connecting Point (Luo)   ● Cleft Point   ● Lower He Point   ● Qi-Source-Point (Yuan)   ● Confluent Point   ● Converging Point

2.4 Further Acupuncture Points (Extraordinary Points)

Extraordinary points are acupuncture points, most of which tend to lie outside the channels and are, therefore, not classified as channels. Their synonyms are "Points outside the Channels" and "Points outside the Meridians" (PoM), "New Points" (NP) or "Additional Points." Various authors and schools have named a large number of extraordinary points that are then classified in different systems. The selection in this atlas comprises the 48 most important generally recognised points. As a result, the numbering and naming of such points deviates somewhat from the authorised standard work published in the People's Republic of China, *The Acupuncture Points*.

In keeping with the current convention the Extraordinary Points will be classified according to the five body regions Head/Neck, Chest/Abdomen, Back, Arm/Hand (upper extremity) and Leg/Foot (lower extremity).

- Extraordinary Points on the Head and Neck   Ex-HN
- Extraordinary Points on the Chest and Abdomen Ex-CA
- Extraordinary Points on the Back   Ex-B
- Extraordinary Points on the Arm and Hand   Ex-AH
- Extraordinary Points on the Leg and Foot   Ex-LF

2.4.1 Extraordinary points on the head and neck (Ex-HN)

Location

The 15 Extraordinary Points on the Head and Neck are located both below and above the hairline and on the nasal mucous membrane and tongue.

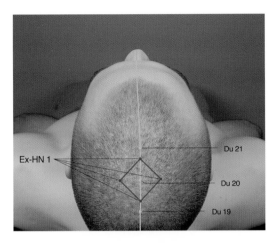

Ex-HN 1

Du 21

Du 20

Du 19

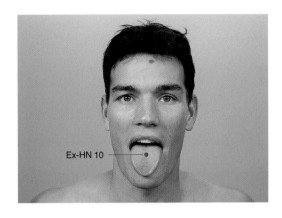

Ex-HN 10

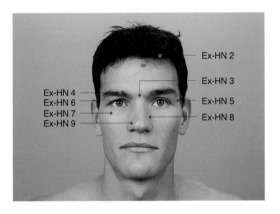

Ex-HN 2

Ex-HN 3

Ex-HN 4
Ex-HN 6
Ex-HN 7
Ex-HN 9

Ex-HN 5

Ex-HN 8

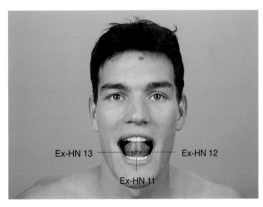

Ex-HN 13

Ex-HN 12

Ex-HN 11

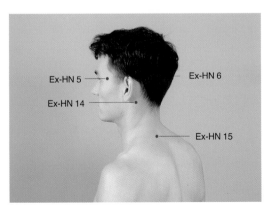

Ex-HN 5

Ex-HN 6

Ex-HN 14

Ex-HN 15

Ex-HN 1 Si Shen Cong Four Alert Spirit

L: four points at the vertex of the scalp, 1 cun anterior, posterior, and lateral to Du 20

T: 0.5–0.8 cun subcutaneously toward Du 20

P: pacifies the heart and spirit, sharpens eyesight and hearing

A: 1. headache, dizziness, and numbness
2. psychic and psychosomatic disorders, epilepsy, insomnia (sedative and cramp-releasing effect)
3. apoplexy

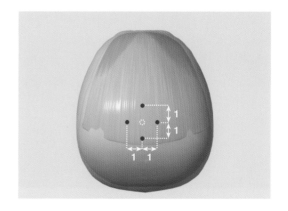

Ex-HN 2 Dang Yang Toward the Yang

L: with the patient staring directly ahead, directly above the pupil, 1 cun within the ideal anterior hairline

T: 0.5–0.8 cun subcutaneously

P: expels wind and clears heat, sharpens eyesight and eliminates dimness of vision

A: 1. "colds," influenza
2. diseases of the eye

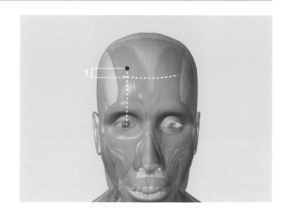

Ex-HN 3 Yin Tang Hall of Impression

L: on the ventral midline, between the eyebrows

T: 0.3–0.5 cun subcutaneously; moxibustion

P: expels wind and alleviates pain, sharpens eyesight and activates the upper body extremities

A: 1. headache, dizziness, and numbness
2. diseases of the eye
3. diseases of the nose, e.g. allergic rhinitis, "blocked nose," sinusitis

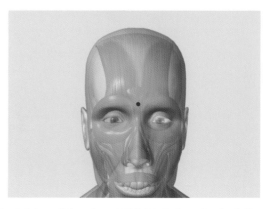

L: Location   T: Insertion Technique   P: Properties   A: Clinical Applications   Pec: Peculiarities

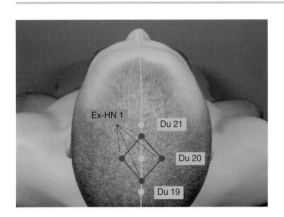

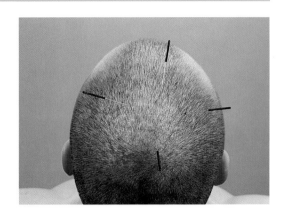

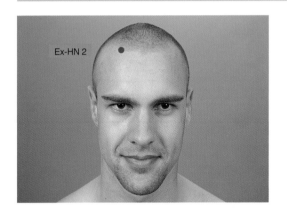

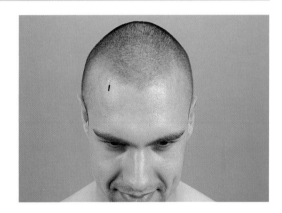

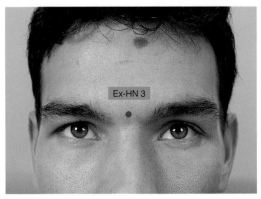

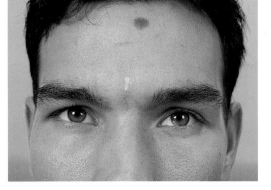

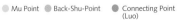

● Mu Point ● Back-Shu-Point ● Connecting Point (Luo) ● Cleft Point ● Lower He Point

● Qi-Source-Point (Yuan) ● Confluent Point ● Converging Point

Ex-HN

Ex-HN 4 Yu Yao Fish Waist

L: with the patient staring straight ahead, directly above the pupil, in the eyebrow

T: 0.3–0.5 cun subcutaneously

P: sharpens eyesight and reduces edema, relaxes the tendons and activates the vessels

A: 1. diseases of the eye
2. tic disorders of the eye
3. oculomotor paresis

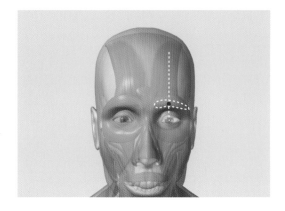

Ex-HN 5 Tai Yang Supreme Yang

L: in the depression approximately one middle finger with dorsal to the midpoint between the lateral border of the eyebrow and the outside corner of the lid

T: 0.3–0.5 cun perpendicular or oblique; prick to bleed

P: clears heat and reduces edema, alleviates pain and activates the vessels

A: 1. all forms of headache
2. acute inflammation of the eye
3. trigeminal neuralgia
4. facial paresis

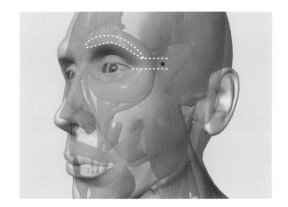

Ex-HN 6 Er Jian Ear Tip

L: with the patient's ear folded laterally, at the auricular apex

T: prick to bleed only;
moxibustion

P: clears heat and alleviates pain, sharpens eyesight, and reduces edema

A: 1. all forms of headache
2. acute inflammation of the eye
3. epidemic parotitis

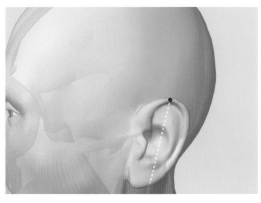

L: Location **T:** Insertion Technique **P:** Properties **A:** Clinical Applications **Pec:** Peculiarities

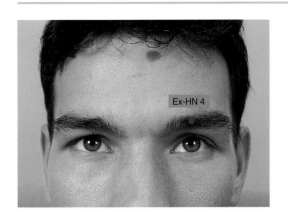

Ex-HN 4

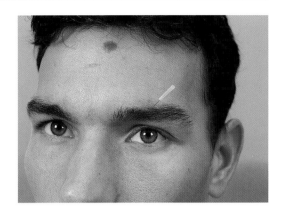

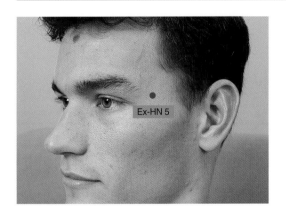

Ex-HN 5

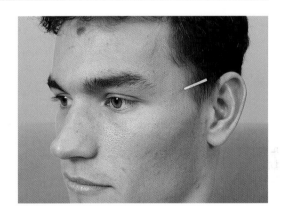

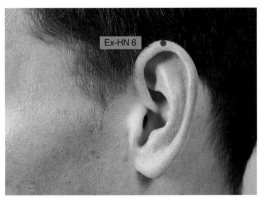

Ex-HN 6

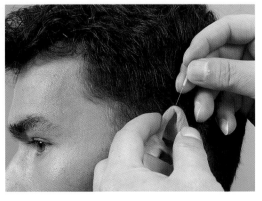

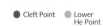

● Mu Point ● Back-Shu-Point ● Connecting Point (Luo) ● Cleft Point ● Lower He Point ● Qi-Source-Point (Yuan) ● Confluent Point ● Converging Point

305

Ex-HN 7 Qiu Hou   Behind the Ball

L: at the intersection of the lateral to the next quarter of the inferior border of the orbit

T: push pupil carefully upwards, 0.5–1 cun perpendicular directly along the inferior border of the orbit; no needle manipulation

P: sharpens eyesight and improves dim eyesight

A: diseases of the eye

Pec: CAUTION, AVOID SPREADING GERMS TO THE ORBIT!

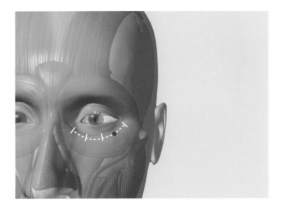

Ex-HN 8 Shang Ying Xiang; also: Bi Tong   Upper LI 20 (Penetrating the Nose)

L: at the superior end of the nasolabial fold, at the junction between the nose bone and nose cartilage, above LI 20

T: 0.3–0.5 cun subcutaneously cranially and medially

P: clears heat and expels wind, sharpens eyesight and activates the upper body orifices

A: 1. sties, acute conjunctivitis
2. diseases of the nose

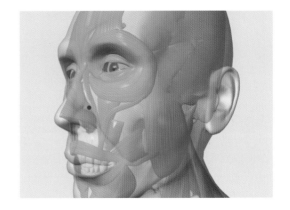

Ex-HN 9 Nei Ying Xiang   Inner LI 20

L: inside the nostril in the mucous membrane, at the junction between the nostril cartilage and the nose muscle

T: prick to bleed only

P: expels wind and clears heat, opens the senses and restores clarity to the brain

A: 1. sudden loss of consciousness (complementary or emergency measure)
2. headache attacks

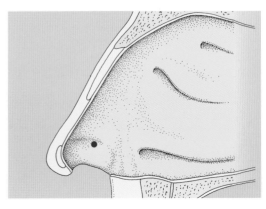

L: Location   **T:** Insertion Technique   **P:** Properties   **A:** Clinical Applications   **Pec:** Peculiarities

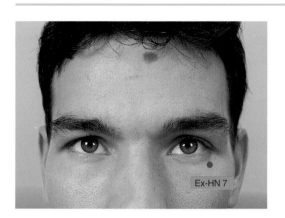

Ex-HN 7

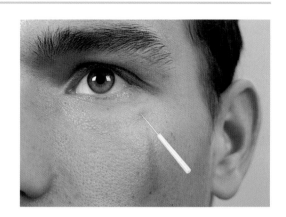

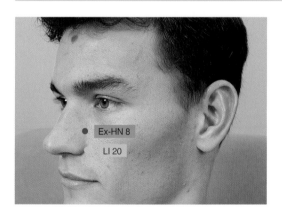

Ex-HN 8

LI 20

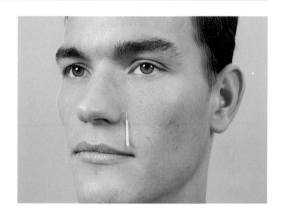

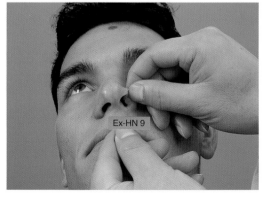

Ex-HN 9

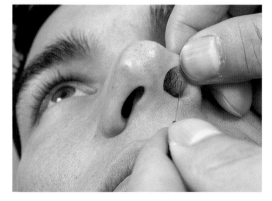

● Mu Point ● Back-Shu-Point ● Connecting Point (Luo) ● Cleft Point ● Lower He Point ● Qi-Source-Point (Yuan) ● Confluent Point ● Converging Point

Ex-HN 10 Ju Quan Gathering Source

L: at the midpoint on the dorsal midline of the tongue

T: 0.1–0.2 cun perpendicular

P: clears heat and promotes body fluids, alleviates coughing and breathing difficulty

A: 1. diabetes mellitus
2. paralysis of the tongue
3. bronchial asthma, bronchitis

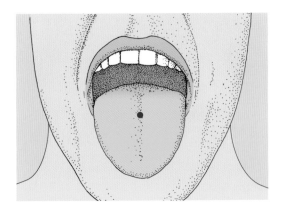

Ex-HN 11 Hai Quan Sea Source

L: at the midpoint of the frenulum of the tongue

T: prick to bleed only

P: promotes body fluids, alleviates thirst, clears heat, and reduces edema

A: 1. diabetes mellitus
2. acute inflammation of the mouth

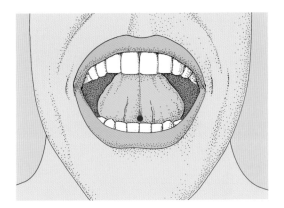

EX-HN 12 Jin Jin Golden Fluid

L: on the vein of the inferior side of the tongue, to the left of the frenulum

T: prick to bleed only

P: clears heat and reduces edema, opens the senses and eliminates muteness

A: 1. acute inflammations of the mouth cavity, e.g. stomatitis aphthosa
2. motor aphasia
3. acute tonsillitis

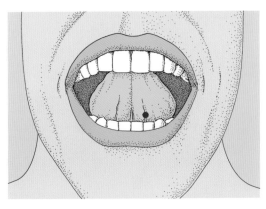

L: Location **T:** Insertion Technique **P:** Properties **A:** Clinical Applications **Pec:** Peculiarities

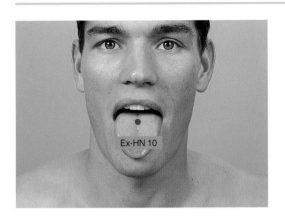

Ex-HN 10

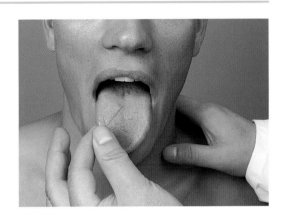

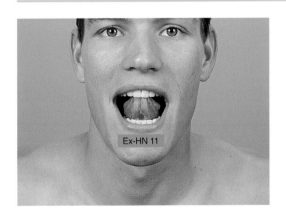

Ex-HN 11

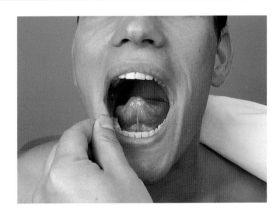

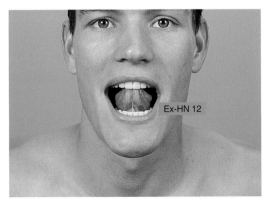

Ex-HN 12

● Mu Point ● Back-Shu-Point ● Connecting Point (Luo) ● Cleft Point ● Lower He Point ● Qi-Source-Point (Yuan) ● Confluent Point ● Converging Point

Ex-HN

Ex-HN 13 Yu Ye Jade Fluid

L: on the vein of the inferior side of the tongue, to the right of the frenulum

T: prick to bleed only

P: clears heat and reduces edema swelling, opens the senses and eliminates muteness

A: 1. acute inflammations of the mouth cavity, e.g. stomatitis aphthosa
2. motor aphasia
3. acute tonsillitis

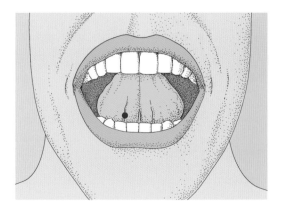

Ex-HN 14 Yi Ming Dim Eyesight Clear (again)

L: behind the earlobe, 1 cun dorsal to SJ 17

T: 0.5–1 cun perpendicular

P: expels wind and sharpens eyesight

A: diseases of the eye

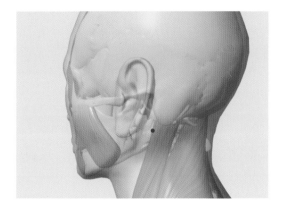

Ex-HN 15 Ying Bai Lao Tuberculosis in the Neck

L: on the neck, 2 cun above the depression below the spinous process C7 (Du 14), 1 cun lateral to the dorsal midline

T: 0.4–0.8 cun perpendicular; moxibustion

P: transforms phlegm and eliminates swelling of the lymph glands, alleviates coughing and breathing difficulty

A: 1. lymphatic discharge disorders in lymphadenitis tuberculosa in the region of the neck
2. bronchitis, bronchial asthma

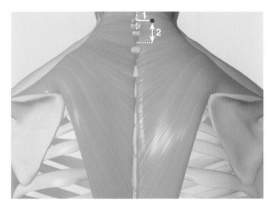

L: Location   T: Insertion Technique   P: Properties   A: Clinical Applications   Pec: Peculiarities

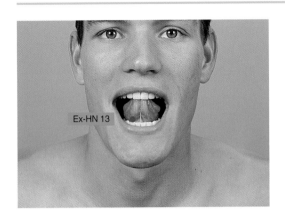

Ex-HN 13

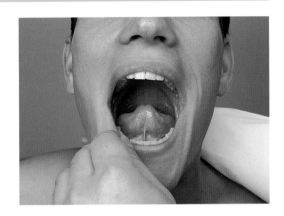

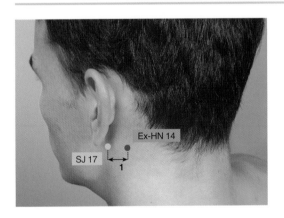

SJ 17 Ex-HN 14 **1**

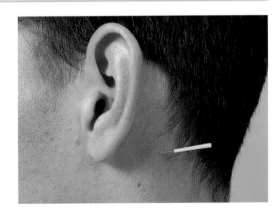

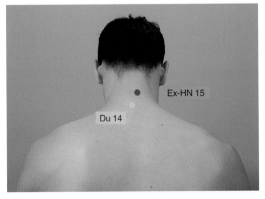

Du 14 Ex-HN 15

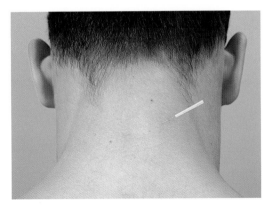

- Mu Point
- Back-Shu-Point
- Connecting Point (Luo)
- Cleft Point
- Lower He Point
- Qi-Source-Point (Yuan)
- Confluent Point
- Converging Point

2.4.2 Extraordinary points on the chest and abdomen (Ex-CA)

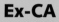

Location

The extra points on the chest and abdomen are located on the thorax and abdomen. The most important point is the Zi Gong point on the lower abdomen.

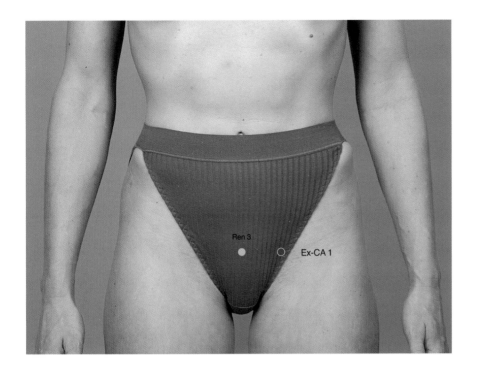

Ex-CA 1 Zi Gong Uterus

L: 4 cun below the umbilicus, 3 cun lateral to Ren 3

T: 0.8–1.2 cun perpendicular

P: regulates menstruation and promotes fertility

A: certain gynecological disorders, e.g. irregular menstruation, uterine prolapse, fertility disorders

Pec: CAUTION IN PREGNANCY!

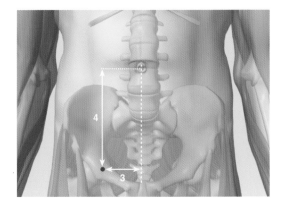

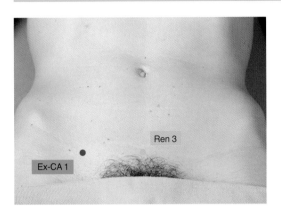

Ren 3

Ex-CA 1

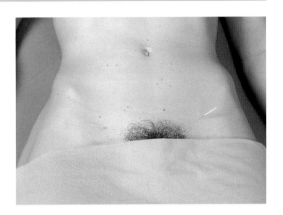

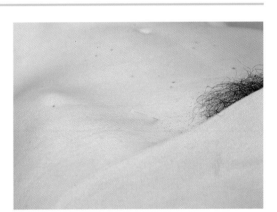

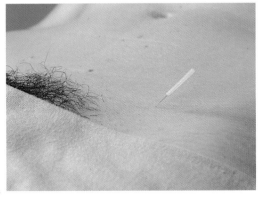

Mu Point　　Back-Shu-Point　　Connecting Point (Luo)　　Cleft Point　　Lower He Point　　　Qi-Source-Point (Yuan)　　Confluent Point　　Converging Point

2.4.3   Extraordinary points on the back (Ex-B)

Location

The nine extra points on the back are dispersed over the back between the neck and the coccyx.

Ex-B

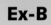

Ex-B

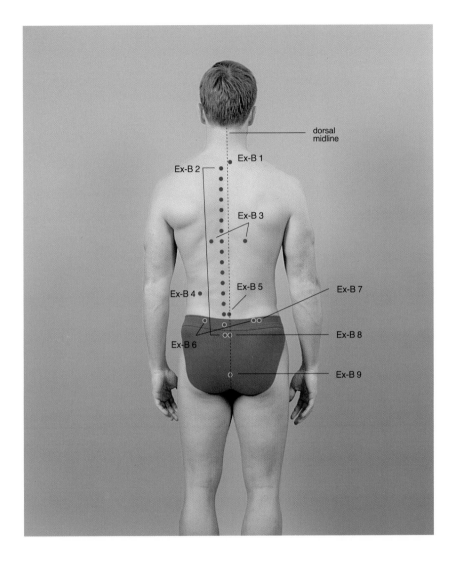

Ex-B 1 Ding Chuan Calm Dyspnoea

L: at the level of the depression below the spinous process C7 (Du 14), 0.5 cun lateral to the dorsal midline

T: 0.5–0.8 cun perpendicular

P: alleviates coughing and breathing difficulty

A: bronchial asthma, bronchitis

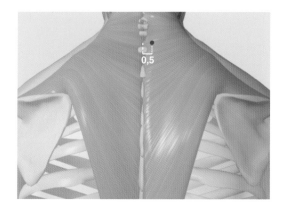

Ex-B 2 Jia Ji (Hua Tuo Jia Ji) Hua Tuo's Paravertrebal Points

L: 17 points at the level of the depression below the spinous processes Th1 – L5, 0.5 cun lateral to the dorsal midline

T: 0.5–1 cun perpendicular; moxibustion

P: restores balance to the Zang (storage) and Fu (palace) organs

A: segmentally in diseases and disorders: Th1–3 (lungs and upper extremity), Th4–7 (heart), Th8–10 (liver and gall bladder), Th11–12 (spleen and stomach), L1–2 (kidneys), L3–5 (bladder, large intestine, small intestine, and lower extremity)

Pec: CAUTION, AVOID PNEUMOTHORAX! FOR THE LUMBER POINTS: CAUTION IN PREGNANCY!

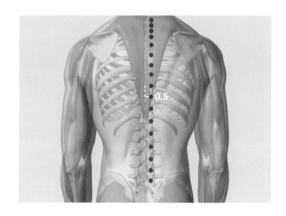

Ex-B 3 Wei Guan Xia Shu Lower Transport Point of the Stomach Cavity

L: one bilateral point at the level of the depression below the spinous process Th8, 1.5 cun lateral to the dorsal midline

T: 0.3–0.5 cun perpendicular or oblique medially; moxibustion

P: alleviates thirst and promotes body fluids

A: diabetes mellitus

Pec: CAUTION, AVOID PNEUMOTHORAX!
Often used in combination with a third point below spinous process Th8

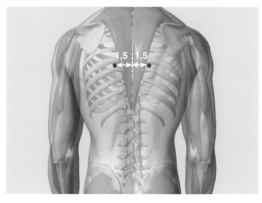

L: Location   T: Insertion Technique   P: Properties   A: Clinical Applications   Pec: Peculiarities

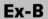

Ex-B

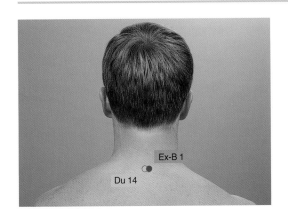

Ex-B 1

Du 14

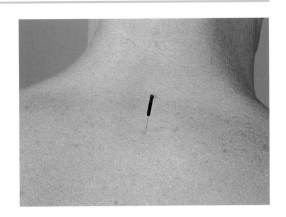

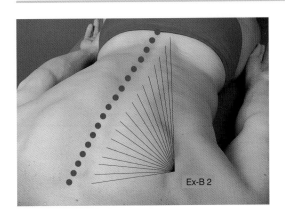

Ex-B 2

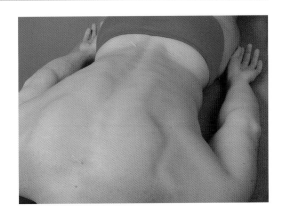

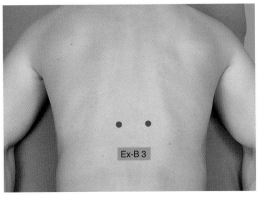

Ex-B 3

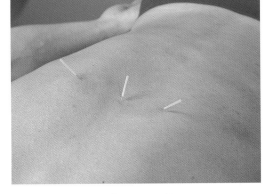

Mu Point ● Back-Shu-Point ● Connecting Point (Luo) ● Cleft Point ○ Lower He Point   ● Qi-Source-Point (Yuan) ● Confluent Point ● Converging Point

Ex-B 4 Pi Gen Root of abdominal swelling

L: at the level of the depression below the spinous process L1, 3.5 cun lateral to the dorsal midline

T: 0.8–1.2 cun perpendicular; moxibustion

P: dispels congestion and eliminates tumours

A: benign abdominal tumours, swelling of the liver and the spleen

Pec: CAUTION, AVOID PNEUMOTHORAX!

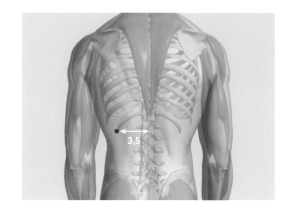

Ex-B 5 Xia Ji Shu Transport Point of the Lower Pole

L: on the dorsal midline, in the depression below the spinous process L3

T: 0.5–1 cun oblique cranially; moxibustion

P: strengthens the spleen and supports the kidney

A: 1. lumbalgia
2. abdominal pain in enteritis
3. urinary incontinence, urinary retention

Pec: CAUTION IN PREGNANCY!

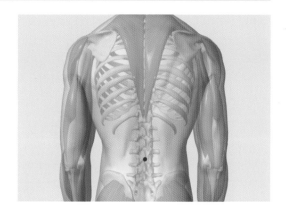

Ex-B 6 Yao Yi Serving the Lumbar Region

L: one bilateral point at the level of the depression below the spinous process L4, 3 cun lateral to the dorsal midline

T: 0.6–0.9 cun perpendicular or 0.3 cun subcutaneously; moxibustion

P: soothes blood and alleviates pain

A: 1. anovulatory dysfunctional uterine bleeding
2. lumbalgia

Pec: CAUTION IN PREGNANCY!
Often used in combination with Du 3

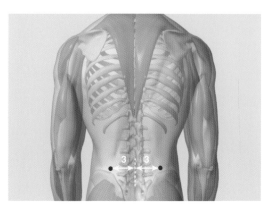

L: Location   T: Insertion Technique   P: Properties   A: Clinical Applications   Pec: Peculiarities

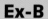

Ex-B

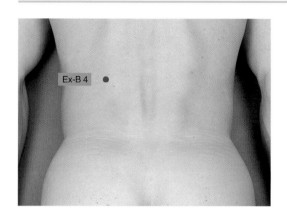

Ex-B 4

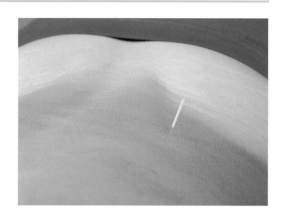

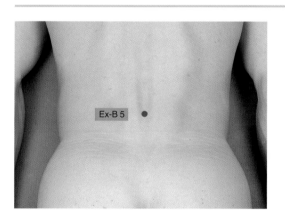

Ex-B 5

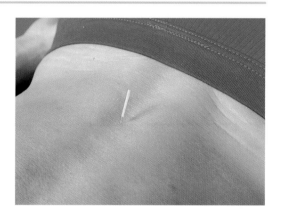

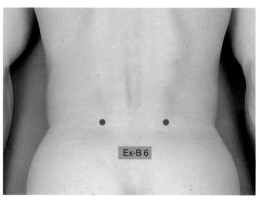

Ex-B 6

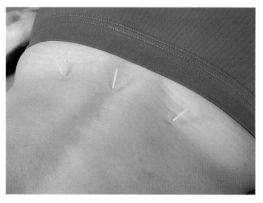

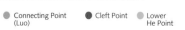

○ Mu Point   ○ Back-Shu-Point   ● Connecting Point (Luo)   ● Cleft Point   ○ Lower He Point   ● Qi-Source-Point (Yuan)   ● Confluent Point   ● Converging Point

Ex-B 7 Yao Yan   Lumbar Eyes

L: at the level of the depression below the spinous process L4, in the depression 3.5 cun lateral to the dorsal midline

T: 0.5–1 cun perpendicular; moxibustion

P: supports the kidney and alleviates pain

A: lumbo-sacral overburdening syndrome

Pec: CAUTION IN PREGNANCY!

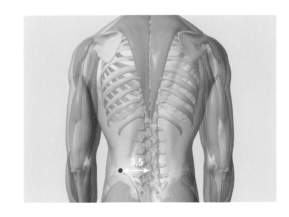

Ex-B 8 Shi Qi Zhui   Seventeenth Vertebra

L: on the dorsal midline, in the depression below the spinous process L5

T: 1–1.5 cun oblique cranially

P: supports the kidney and promotes urination

A: 1. urinary retention
2. lumboischialgia

Pec: CAUTION IN PREGNANCY!

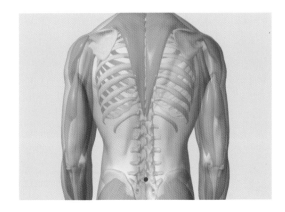

Ex-B 9 Yao Qi   Peculiar to the Lumbar Region

L: on the dorsal midline, 2 cun above the coccyx, in the depression between the two cornua sacralia

T: 1.5–2 cun oblique cranially; moxibustion

P: suppresses cramps and stops vertigo

A: 1. epilepsy
2. headache

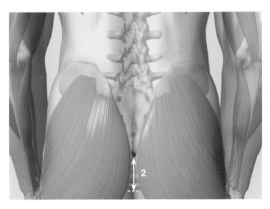

L: Location   T: Insertion Technique   P: Properties   A: Clinical Applications   Pec: Peculiarities

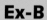

Ex-B

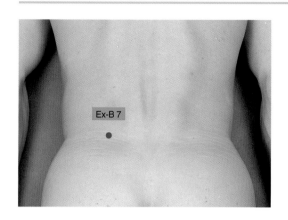

Ex-B 7

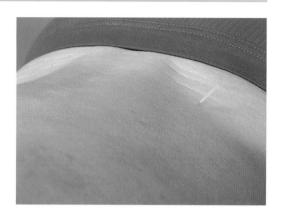

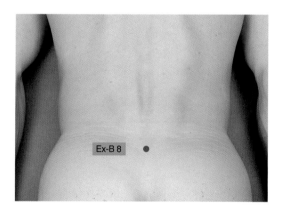

Ex-B 8

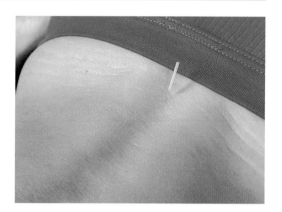

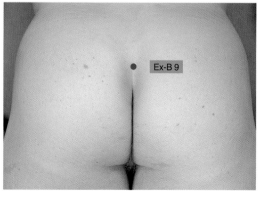

Ex-B 9

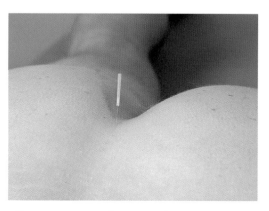

○ Mu Point ○ Back-Shu-Point ○ Connecting Point (Luo) ● Cleft Point ○ Lower He Point ● Qi-Source-Point (Yuan) ● Confluent Point ● Converging Point

2.4.4 Extraordinary points on the arm and hand (Ex-AH)

Location

The eleven extraordinary points of the upper extremity (also known as the Extra Points of the Upper Extremity: Ex-UE) are located on the olecranon, the inside of the lower arm and the hand.

Ex-AH

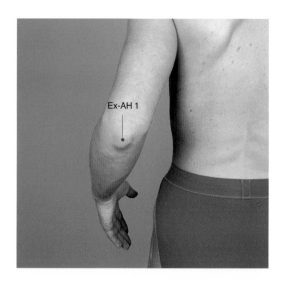

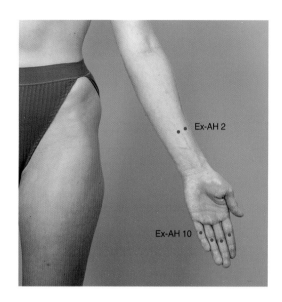

Ex-AH

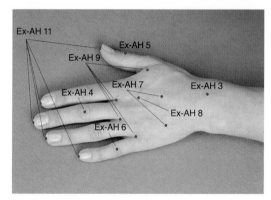

Ex-AH 1 Zhou Jian Elbow Tip

L: with the patient's elbow flexed at 90 degrees, on the tip of the olecranon

T: 0.1 cun perpendicular or 0.5 cun subcutaneously; moxibustion

P: transforms phlegm and reduces edema

A: 1. lymphatic discharge disorders in lymphadenitis tuberculosa in the region of the neck and axilla
2. acute appendicitis

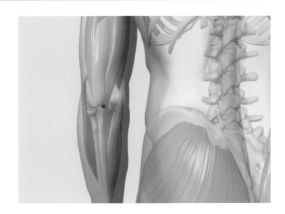

Ex-AH 2 Er Bai Two Whites

L: 2 points 4 cun proximal to the distal wrist crease radial and ulnar to the flexor carpi radialis tendon

T: 0.5–1 cun slightly oblique proximally

P: firms prolapses and eliminates hemorrhoids

A: 1. hemorrhoids
2. anal and rectal prolapse

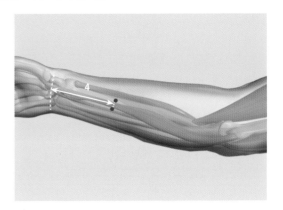

Ex-AH 3 Zhong Quan Middle Source

L: on the dorsal wrist crease, in the depression radial to the extensor digitorum communis muscle

T: 0.2–0.3 cun slightly oblique proximally; moxibustion

P: descends Qi and alleviates pain

A: 1. thoracic pain
2. stomach pain, nausea, vomiting

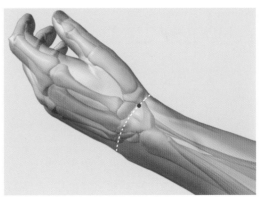

L: Location   **T:** Insertion Technique   **P:** Properties   **A:** Clinical Applications   **Pec:** Peculiarities

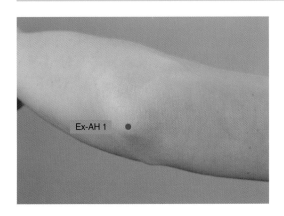

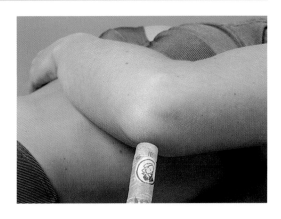

Ex-AH

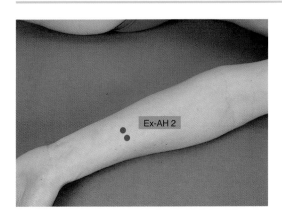

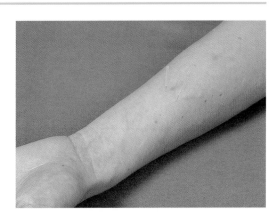

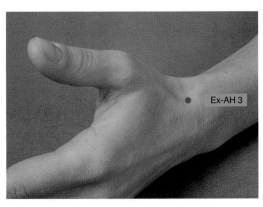

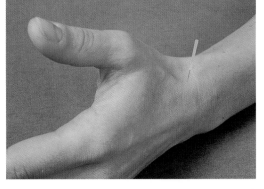

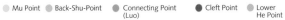

⬤ Mu Point ⬤ Back-Shu-Point ⬤ Connecting Point (Luo) ⬤ Cleft Point ⬤ Lower He Point ⬤ Qi-Source-Point (Yuan) ⬤ Confluent Point ⬤ Converging Point

Ex-AH 4 Zhong Kui   Ringleader in the Centre

L: on the extensor side of the middle finger, in the middle of the proximal interphalangeal joint

T: 0.2–0.3 cun perpendicular; moxibustion

P: descends inverted Qi and harmonizes the stomach

A: nausea and vomiting in esophagitis, gastritis

Pec: CAUTION, AVOID SPREADING GERMS TO THE INTERPHALANGEAL JOINT!

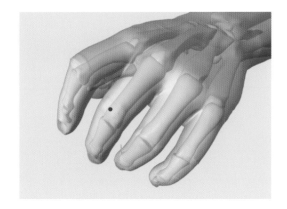

Ex-AH

Ex-AH 5 Da Gu Kong   Great Crevice

L: on the extensor side of the thumb in the middle of the interphalangeal joint

T: moxibustion only

P: corrects dim vision and sharpens eyesight

A: diseases of the eye

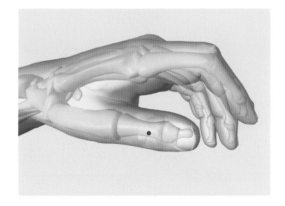

Ex-AH 6 Xiao Gu Kong   Little Crevice

L: on the extensor side of the little finger in the middle of the proximal interphalangeal joint

T: moxibustion only

P: corrects dim vision and sharpens eyesight

A: diseases of the eye

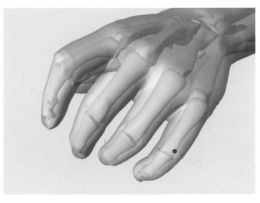

L: Location   **T:** Insertion Technique   **P:** Properties   **A:** Clinical Applications   **Pec:** Peculiarities

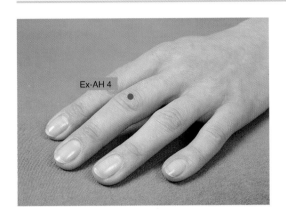

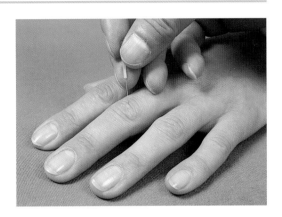

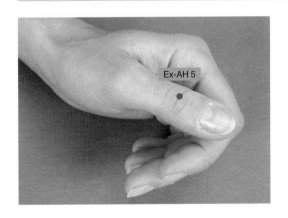

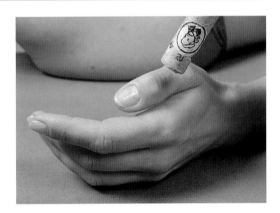

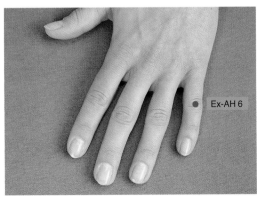

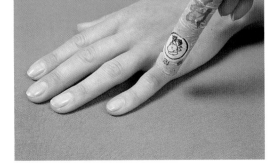

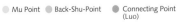

Mu Point   Back-Shu-Point   Connecting Point (Luo)   Cleft Point   Lower He Point   Qi-Source-Point (Yuan)   Confluent Point   Converging Point

Ex-AH 7 Yao Tong Dian Lumbago Points

L: two points on the dorsum of the hand, one in the proximal angle between the second and third metacarpal bones and the other in the proximal angle between the fourth and fifth metacarpal bones, each at the midpoint between the dorsal wrist crease and the metacarpo-phalangeal joints

T: 0.3–0.5 cun perpendicular

P: activates the channels and alleviates pain

A: lumbalgia, lumbago

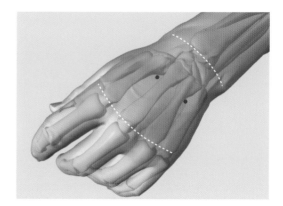

Ex-AH 8 Wai Lao Gong (Laozhen) Outside Pe 8 (Stiff Neck)

L: on the dorsum of the hand between the second and third metacarpal bones, 0.5 cun proximal to the metacarpo-phalangeal joints

T: 0.5–0.8 cun perpendicular or oblique; moxibustion

P: reduces edema and alleviates pain

A: 1. acute stiffness of the neck
2. pains in the dorsum of the hand

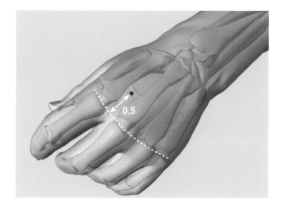

Ex-AH 9 Ba Xie Eight (against) Pathogens

L: four points between the metacarpo-phalangeal joints, at the dividing line between red and white flesh, at the border of the interdigital skin

T: 0.5–0.8 cun oblique towards the middle of the palm; prick to bleed; moxibustion

P: decongests and activates the channels and their vessels

A: pains, paraestheses, and restricted movement of the hand

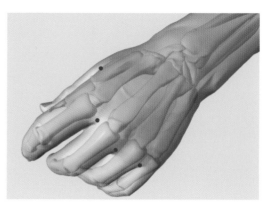

L: Location   T: Insertion Technique   P: Properties   A: Clinical Applications   **Pec:** Peculiarities

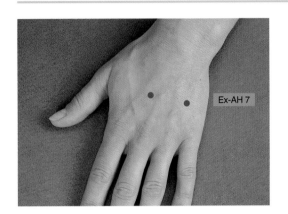

Ex-AH 7

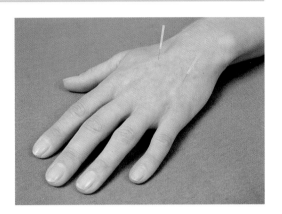

Ex-AH

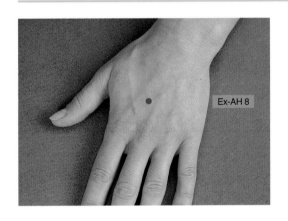

Ex-AH 8

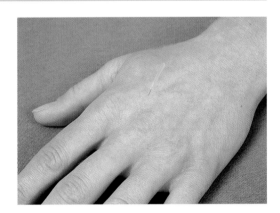

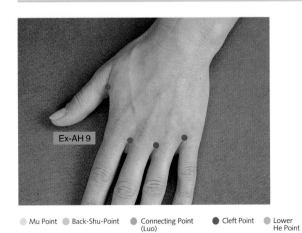

Ex-AH 9

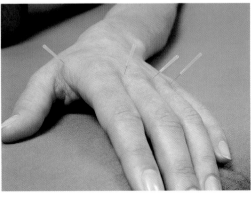

⬤ Mu Point ⬤ Back-Shu-Point ⬤ Connecting Point (Luo) ⬤ Cleft Point ⬤ Lower He Point ⬤ Qi-Source-Point (Yuan) ⬤ Confluent Point ⬤ Converging Point

331

Ex-AH 10 Si Feng Four Seams

L: four points on the bending side of the fingers in the middle of the interphalangeal joints

T: 0.1–0.2 cun subcutaneously; squeeze until a small amount of tissue fluid or blood appears

P: strengthens the spleen and eliminates congestion

A: loss of appetite, digestive, and eating disorders in children

Pec: CAUTION, AVOID SPREADING GERMS TO THE INTERPHALANGEAL JOINTS!

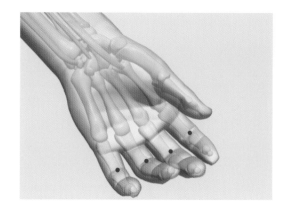

Ex-AH 11 Shi Xuan Ten Diffusions

L: five points, each in the centre of each finger tip 0.1 cun from the free end of the nails

T: 0.1–0.2 cun subcutaneously; prick to bleed

P: opens the senses and restores clarity to the brain, drains and expels heat and suppresses cramp

A: 1. sudden loss of consciousness (complementary or emergency measure)
2. fever cramps
3. parestheses of the finger tips

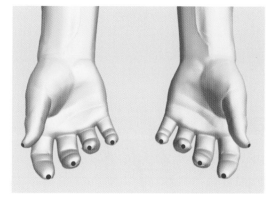

Ex-AH

L: Location   T: Insertion Technique   P: Properties   A: Clinical Applications   Pec: Peculiarities

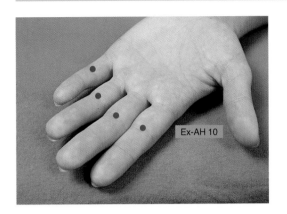

Ex-AH 10

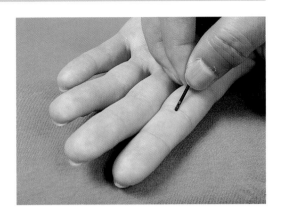

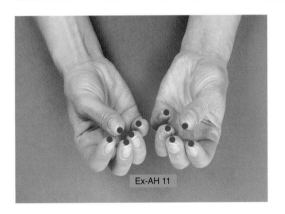

Ex-AH 11

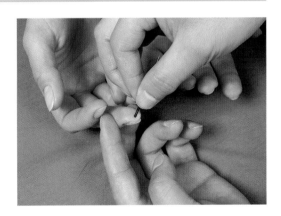

Mu Point ● Back-Shu-Point ● Connecting Point (Luo) ● Cleft Point ● Lower He Point ● Qi-Source-Point (Yuan) ● Confluent Point ● Converging Point

2.4.5 Extraordinary points on the leg and foot (Ex-LF)

Location

The twelve extra points of the lower extremity (also known as the Extra Points of the Lower Extremity: Ex-LE) are located on the distal upper leg, in the region of the knee, on the proximal lower leg and at the front of the foot

Ex-LF

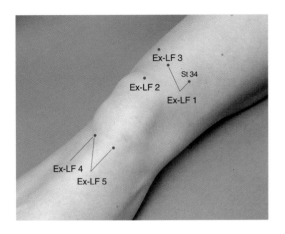

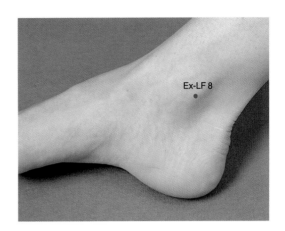

Ex-LF

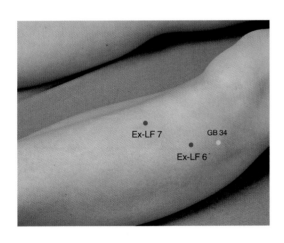

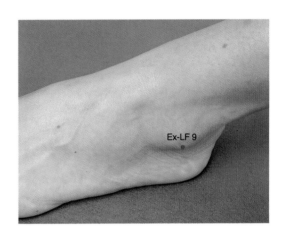

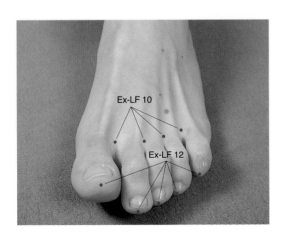

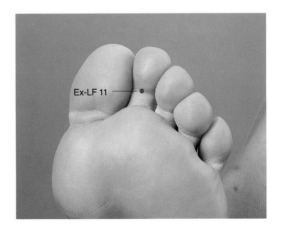

Ex-LF 1 Kuan Gu   Hip Bone

L: two points above the knee joint, each 1.5 cun lateral/medial from St 34

T: 0.5–0.8 perpendicular; moxibustion

P: relaxes the tendons and alleviates pain

A: leg pain

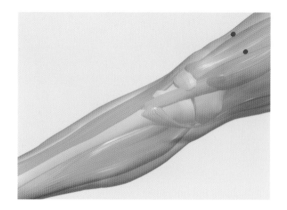

Ex-LF 2 He Ding   Crane's Summit

L: in the depression in the middle of the superior border of the patella

T: 0.3–0.5 perpendicular; moxibustion

P: activates the vessels and alleviates pain

A: 1. knee joint pain
2. restricted movement of the lower extremity

Pec: CAUTION, AVOID SPREADING GERMS TO THE KNEE JOINT!

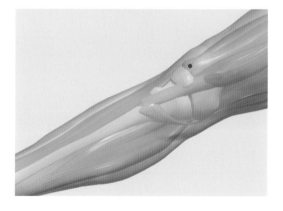

Ex-LF 3 Bai Chong Wo   Hundred Insect Burrow

L: with the patient's knee flexed, 3 cun above the medial superior border of the patella, that is 1 cun above Sp 10

T: 0.5–1.2 perpendicular; moxibustion

P: clears heat and cools the blood, dispels wind and overcomes damp

A: skin diseases, e.g. rubella, urticaria, pruritus

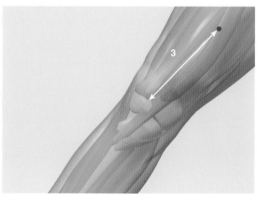

L: Location   T: Insertion Technique   P: Properties   A: Clinical Applications   Pec: Peculiarities

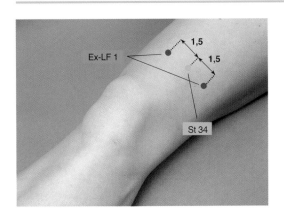

Ex-LF 1

1,5

1,5

St 34

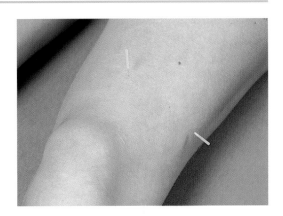

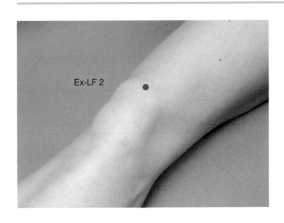

Ex-LF 2

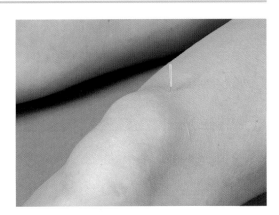

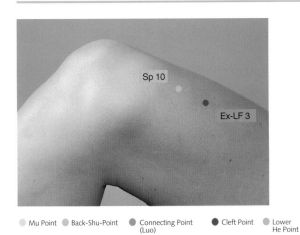

Sp 10

Ex-LF 3

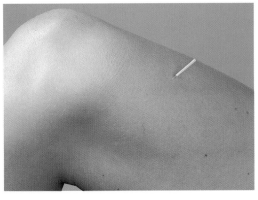

○ Mu Point　　○ Back-Shu-Point　　○ Connecting Point (Luo)　　● Cleft Point　　○ Lower He Point　　　　　● Qi-Source-Point (Yuan)　　● Confluent Point　　● Converging Point

Ex-LF 4 Nei Xi Yan   Inner Eye of the Knee

L: with the patient's knee flexed, in the depression medial to the patellar ligament opposite St 35

T: 0.5–1 oblique towards the centre of the knee joint; moxibustion

P: relaxes the tendons and alleviates pain

A: pain in the knee joint

Pec: CAUTION, AVOID SPREADING GERMS TO THE KNEE JOINT!

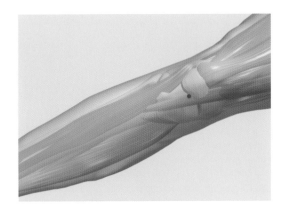

Ex-LF 5 Xi Yan   Eyes of the Knee

L: with the patient's knee flexed, two points in the depression medial (Nei Xi Yan corresponds to Ex-LF 4) and lateral (Wai Xi Yan corresponds to St 35) to the patellar ligament

T: 0.5–1 oblique towards the centre of the knee joint; moxibustion

P: relaxes the tendons and alleviates pain

A: pain in the knee joint

Pec: CAUTION, AVOID SPREADING GERMS TO THE KNEE JOINT!

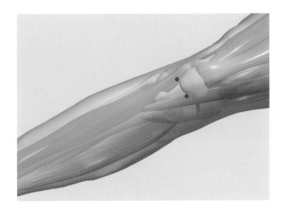

Ex-LF 6 Dan Nang   Gall Bladder Point

L: 2 cun below GB 34 on the gall bladder channel

T: 0.8–1.2 perpendicular

P: clears heat and promotes the gall bladder

A: acute and chronic cholecystitis

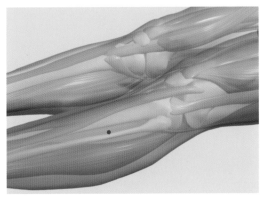

L: Location   T: Insertion Technique   P: Properties   A: Clinical Applications   Pec: Peculiarities

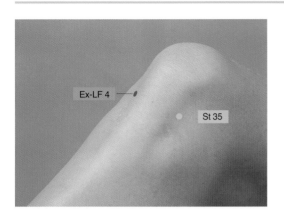

Ex-LF 4

St 35

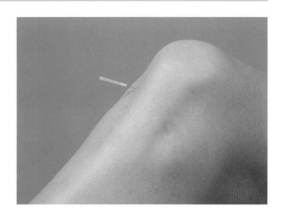

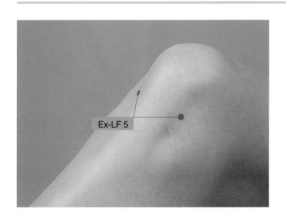

Ex-LF 5

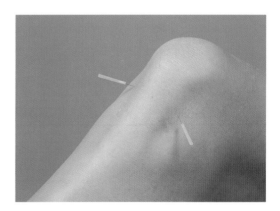

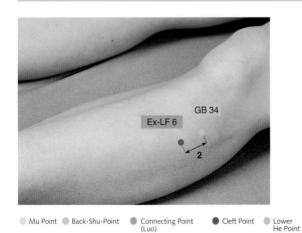

GB 34

Ex-LF 6

2

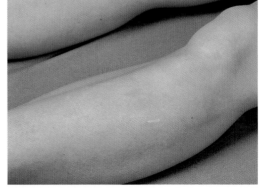

○ Mu Point ○ Back-Shu-Point ○ Connecting Point (Luo) ● Cleft Point ○ Lower He Point   ● Qi-Source-Point (Yuan) ● Confluent Point ● Converging Point

Ex-LF 7 Lan Wei Appendix

L: 5 cun below St 35, 2 cun below St 36 on the stomach channel

T: 0.5–1.5 perpendicular;
moxibustion

P: clears heat and alleviates pain

A: acute and chronic appendicitis

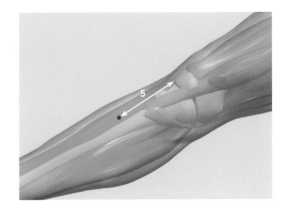

Ex-LF 8 Nei Huai Jian Tip of the Inside Ankle

L: at the highest prominence of the medial malleolus

T: prick to bleed only;
moxibustion

P: activates the vessels and alleviates pain

A: 1. calf cramps
2. toothache

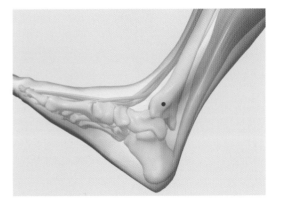

Ex-LF 9 Wai Huai Jian Tip of the Outside Ankle

L: at the highest prominence of the lateral malleolus

T: prick to bleed only;
moxibustion

P: promotes urination and activates the urinary tract, clears heat and alleviates pain

A: 1. acute infections of the urinary tract

2. muscle cramp on the outside of the foot

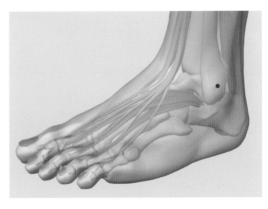

L: Location **T:** Insertion Technique **P:** Properties **A:** Clinical Applications **Pec:** Peculiarities

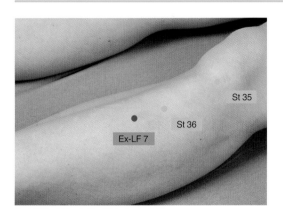

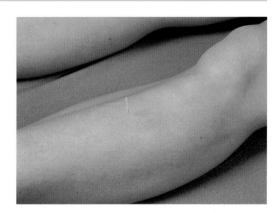

Ex-LF

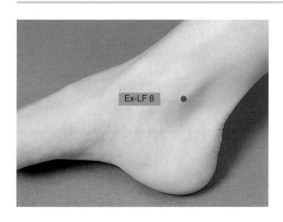

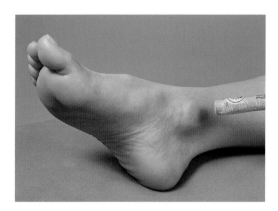

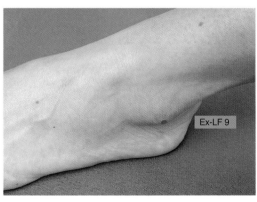

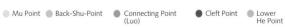

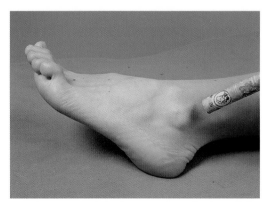

Mu Point ● Back-Shu-Point ● Connecting Point (Luo) ● Cleft Point ● Lower He Point ● Qi-Source-Point (Yuan) ● Confluent Point ● Converging Point

Ex-LF 10 Ba Feng   Eight (against) Winds

L: four points between the metatarso-phalangeal joints, at the dividing line between red and white flesh, at the border of the interdigital skin

T: 0.5–0.8 cun oblique towards the centre of the sole; moxibustion

P: activates the vessels and alleviates pain

A: 1. redness, swelling, and pain on the dorsum of the foot and toes
2. paraestheses and restricted movement of the lower extremity

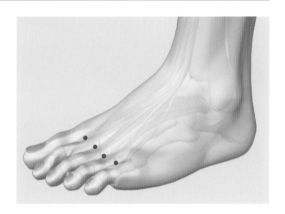

Ex-LF 11 Du Yin   Only Yin

L: on the bending side of the second toe in the middle of the distal interphalangeal joint

T: 0.1–0.2 perpendicular; moxibustion

P: mobilises the blood and regulates menstruation

A: gynecological and obstetric disorders, e.g. protracted labour, retention of the placenta, irregular menstruation

Pec: CAUTION, AVOID SPREADING GERMS TO THE INTERPHALANGEAL JOINT!

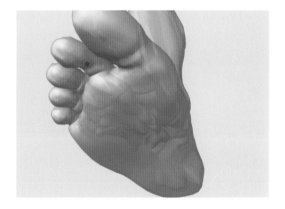

Ex-LF 12 Qi Duan   Qi Ends

L: five points, each on the tip of each toe, 0.1 cun from the free ends of the nail borders

T: 0.1–0.2 cun perpendicular; moxibustion

P: relaxes the tendons and activates the vessels

A: foot pain, paraestheses of the toes

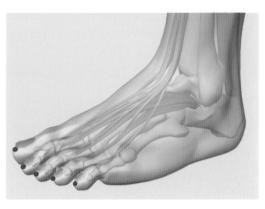

L: Location   T: Insertion Technique   P: Properties   A: Clinical Applications   Pec: Peculiarities

Ex-LF

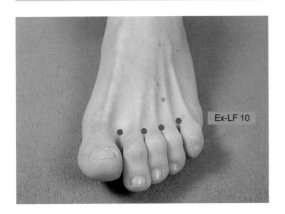

Ex-LF 10

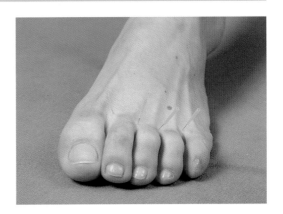

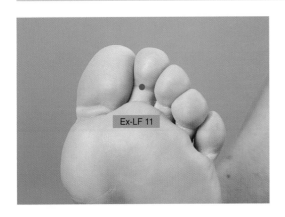

Ex-LF 11

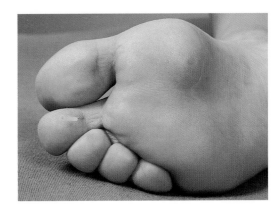

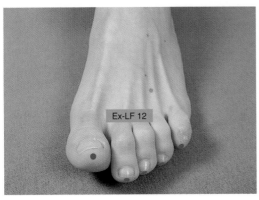

Ex-LF 12

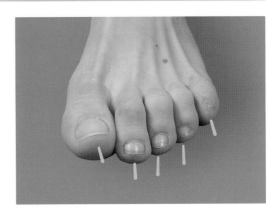

● Mu Point   ● Back-Shu-Point   ● Connecting Point (Luo)   ● Cleft Point   ● Lower He Point   ● Qi-Source-Point (Yuan)   ● Confluent Point   ● Converging Point

Nomenclature

Term used in this atlas	Chinese name	Alternative synonymous terms
Back-Shu-Point	Bei Shu Xue	• Applause Point • Back (Shu) Transport Point • Concordance Point • Dorsal Segment Point • Influence Point in the Back • Yu-Point
Channel	Jing	• Meridian
Cleft Point	Xi Xue	• Acute Point • Border Point
Confluent Point	Ba Mai Jiao Hui Xue	• Cardinal Point • Connecting Point • Opening Point • Reunion Point • Tuning Point
Connecting Point (Luo)	Luo Xue	• Crossing Point • Passage Point
Dampness	Shi	• Cold-Dampness
Du Mai	Du Mai	• The Channel • The Governing Vessel • The Vessel
Emptiness	Xu	• Energy Deficiency • Underfunctioning • Weakness
Extraordinary Vessels	Qi Jing Ba Mai	• Extraordinary Meridians • Unpaired Channels • Unusual Meridians • Wonder Meridians
Extraordinary Points	Jing Wai Qi Xue	• Extra Points • New Points (NP) • Points outside the Meridians

Term used in this atlas	Chinese name	Alternative synonymous terms
Five Shu-Points	Wu Shu Xue	• Five Ancient Points • Five Inductoria
Fullness	Shi	• Energy Redundancy • Overburdening • Overfunctioning
Fu (Palace) Organs	Fu	• Empty Organ • Passage Orbis
He (Sea) Point (5th Shu-Point)	He Xue	• 5th Ancient Point • He Point (Delta, Mouth) • Ho (Sea) Point • Union Point/ Discharge Point
Jing (River) Point (4th Shu-Point)	Jing Xue	• 4th Ancient Point • Crossing Point • Discharge Point • Jing(River) Point • King (Stream) Point
Jing (Well) Point (1st Shu-Point)	Jing Xue	• 1st Ancient Point • Jing Point (Source) • Source/Well-Point • Ting-Point (Source) • Tsing Point • Well-Point
Lower He (Sea) Point	Xia He Xue	• Lower Point of Influence
Mu (Front) Point	Mu Xue	• Herold Point • Mo-Point • (Segmental) Alarm Point

Term used in this atlas	Chinese Name	Alternative synonymous terms
Pericardium	Xin Bao	• Bag/Heart-Master • Circulation/Sexuality • Girdling Network of the Heart • Heart • Heart Cover • Master of the Heart • Pericardium/Circulation
Qi-Source-Point	Yuan Xue	• Source Point • Qi-Point
Ren Mai	Ren Mai	• Conception Vessel • Servant Vessel • Vessel of Conception
Sanjiao	San Jiao	–
Sedate	Xie	–
Shu (Stream) Point (3rd Shu-Point)	Shu Xue	• 3rd Ancient Point • Inductorium (Point of Particular Influence) • Shu-Point (Small River) • Yu/Yunn Point
Spleen-Channel	Pi	• Spleen/Pancreas Channel
Surface	Biao	• Outside
Tonify	Bu	–
Xing (Spring) Point (2nd Shu-point)	Xing Xue	• 2nd Ancient Point • Ying (Brook) Point • Ying (Spring) Point • Yong (Brook) Point • Point of Outpouring
Zang (Storage) Organ	Zang	• Parenchymatous Organ

Needle Material Used

The following SEIRIN needles were used in this atlas:

B-Type 0.2 x 15

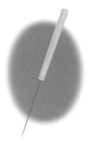

Soft Needle 0.3 x 30

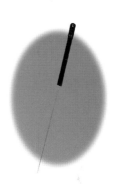

Recommended Needle Sizes

	Body	Head	Ear
Adult	0.25 x 40 mm 0.30 x 30 mm 0.35 x 50 mm	0.16 x 30 mm 0.20 x 15 mm 0.30 x 30 mm	0.20 x 15 mm
Children *	0.20 x 15 mm 0.25 x 40 mm 0.30 x 50 mm	0.16 x 30 mm 0.20 x 15 mm	0.20 x 15 mm
Small Children *	0.16 x 30 mm 0.20 x 15 mm	0.16 x 30 mm 0.20 x 15 mm	0.20 x 15 mm
Patients afraid of needles *	0.16 x 30 mm 0.20 x 15 mm 0.25 x 40 mm	0.16 x 30 mm 0.20 x 15 mm	0.20 x 15 mm

* Acupressure and soft-laser therapy can be used as atraumatic alternatives in children, small children, and patients afraid of needles.

Index

Reference Works and Recommended Literature

[1] **Beijing College of Traditional Chinese Medicine, Shanghai College of Traditional Chinese Medicine, Nanjing College of Traditional Chinese Medicine, The Acupuncture Institute of the Academy of Traditional Chinese Medicine [eds.]:** Essentials of Chinese Acupuncture. Foreign Languages Press, Beijing 1980

[2] **Cheng Xin-nong [eds.]:** Chinese Acupuncture and Moxibustion. Foreign Languages Press, Beijing 1987

[3] **Institut für Akupunktur und Moxibustion an der Chinesischen Akademie für Traditionelle Chinesische Medizin:** Die Akupunkturpunkte. Das Standardwerk aus China. Verlag für fremdsprachige Literatur, Beijing 1993

[4] **Li Ding:** Acupuncture, Meridian Theory and Acupuncture Points. Foreign Languages Press, Beijing 1991

[5] **Li Shi-hua [eds.]:** Yue Han-zhen (Qing): Jingxuejie. Zhang Can-jia, Zha Chang-hua dianjiao. Renmin weisheng chubanshe, Beijing 1990

[6] **Liu Gong-wang, Akira Hyodo [eds.]:** Fundamentals of Acupuncture & Moxibustion. Tianjin Science & Technology Translation & Publishing Corporation, Tianjin 1994

[7] **Sun Yong-xian:** Jingluo kaobian. Qingdao chubanshe, Qingdao 1989

[8] **Yang Jia-san [eds.]:** Zhenjiuxue. Renmin weisheng chubanshe, Beijing 1989

[9] **Zhongguo zhongyi yanjiuyuan zhenjiu yanjiusuo:** Biaozhun zhenjiu xuewei tuce. Qingdao chubanshe, Qingdao 1990

Editors

Dr. Hans P. Ogal, M.D.
Consultant anaesthesiologist, trained in pain management (Department of Anaesthesiology and Intensive Care Medicine at Justus-Liebig University in Giessen, Germany, by Professor H. F. Herget, M.D.); lecturer in acupuncture, body energetic balance and pain treatment at Philipps University in Marburg, Germany; lecturer for the German Medical Society for Acupuncture (DÄGfA) and other professional organisations; director of the Pain Clinic at Aeskulap-Klinik Dr. Brander, Centre for Holistic Medicine, Brunnen, Lake Lucerne, Switzerland.

Dr. Wolfram Stör
Consultant General Practitioner, Natural Healing Techniques, Homeopathy; guest teaching fellow for acupuncture at the Ludwig-Maximilian University in Munich, coordinator of the Further Education Center, and member of the Governing Council of the German Medical Society for Acupuncture (DÄGfA).

Authors

Prof. Yu-Lin Lian
Professor of acupuncture at the First Teaching Hospital of the University for Traditional Chinese Medicine in Tianjin – the national Acupuncture Research Centre of China. Collaborating member in research project devoted to acupuncture in pain therapy in Bad Birnbach in cooperation with the Neurological Clinic at The Technological University of Munich.

Dr. Chun-Yan Chen
Physician and human biologist; studied medicine and trained in TCM in China; clinical activity in the Centre for Acupuncture and Traditional Chinese Medicine (TCM) in Regensburg; lectures on acupuncture and TCM.

Dr. med. Michael Hammes
Four-year study of TCM in China sponsored by the DAAD and one year as physician at the Teaching Hospital at Beijing University, guest physician in Nanjing, Shanghai, Quandong, and Tianjin; training in neurology and pain therapy at the Technological University in Munich; currently in the Neurological Clinic Lippe-Lemgo; lecturer for the German Medical Society for Acupuncture (DÄGfA).

Dr. Bernard C. Kolster
Physician and physiotherapist, specialist clinical training in gynecology, obstetrics, and physical medicine; specialist training in acupuncture at the German Medical Society for Acupuncture (DÄGfA) amongst others; author and editor of medical journals.